The Trigger Point Therapy Workbook

SECOND EDITION

YOUR SELF-TREATMENT GUIDE FOR PAIN RELIEF

Clair Davies, NCTMB
with Amber Davies, NCTMB

Foreword by David G. Simons, MD

New Harbinger Publications, Inc.

Publisher's Note

Distributed in Canada by Raincoast Books

Copyright © 2004 by Clair Davies
                New Harbinger Publications, Inc.
                5674 Shattuck Avenue
                Oakland, CA 94609

Cover design by Amy Shoup
Illustrations by Clair Davies
Text design by Michele Waters

ISBN-10 1-57224-375-9
ISBN-13 978-1-57224-375-0

All Rights Reserved

Printed in the United States of America

New Harbinger Publications' website address: www.newharbinger.com

10   09   08

15   14   13   12   11

This book is dedicated to my daughter Amber Davies. I could not have written it without her steady faith in me. Her patience, constant encouragement, tactful criticism, and undying enthusiasm for trigger point therapy continually renewed my faith in myself and in the value of this project.

Amber has been my number one disciple. As a longtime sufferer of debilitating chronic pain, she was highly motivated to test and validate every new idea regarding self-treatment. My greatest reward has been in seeing her become relatively pain free and self-reliant due to our combined efforts. Amber has gone on to become a skilled massage therapist and is now devoted to helping bring the benefits of trigger point therapy to others.

Contents

Illustrations

Foreword

By David G. Simons, M.D.

Clair Davies possesses a fortunate combination of attributes: He is a skilled practitioner, has good writing skills, and shows a remarkable determination to help relieve mankind of unnecessary suffering. The message of this book is a voice in a wilderness of neglect. Muscle is an orphan organ. No medical specialty claims it. As a consequence, no medical specialty is concerned with promoting funded research into the muscular causes of pain, and medical students and physical therapists rarely receive adequate primary training in how to recognize and treat myofascial trigger points. Fortunately, massage therapists, although rarely well trained medically, are trained in how to find myofascial trigger points and frequently become skilled in their treatment.

Since there is no well-established body of research on this subject, there is no well-recognized etiology. Nevertheless, a credible hypothesis based on solid scientific research is available to serve as a model for further research to clarify the nature of myofascial trigger points. Much research needs to be done on this neglected subject.

It is becoming increasingly clear that nearly all fibromyalgia patients have myofascial trigger points that are contributing significantly to their total pain problem. Some patients are diagnosed as having fibromyalgia when in fact they only have much more treatable multiple trigger points. Inactivation of the trigger points of fibromyalgia patients requires especially delicate and skilled treatment.

Skilled clinicians recognize myofascial trigger points as the most common cause of ubiquitous enigmatic musculoskeletal pain, but finding a truly skilled practitioner can be frustratingly difficult. The guidance in this book can serve practitioners who have yet to understand the nature of their own musculoskeletal pain and can also benefit patients who are unable to find a practitioner adequately skilled in this neglected subject.

There is no substitute for learning how to control your own musculoskeletal pain. Treating myofascial trigger points yourself addresses the *source* of that kind of common pain and is not just a way of temporarily relieving it.

Acknowledgments

I'm fortunate to have been influenced by so many good people during the development of this book and throughout my own evolution. The following deserve special notice:

Ann Luray Hatton of Lubbock, Texas (formerly Ann Gyor of Lexington, Kentucky), my first massage therapist, "the one I liked so much," the wondrous woman who introduced me to trigger points and then moved away, making it necessary for me to draw on my own resources and ultimately produce this method of self-treatment. If all health-care practitioners had Ann's mind, hands, and heart, there would be very little pain in the world.

Barbara G. Cummings, the illustrator for Travell and Simons's *Myofascial Pain and Dysfunction: The Trigger Point Manual*, whose insight, imagination, and graphic skills made it possible to comprehend the reality of trigger points for the first time. The complex medical innovations of Janet Travell and David Simons would have been virtually incomprehensible without Barbara's drawings. She made the *Trigger Point Manual* work. Her illustrations were a constant inspiration while I was struggling to create my own illustrations for this book.

All my friends in the Piano Technicians Guild, who fostered my growth, not only as a piano technician, but also as a writer and illustrator in the *Piano Technicians Journal*. I continue to feel their support, even after leaving the fold and taking on this disconcerting new identity.

My instructors and classmates at the Utah College of Massage Therapy, who helped bear the "old man" into a new world of caring and healing. So many new experiences! What a trip!

My daughter Maria, my son-in-law (and former apprentice) Wayne Worley, my former wife (and best friend) Janice Lipuma, her son Will Drane, my mother-in-law Ruth Quigley Smith, and my grandsons Michael and Adam, who were all always in my corner, even when I was too preoccupied to notice.

The editors and staff at New Harbinger Publications, who know exactly what they're doing in putting a book together and caring for an ignorant and apprehensive new author. Special thanks to Clancy Drake, Heather Garnos, Kasey Pfaff, Spencer Smith, Amy Shoup, and Michele Waters.

To avoid the disgrace of forgetting someone, I won't try to name the numerous clients and personal friends who have given me so much of their confidence and trust as I rediscovered myself in the transition from piano mechanic to massage therapist and teacher of self-care.

Introduction

Jennifer, twenty-eight, who loved to run for her health every day in the fresh morning air, has had to stop running and is reluctant even to walk any distance because of relentless pain in her knees and heels.

Larry, fifty-two, can think of little else but the constant pain in his back. It's hard to get in and out of bed. His back hurts whether he's sitting, standing, or lying down. It makes him hate his job and has ruined his love life.

Melanie, thirty-six, spends her days at a computer keyboard and her nights worrying about her future and the unremitting pain and numbness in her arms and hands. As a single mother, she has to keep working no matter what.

Jack, forty-five, has shoulder pain that wakes him up at night. He can't raise his arm to comb his hair. Reaching up to scratch his back is impossible. A sudden movement brings a jolt of pain that feels like an electric shock and doubles him over, grimacing and breathless. Is this the start of the inevitable decline into old age, disability, and death?

Howard, twenty-three, is a gifted violin student. After years of hard work under some of the best teachers in the country, he now fears a professional career is out of reach because of constant pain and an unexplained, increasing stiffness in his fingers.

Do you know anybody like these people? They're everywhere—on every job, in every office, in every home. The thing all these people have in common, other than chronic pain, is that they aren't getting the help they need. It's not that they haven't looked. They've gone the rounds. They've seen doctors, had tests, done physical therapy, and filled out insurance forms, or—sick at heart—have paid the exorbitant bills themselves.

They've tried chiropractic, acupuncture, magnets, pain diets, and herbal therapy. They take their pain medicine and dutifully do their stretching exercises. Sometimes they feel better for a while, but the pain always comes back. Nothing really seems to get to the bottom of the problem. They fear surgery may be the only solution, despite being told there are no guarantees of success. They're beginning to wonder if anybody really knows anything about pain.

If all this describes your own situation or that of someone you care about, this book may provide the help you've been seeking. It proposes to give you a sensible explanation of what's wrong and help you find the real cause of your pain. Even better, it may well show you how to get rid of the pain yourself, hands on. No doctors. No pills. No bills.

The daily clinical experience of thousands of massage therapists, physical therapists, and physicians strongly indicates that most of our common aches and pains—and many other puzzling physical complaints—are actually caused by *trigger points*, or small contraction knots, in the muscles of the body. Pain clinic doctors skilled at detecting and treating trigger points have found that they're the primary cause of pain roughly 75 percent of the time and are at least a part of virtually every pain problem. Even fibromyalgia, which is known to afflict millions of people, is thought in many instances to have its beginning with trigger points (Travell and Simons 1999, 12–19; Gerwin 1995, 121; Fishbain et al. 1986, 181–197).

Trigger points are known to cause headaches, neck and jaw pain, low back pain, the symptoms of carpal tunnel syndrome, and many kinds of joint pain mistakenly ascribed to arthritis, tendinitis, bursitis, or ligament injury. Trigger points cause problems as diverse as earaches, dizziness, nausea, heartburn, false heart pain, heart arrhythmia, tennis elbow, and genital pain. Trigger points can also cause colic in babies and bed-wetting in older children, and may be a contributing cause of scoliosis. They are a cause of sinus pain and congestion. They may play a part in chronic fatigue and lowered resistance to infection. And because trigger points can be responsible for long-term pain and disability that seem to have no means of relief, they can cause depression.

The problems trigger points cause can be surprisingly easy to fix; in fact most people can do it themselves if they have the right information. That's good, because the time has come for ordinary people to take things into their own hands. The reason for this is that an appallingly high percentage of doctors and other practitioners are still pretty much out of the loop regarding trigger points, despite their having been written about in medical journals for over sixty years. There has been, and continues to be, great resistance to the whole idea that trigger points are real and should be taken seriously.

Why has the medical profession not embraced the idea of trigger points? Partly it's because trigger points are commonly confused with acupressure points. Acupressure, which has come down to us from ancient Chinese medicine, is alleged to have a positive effect on supposed flows of energy throughout the body. Although acupressure and other Eastern methods of healing do seem to have a beneficial effect, they're very resistant to solid scientific investigation and are viewed by many doctors and a large segment of the public as quack medicine with no proven results. If you don't know the difference, the claims about trigger points sound like quack medicine too.

Our knowledge of trigger points, however, comes right out of Western medical research. Trigger points are real. They can be felt with the fingers. They emit distinctive electrical signals that can be measured by sensitive electronic equipment. Trigger points have also been photographed in muscle tissue with the aid of the electron microscope (Travell and Simons 1999, 57–70).

Most of what is known about trigger points is very well documented in the two-volume medical text *Myofascial Pain and Dysfunction: The Trigger Point Manual*, by Janet Travell and David Simons. These books tell virtually all that is known about trigger points, and the prospects for pain relief are very exciting. Much of the information in *The Trigger Point Manual* is couched in difficult scientific terms, but basic trigger point science isn't hard to grasp if it's put into everyday language.

Travell and Simons describe a trigger point as simply a small contraction knot in muscle tissue. It often feels like a partly cooked piece of macaroni, or like a pea buried deep in the muscle. A trigger point affects a muscle by keeping it both tight and weak. At the same time, a trigger point maintains a hard contraction on the muscle fibers that it is a part of. In turn, these taut bands of muscle fiber keep constant tension on the muscle's attachments, often producing symptoms in adjacent joints. The constant tension in the fibers of the trigger point itself restricts circulation in its immediate area. The resulting accumulation of the by-products of metabolism, as well as deprivation of the oxygen and nutrients needed for metabolism, can perpetuate trigger points for months or even years unless some intervention occurs. It's this self-sustaining vicious cycle that needs to be broken (Travell and Simons 1999, 71–75).

The difficulty in treating trigger points is that they typically send pain to some other site. Most conventional treatment of pain is based on the assumption that the cause of pain will be found at the site of the pain. But trigger points almost always send their pain elsewhere. This referred pain is what has always thrown everybody off, including most doctors and much of the rest of the health-care community. According to Travell and Simons, conventional treatments for pain so often fail because they focus on the pain itself, treating the site of the pain while overlooking and failing to treat the cause, which may be some distance away.

Even worse than routinely treating the site of the pain is the pharmaceutical treatment of the whole body for what is usually a local problem. Painkilling drugs, the increasingly expensive treatment of choice these days, give us the illusion that something good is happening, when in reality they only mask the problem. Most common pain, like headaches, muscle aches, and joint pain, is a warning—a protective response to muscle overuse or trauma. Pain is telling you that something is wrong and needs attention. It's not good medicine to kill the messenger and ignore the message. When pain is seen in its true role as the messenger and not the affliction itself, treatment can be directed to the *cause* of pain.

Luckily, referred pain is now known to occur in predictable patterns. The valuable medical advance made by Travell and Simons and their brilliant illustrator, Barbara Cummings, has been in delineating these very patterns. Once you know where to look, trigger points are easily located by touch and deactivated by any of several methods.

Unfortunately, the two clinically oriented methods put forth in *The Trigger Point Manual* don't lend themselves to self-treatment. The goal of this book is to build on the work of Travell and Simons and provide a more practical and cost-effective approach to pain therapy: a classic do-it-yourself approach, rather than a reliance on multiple professional office visits. This new approach is a system of self-applied massage directed specifically at trigger points. Significant relief of symptoms often comes in just minutes. Most problems can be eliminated within three to ten days. Even long-standing chronic conditions can be cleared up in as little as six weeks. Results may be longer in coming for those who suffer from fibromyalgia, chronic fatigue, or widespread myofascial pain syndrome, but even they can experience continuing progress and can have genuine hope of significant improvement in their condition.

Self-applied trigger point massage works by accomplishing three things: it breaks into the chemical and neurological feedback loop that maintains the muscle contraction; it increases circulation that has been restricted by the contracted tissue; and it directly stretches the trigger point's knotted muscle fibers. The illustrations in this book show you how to find the trigger points that are generating your specific problems, as well as the exact hands-on techniques for deactivating them. Special attention has been given to designing methods of massage that do no damage to hands that may already be in trouble from overuse.

This book's primary use is as a self-instruction manual, but it can also be used as a text-book for classroom use. This simplified and direct approach to treating pain with self-applied massage can constitute a foundational course in trigger point therapy in any professional training curriculum. Students in chiropractic colleges, physical therapy depart-ments, and massage schools will derive particular benefit. (A new chapter has been added—chapter 11, "Clinical Trigger Point Massage"—to help the professional therapist adapt the book's technical content to the treatment of others.) If student therapists can learn how to interpret their own referred pain and how to find and treat their own trigger points, they will know exactly what to do when they encounter similar problems in their future clients.

A class in self-applied trigger point massage would be a boon in medical schools for exactly the same reasons. When new doctors can learn how to fix their own pain with self-applied massage, they are in better touch with the realities of pain and with the great potential in the treatment of trigger points. Such an addition to medical education would profoundly improve the treatment of pain and significantly lower its cost.

And it's not too late for physicians already in practice to learn about trigger points and myofascial pain and put the knowledge to good use. They will find this book a quick and practical introduction to the magnificent work of Travell and Simons and this neglected branch of medicine. Hopefully, many will be encouraged to go to Travell and Simons's *Trig-ger Point Manual* for a deeper scientific understanding and for even greater benefit to their practice. A large segment of the public needs help and encouragement in learning how to deal with their trigger point–induced pain. No one is better positioned to provide this help than the medical community.

The medical profession is not unaware of the deficiencies of current methods of treating pain. Doctors hurt too. Many of them worry like the rest of us about the relentless popping of pills, and many experience frustration with their inability to offer better solutions to their patients. Trigger point therapy, whether self-applied or administered by a professional, has the potential to truly revolutionize pain treatment throughout the world.

CHAPTER 1

A New Life

I was sixty years old when, at the height of my success in a business I'd pursued for almost four decades, I decided to dump it all and start at the bottom in a completely new field.

Piano rebuilding had been my trade and it had been a good one. My income had exceeded one hundred thousand dollars in some years; as a massage therapist, I knew I'd be lucky to make twenty thousand. The old life was full of rewards, not the least of which was intense satisfaction in the work itself, great prestige in my community, and unquestioned status among my peers. The new life would be full of anxieties and uncertainties, with little likelihood of ever equaling the success I'd enjoyed in the old one. What was my motive for making such a wrenching change?

In a word, the motive was pain. Through a difficult personal struggle with pain, I believed I had learned something worth sharing with the world. I believed I'd discovered something new in the treatment of pain that could change lives as it had changed mine. I couldn't be content with keeping it to myself.

You wouldn't be reading this book if you weren't in the midst of your own unresolved struggle with pain—or if you weren't searching for a better way to help those who hurt. I hope my story will show you what can be done when there seems to be no help.

Vladimir Horowitz's piano tuner taught me to tune pianos. It was 1960 and I was an apprentice at Steinway & Sons in New York. It was a great start. After I left Steinway, I had my own business in New York for several years, tuning in homes, churches, concert halls, recording studios, and theaters all over town. New York was cheap, a lot of really famous people knew my name, I rode a motorcycle, I had girlfriends—life was good.

In the late sixties, I moved to Kentucky, seeking cleaner air and a place to park my new car. I settled down, got married, and started raising two spunky daughters. In succeeding years, I rebuilt and refinished hundreds of grand pianos and tuned tens of thousands of pianos of all kinds. The business was full of rewards for a restless, creative spirit: I invented dozens of new tools for the piano trade, and through the many articles I wrote for the *Piano Technicians Journal*, piano tuners all over the world became acquainted with my tools, my methods, my name. I gained a reputation as someone who was good at finding simple solutions for difficult problems.

But during my time in the piano business I had a lot of trouble with pain—neck pain, back pain, every kind of pain you'd expect to get from hard physical work. As time went by, I grew increasingly concerned about how long I could continue. I had gradually become aware that the happiness and the very livelihood of virtually every piano technician I'd ever known had been threatened at one time or another by work-related pain. I remembered one of my teachers at Steinway had once been so crippled by a bad shoulder that he could hardly do his work.

When I eventually came down with a bad shoulder of my own, I had to face the fact that there really weren't any good solutions for pain. Basically, you popped a pill and tried to live through it. I discovered that the worst thing about pain was that doctors and others who were supposed to help didn't really help; many almost seemed to be faking an understanding. And they all charged an arm and a leg whether they helped you or not. The situation made me so mad and desperate that I made up my mind to fix my shoulder myself, if there was any possible way.

Before I was done, I had not only gotten rid of my shoulder problem, but I had retired from my work with pianos and had graduated from massage school. Instead of tuning pianos I was now tuning people. I had discovered the most important work of my life.

Nobody Understood Shoulders

Ironically, my life-changing crisis with pain wasn't caused directly by piano work—though I'm sure my job set me up for it. The trouble began one January morning when I came in from shoveling snow in my driveway with an oppressive little pain in my shoulder. As I went on with my shop work that day and in the days that followed, I favored the shoulder more and more. Everything I did irritated my condition—whatever that condition was. Before long, I could hardly raise my arm. Soon, I couldn't pick up my grandson, reach across to get my seat belt, or crawl under a grand piano to do a repair without excruciating pain. It got so bad that a sudden move would give me a jolt of pain that felt like an electric shock, doubling me over, grimacing and breathless, for several minutes. I couldn't sleep. I'd get up in the night seeking relief with ice rubs and hot showers, but nothing I did had any lasting effect. The ice would dull the pain long enough to let me get back to sleep, but in the morning the pain was back in full force.

Some years earlier, I had gone to a massage therapist for a back spasm. I had gone as a last resort, not really hoping for or expecting much. But she fixed me, and then went on to fix the chronic pain I had in my arms and hands. I couldn't have been more pleased—or surprised. I had barely been aware that massage therapy existed, let alone having any notion that it actually worked. I had figured the pain in my arms and hands was just the inevitable and all-too-precipitous decline of old age. But in only three sessions, my massage therapist succeeded in ridding me of an affliction that had possessed me for as long as I could remember. Unfortunately, I was at a loss with the new shoulder problem. This wondrous woman had moved away and I had no choice but to try to find someone else with a similar gift for healing. It was a fruitless search. Variations on the theme of "exercise and stretch" were all I heard, despite my protests that stretching made my pain worse, not better. At one point, I realized that the physical therapist who was treating me for my frozen shoulder was herself secretly suffering from exactly the same affliction! She couldn't fix herself and she couldn't fix me, but she expected payment just the same.

I had a sense that nobody really understood shoulders. I tried a series of massage therapists, looking for the grand results I'd had before, but they all just seemed to tinker with my shoulder problem. From previous experience, I had no faith in chiropractic for this problem. I also had no reason to think doctors would offer me anything but painkillers or, worse, surgery. You also hear about doctors forcibly manipulating frozen shoulders. Not in this lifetime, I thought; thanks just the same.

In the midst of my frustrating search for effective treatment, I decided to go to the annual convention of the Piano Technicians Guild. There were classes all week on various aspects of piano technology, and I had always felt revitalized by the dynamic exchange of ideas there. I was determined to go despite my disability and was hoping a break from work would help. But sitting all day in classes holding my arm defensively and motionless at my side only seemed to aggravate the problem. I rubbed at my shoulder continuously; I squeezed it; I tried to relax it; I tentatively and cautiously flexed it. The only result was an ache that rose in intensity throughout the week. My every thought was of pain.

On the last night, the pain was so unremitting that not even the ice treatments had any effect. I lay in bed in my hotel room at two o'clock in the morning and cried like a baby. Evidently, all I could hope for was to somehow outlive the problem. I had heard that it took about a year for a shoulder to heal itself—if it *did* heal itself.

Lying there in my misery, I happened to remember a pair of medical books I had seen years earlier on the desk of that first massage therapist I'd liked so much. She told me she referred to those books constantly, and she had been the only person who really seemed to know what she was doing in regard to pain. I realized I was going to have to find a way to take care of this problem myself and those medical books might at least be a place to start. It was a spark of hope.

A New Technology

When I got home from the convention, I ordered the books: volumes 1 and 2 of *Myofascial Pain and Dysfunction: The Trigger Point Manual*, by Janet Travell and David Simons. The price of medical books was a shock and I bridled a bit, but I finally had to ask myself: What is this knowledge worth? My shoulder answered the question for me.

When the books came, I entered a world I hadn't known existed. As soon as I began to read, the mystery of my shoulder problem began to clear. In *The Trigger Point Manual*, I found hundreds of beautifully executed illustrations of the muscles of the body. They showed the likely trigger points for every muscle and the patterns of pain they predictably touched off.

I found that, although the physiology of a trigger point was extremely complex, a trigger point for practical purposes could be viewed as what most people call a "knot": a wad of muscle fibers staying in a hard contraction, never relaxing. A trigger point in a muscle could be actively painful or it could manifest no pain at all unless touched. More often, though, it would sneakily send its pain somewhere else. I gathered that much of my pain, perhaps all of it, was probably this mysterious displaced pain, this referred pain. I had never been able to figure out why all the rubbing I had been doing had never done any good. It was a mistake to assume the problem was at the place that hurt!

The pain in the front of my shoulder was actually coming from behind it, from trigger points in the infraspinatus, a muscle that covered part of the outside of my shoulder blade. The deep aching behind my shoulder was coming from trigger points in the subscapularis, a muscle on the underside of my shoulder blade, sandwiched between the shoulder blade and the ribs. The unrelenting pain at the inner edge of my shoulder blade was being sent by trigger points in the scalene muscles, in the front and sides of my neck. It was no wonder nobody knew what to do for me!

It was clear to me that all I had was a massive number of trigger points in the muscles in my shoulder—trigger points in over *twenty* muscles, as it turned out. That first massage therapist, the one I liked so much, had treated me very successfully with ordinary massage techniques and I understood now that it was trigger points she was dealing with. Perhaps I could deal with the trigger points myself using massage. I began to think that this might be a job for someone with a technician's mentality—maybe someone who was smart enough to take on the complexities of a grand piano would be well equipped to fix trigger points.

Driven by my misery and by my excitement about these new ideas, I studied Travell and Simons night and day. I found that my trigger points would yield under the touch of my own hands if I persisted. After only about a month of assiduously applying what I was learning chapter by chapter, I had succeeded in fixing my shoulder . . . *my own shoulder!* I was astounded. The pain was gone. I could raise my arm. I could sleep through the night. This stuff really worked!

Given the innately optimistic cast of my mind, I immediately took a larger view. I saw that I had in my hands the tools to take effective care of myself, at least when it came to any kind of myofascial pain. I supposed that I might be able to treat any trigger point I could reach and extinguish virtually any pain I might have. I could develop a complete system, a kind of new technology, and maybe other people would be helped by it.

Mechanical Ingenuity

Travell and Simons had done a wonderful thing in giving the science of myofascial pain to the medical community. The illustrations by Barbara Cummings brilliantly clarified every aspect of the subject. Without these dedicated people, the science of trigger points and referred pain would still be an impossible jumble, largely unknown and inaccessible.

Unfortunately, Travell and Simons's two main methods for deactivating trigger points weren't oriented toward self-treatment. They were designed specifically for the doctor's office or the physical therapy clinic: a doctor could inject trigger points with procaine, a local anesthetic; and a physical therapist could presumably stretch trigger points out of existence. It bothered me, however, that the physical therapy protocol, which Travell and Simons called their "workhorse" method, involved the muscle stretching that I had found so ineffective and even dangerous, in that it had made my shoulder problem dramatically worse. To be sure, Travell and Simons had made stretching safer by using a refrigerant spray on the skin. "Distracting" the nervous system with the spray meant the underlying muscles were less likely to tighten up in defense. Nevertheless, safe or not, I felt that the spray and stretch method was too elaborate to be practical for self-treatment, and that it would be impossible to use on areas that were hard to reach.

In addition, trying to get at the relatively small trigger points by stretching whole groups of recalcitrant muscles seemed unnecessarily indirect and inefficient. The problem was not with the generalized tension in the muscle, but rather with the trigger point, a very specific, circumscribed place within the muscle. The trigger point's knotted up muscle fibers obviously needed to relax and let go, but why not go straight to the trouble spot and deal with it directly? Massage seemed to me the natural approach, and it obviously worked with trigger points—that good massage therapist had proven that much to me.

I wanted to find simple ways to use massage for self-treatment. I wanted to develop a comprehensive method for dealing with trigger points anywhere in the body. I wanted something that a regular person like me could immediately understand and use. I was sure all this could be done.

Among the old-time piano men at Steinway, the highest compliment was to be called "a good mechanic." A good mechanic cared about the details and he stuck with the job until he got it right; he could find the solution to a problem even if it wasn't in the book. My life up to that point had been built around being a good mechanic, and being able to find the simple solution. That's certainly what I had to do in devising ways to self-treat trigger points. For the purposes of treating trigger points, I felt the body was best thought of as a machine, a mechanical system of levers, fulcrums, and forces, especially in regard to the bones and muscles. I could understand such a system. A lifetime of working with my hands was about to begin to pay off in a new and unexpected way.

My first challenge was to learn the exact location of each muscle, to visualize how it attached to the bones, and to understand the job the muscle did. Finding the precise massage technique that a trigger point would respond to was where the art would come in. The difficulty here was in figuring out how to reach unreachable places and get effective leverage in awkward positions without hurting my hands and fingers, which were already being overused in the course of an ordinary workday.

The project became an obsession. I studied Travell and Simons the first thing in the morning and the last thing at night. I studied in the parking lot at McDonald's. Using my own body as the laboratory, I discovered something new every day. I found trigger points everywhere and became aware of pain that I didn't know I had. I only wanted to talk about trigger points and often greeted family members excitedly with the exclamation, "I found another one! I found another one!" Over a period of three years, I learned how to find and deactivate trigger points in 120 pairs of muscles, which enabled me to cope with every trigger point that Travell and Simons dealt with in their books except those inside the pelvis.

A World of Pain

The misdiagnosis of pain is the most important issue taken up by Travell and Simons. Referred pain from trigger points mimics the symptoms of a very long list of common maladies; but physicians, in weighing all the possible causes for a given condition, have rarely even conceived of there being a myofascial source. The study of trigger points has not historically been a part of medical education. Travell and Simons hold that most of common everyday pain is caused by myofascial trigger points and that ignorance of that basic concept could inevitably lead to false diagnoses and the ultimate failure to deal effectively with pain (Travell and Simons 1999, 12–14).

From the beginning, I had a sense that for some reason the great work of Janet Travell and David Simons had fallen into a deep pit and was in danger of being buried and forgotten. Surely by now Travell's discoveries about pain should have swept the country and changed the world of health care. The first volume of *The Trigger Point Manual* had been published in 1983, but I couldn't find anything about trigger points in the public library. None of the popular family medical guides even mentioned trigger points. Nothing truly informative was to be found in bookstores. Doctors were still using drugs as the primary treatment for pain. Many were actively hostile to the concept of trigger points, discounting the idea as just more bogus medicine, something purely imaginary.

Only massage therapists seemed to be informed about trigger points and referred pain, and only exceptional individuals among them (in my own experience at least) were treating trigger points effectively. What's more, the burgeoning variety of unproven modalities offered by massage therapists gave the profession such an aura of flakiness that the elegant science of myofascial pain treatment got unfairly confused with treatments whose results could easily be attributed to the placebo effect. With such an identity, how could the medical profession or the public ever consider massage a legitimate therapy for pain?

Clearly, there was a world of pain out there in need of the simple and genuine solutions I felt I had in hand. I despaired of doctors ever listening to me about trigger point therapy. Taking the facts about myofascial pain directly to the public seemed the more logical tack. I began to think about leaving the piano business behind. There was something more important for me to do.

The first thing I wanted to do was to write about the self-treatment of pain for all my ailing friends in the Piano Technicians Guild. Previous articles in the *Piano Technicians Journal* had given me a following. I guessed that my ideas about pain had a better chance of publication in this journal than almost anywhere else.

I also conceived of giving seminars and workshops about the self-treatment of pain, and I thought that getting a massage school diploma might give me more credibility. But I had an even better motive for going to massage school. My daughter Amber had had chronic back pain ever since lifting a heavy chair during a scene change while she was working in summer theater. Employing my new knowledge about trigger points, I'd been trying to give her massage, but I just wasn't very good. I didn't know the time-tested manual techniques used by massage therapists. It would be worth learning to do massage right, if only to help my daughter; and anything I learned that benefited my method of self-treatment would be a plus.

I applied to the biggest massage school I could find, one with a busy, well-managed student clinic where I could get a great deal of experience in the shortest time possible. At that moment, I couldn't imagine becoming a professional therapist, but I definitely wanted the skills. With the help of my son-in-law, who I had trained to take over my piano business, I plowed through a backlog of half a dozen rebuilding jobs. We cleared my calendar in time for me to start a six-month clinical course at the Utah College of Massage Therapy.

Massage School

There were forty-nine of us in the class: thirty-six women and thirteen men. We were a greatly varied group of all backgrounds, from many states and foreign countries, and ranging in age from seventeen to sixty. It soon became apparent that, although I was the oldest in the class (and possibly prejudged by most of the others to be a creaking fuddy-duddy), I was the only one who could claim to be free of pain. All the others—young and old, male and female—had some kind of enduring problem with pain. I found that it was almost a cliché that people go to massage school because they have chronic pain and they're looking for the solution they haven't found elsewhere.

It seemed ironic to me that I arrived in Utah having read both volumes of Travell and Simons's *Trigger Point Manual* and having gone a long way toward developing my method of self-healing, yet I couldn't get anyone to listen. I had just left a business where my word was taken as gospel. People were eager to hear what I had to say about pianos. In the role of student, my accustomed authority was reduced to nil. Nobody wanted to hear what I knew about trigger points. I could only stand and watch as a fellow student would have a pain crisis, usually bad neck pain or a back spasm, and run off to a chiropractor or to the emergency room. I kept offering help and being turned down.

It was even harder to approach the instructors about do-it-yourself massage, but the anatomy teacher apparently felt less threatened than the others. He was a big, self-confident guy with a great sense of humor, who didn't fear losing his authority with the students. During a break one day, he heard me talking to a classmate about trigger points and asked if I knew how to fix pain. He said he often had pain that shot diagonally across one side of his chest. He was having it again just that morning. It wasn't his heart, he said; he'd had it checked. While he explained, I reached up and began pressing on his neck just above his collarbone. He suddenly stopped talking and winced, then exclaimed, "Hey, that's it! That's my pain! How did you do that?" A trigger point in a scalene muscle was causing the pain in his chest. I showed him how to work the trigger point himself and he told me later that the pain had gone away and hadn't come back.

I couldn't get over it. This man was a registered nurse and a gifted teacher of anatomy who knew his muscles but didn't know about his own trigger points. He was a product of the same system that turns out physicians with the same astounding gap in their knowledge.

After my classmates saw me go hands on with our anatomy teacher's trigger points, they began letting me show them some of my tricks. I showed one student how to kill her sinus pain by working on her jaw muscles, another how to stop his feet from hurting by massaging his calves, and another how to get rid of her dizzy spells with attention to trigger points in the front of her neck. Several eventually came to me for back pain of various kinds. Near the end of the course, I got to show the whole class my techniques for getting rid of arm and hand pain, something we all experienced working in the clinic. Several classes of budding massage therapists worked in the weekend clinic where it was not unusual for us to give twelve hundred massages on a Saturday and Sunday.

I saw the same pain patterns in the clinic that I had seen with my fellow students: lots of back trouble, plus a broad selection of every other kind of pain you could think of. I saw pain in every part of the body and every joint: shoulders, elbows, wrists, knuckles, hips, knees, and ankles. Typically, the client had already been the rounds of doctors, chiropractors, physical therapists, and so on, looking for the magician in the white coat. They'd tried yoga, magnets, pain diets, herbal therapies, and acupuncture. Some had had their problem for ten years and more. Many guessed they were just getting arthritis and so were habitually popping pills. They felt older than their years, handicapped by pain. They felt their careers in danger. Depression due to constant pain was a prevailing theme.

It was exasperating to hear the same stories repeatedly, to know both how simple their problems were and just what to do for them, and to know many clients were coming for massage only as a last resort. In my view, massage was the only thing that worked for these kinds of pain, and should be the first thing tried, not the last. I consistently found trigger points to be the cause of my clients' problems, and clients nearly always got off my table feeling better. Many left my booth feeling they'd finally found something that worked. I felt more and more that I also had found something that worked. I liked giving massage a great deal—I was surprised at how much. I asked for extra shifts and accumulated almost twice as many hours as were required.

Until I was working regularly in the clinic, I hadn't seen that giving massage to others was a way of taking care of myself. I'd only been thinking of getting a diploma from a good school so I would have a bit of credibility when I went on to teach self-massage. Unexpectedly, I got as much from the massages as my clients did, maybe more. I felt myself becoming kinder and more empathic. Knowing how to take care of my own pain had made me more fit for taking care of others, which made me more fit for taking care of myself. My six months at the Utah College of Massage Therapy was transformational. I regretted I hadn't done it sooner.

Recurrent Themes

While in massage school, I finished writing my series of eight articles on self-applied trigger point massage for the *Piano Technicians Journal*. Publication began two months after I graduated. When the first article appeared, desperate piano tuners began calling me for advice from all over the United States and Canada. They didn't want to wait until the article on their particular problem came out. Many were on the verge of quitting piano work because of chronic pain. Some had been in pain for as long as twenty years, repeatedly going the rounds of the health care community just like I had, with the same frustrating results.

One tuner from New England had been afflicted with severe recurrent pain in both knees since climbing Mount Katahdin, the highest point in Maine, twelve years earlier. The pain had started as he descended the mountain and his friends had had to carry him most of the way to the bottom. Now he couldn't even go out and mow his lawn without being crippled for days by the effort. Working with me over the phone, he was able to find and massage the horribly painful trigger points in his thigh muscles that were causing the pain in his knees. Before we hung up, the pain was gone. There had been no way for him to know that his trouble was not in his knees but in his thigh muscles, strained by the unaccustomed mountain climbing: his doctors, physical therapists, and chiropractors hadn't known. At the Piano Technicians Guild National Convention a couple of months later, he happily told me he'd continued working on his trigger points and hadn't had any more trouble with his knees. I was as pleased as he was.

I was scheduled to give a workshop on the self-treatment of pain at that convention and was worried that nobody would come. From the number of sufferers who had called me on the phone, I should've known better. One hundred and ten people showed up, and it was standing room only in the modest-sized meeting room. I knew at least one thing about every person in the room before we even began: they all hurt.

Piano technicians are the most diverse, intelligent, creative group of people I've ever had the privilege to know, and at the same time they're the most assertively independent. Some literally would rather die than ask for help. If I could tell them something about the treatment of pain that they could do themselves, they wanted to hear it. They were all in such need that no one so much as looked away throughout the whole program. I was very encouraged.

That was the first convention I went to not as a piano tuner, but as a massage therapist. I didn't go to classes at all that week. I didn't go to committee meetings. I didn't even party at night. I had something better to do. I spent every day, from eight in the morning until ten at night, troubleshooting trigger points and giving massages, only leaving my room to get a quick meal. They weren't all piano tuners who came to me; spouses needed help too. Although there were some recurrent themes, like shoulder pain, they brought me all kinds of problems—back pain, neck pain, headaches, numb hands—just like in the massage school clinic. People at the convention had come from all over North America, even from several foreign countries. No matter where these people lived, they all had the same story: they'd had trouble getting effective treatment. Nobody seemed to know what caused their pain and nobody could help.

Back in Kentucky, as I began my private practice, again I saw all the by now familiar patterns. All the people who came for massage had already been to a physician or a pain clinic. Almost all had experimented with chiropractic. Many had been to the emergency room for their pain. Most had been through physical therapy. They had tried everything, including various forms of alternative medicine. Some had even tried massage but hadn't been impressed. It had been "feel-good" massage: it had been relaxing but hadn't put a dent in their pain.

Interestingly, almost all the people who came to me had some kind of back pain along with whatever other pain complaint they had. Their previous treatments for back pain had always focused on the spine. I heard about injections of papaya or cortisone. People had usually been told they had arthritis or bad disks, or that their cartilage had been worn away. They'd been shown X-rays that purported to prove it. One woman was on her doctor's schedule to have her vertebrae fused. Some had already had surgery, and frequently had as much pain after surgery as before. Typically, the surgeon's last word was always that he was sorry but he'd done all he could. Then he'd renew their prescription for painkillers and dump them off on a physical therapist. I heard these stories over and over again. And over and over, I found that trigger point therapy gave them the relief they'd been seeking for so long. Had trigger points been the problem in the first place? Arthritis? Bad disks? In Travell and Simons's *Trigger Point Manual*, I had read that you can have herniated disks and arthritis of the spine and still find that myofascial trigger points are the primary cause of your back pain.

One client said her doctor confided sympathetically that he had back pain too. He wore magnets under his clothing just like she did. Many of my clients had tried magnets and were often a little embarrassed to say so. Yes, the magnets did seem to help, they said, but the pain always came back. It was the same with TENS units: when you took them off, you still had your problem. (A transcutaneous electrical nerve stimulation [TENS] unit gives you little shocks that interfere with pain signals, but has no effect on the cause of the pain.)

Nearly everyone I treated was on pain medication of some kind, although few had the illusion that painkillers were a real cure. People seem to know intuitively that throwing a cloak over the pain only keeps you from seeing the real problem. When you hide the problem, you never get the opportunity to address it. Looked at in this way, painkillers actually perpetuate pain. People want real solutions; they don't want to dope the problem away.

Another common theme among the people who came to me was numbness and pain in the hands and fingers. I began to get the impression that the computer keyboard was crippling the country. I saw wrist braces of all kinds. A doctor had wanted to put one woman's wrists in casts to heal her numb hands. While many clients feared they had carpal tunnel syndrome or had even been given the diagnosis, massage of trigger points in the forearms, shoulder, and neck always took the pain and numbness away. This outcome was usually a surprise to the client. It soon ceased to be a surprise to me. Good results were so consistent with "carpal tunnel" symptoms that I began to wonder whether true carpal tunnel syndrome really existed.

What did all this mean for me? I knew how to help myself and it was clear I could help other people, but what was the best use of my newfound skills? There was indeed a world of pain out there, but I'd started too late as a massage therapist to hope to help very many people one-on-one. At my age I wasn't going to have a long career as a healer. What could I do for the world of pain with the time and energy I had left? It became increasingly clear that I had to write a book about trigger point therapy and get this information out to as many people as possible.

Casting a Wider Net

A doctor should have written this book. It should've been written by a bona fide, credentialed expert in a white coat with years and years of experience and scores of articles published in medical journals. If "M.D." followed my name on the cover of this book, I wouldn't have had to write this chapter. This chapter is meant to give you some reason to trust what I have to say about pain, some reason to suspend your disbelief long enough to give my methods a fair try. The best evidence of whether my method is a good one for you will come from your own personal experience with it. Trying it is the only way you can truly validate my claims about its success.

I don't claim to be an authority on pain. Travell and Simons are the pain experts. In writing this book, my job has primarily been to put their vast knowledge into more understandable form and transmit it to you. Having figured out how to fix my own pain counts for something, though. Being a massage therapist counts too, because I've proven to myself and to my clients that I know how to fix pain for other people.

I thought you might be interested in my shoulder story. I thought you might be interested in how the wisdom of Janet Travell and David Simons got me through my difficulties and how they truly gave me a new life. From my success in defeating pain, I thought you might gain a smidgen of hope: my new life offering the possibility of a new life for you. My own hope is that this book will be a useful one. It's you who will prove me right or wrong.

CHAPTER 2

All about Trigger Points

In the four introductory chapters of *Myofascial Pain and Dysfunction: The Trigger Point Manual* (1999), Travell and Simons give a detailed presentation of everything that is known about the science of trigger points and referred pain. They substantiate their assertions with references to several hundred scientific articles that pertain to the subject. The personal authority of Janet Travell and David Simons is impressive in itself.

Janet G. Travell, M.D. (1901–1997)

Among those who recognize the reality and importance of myofascial pain, Janet Travell is generally recognized as the leading pioneer in diagnosis and treatment. Few would deny that she single-handedly created this branch of medicine. At the time the first volume of her book went to press in 1983, she had been studying and treating trigger points and referred pain for over forty years. She had already published more than forty articles about her research in medical journals, the first appearing in 1942. Her revolutionary concepts about pain have improved the lives of millions of people. Trigger point massage, the most effective modality used by massage therapists for the relief of pain, is based almost entirely on Dr. Travell's insights. The innovative clinical techniques for the treatment of myofascial pain that are beginning to be used by physicians and physical therapists all over the world wouldn't have existed without Dr. Travell's dedicated energy and intelligence.

Dr. Travell's personal success with one particular patient had a far-reaching effect on history. Not many people remember that Janet Travell was the White House physician during the Kennedy and Johnson administrations. President Kennedy honored her with that position in gratitude for her treatment of the debilitating myofascial pain and other ailments that had threatened to prematurely end his political career. It's a stunning example of how trigger point therapy can change someone's life and destiny.

Although she was in her sixties at the end of her duties at the White House, Dr. Travell had no intention of retiring or even slowing down. She went on developing and teaching her methods with vigor and enthusiasm for the next thirty years. She was past eighty when the first volume of *The Trigger Point Manual* was published, and past ninety when the second volume appeared. She refused to rush into print: she wanted to get it right.

David G. Simons, M.D. (b. 1922)

David Simons lends authority to the study of myofascial pain with his long experience as a research scientist. In his early career, Dr. Simons worked as an aerospace physician, developing improved methods of measuring physiological responses to the stress of weightlessness. A fascinating sidelight to his career is the world altitude record for manned balloon flight he set in 1957 as a young Air Force flight surgeon. In point of fact, he beat Sputnik into space. He was featured on the cover of *Life* magazine that year and subsequently wrote a book, *Man High* (1960), about his adventure.

Drs. Travell and Simons first met when she lectured about trigger points and myofascial pain at the Air Force's School of Aerospace Medicine. Simons was so intrigued by Travell's work that he eventually retired from the Air Force and began a long informal apprenticeship under her wing. An intense synergy developed between the two over the next twenty years, culminating at last in the production of *The Trigger Point Manual*, an inspiring testament to the transcendent power generated when two minds of uncommon intelligence work together.

Dr. Simons's strict attention to detail and adherence to scientific method helped him bring rigorous objectivity to the documentation of myofascial pain. He was the driving force in getting the Travell and Simons books written, doing most of the actual writing himself, with Dr. Travell's vast knowledge and experience as his primary resource. One day, when ordinary people know about trigger points and the diagnosis and treatment of myofascial pain is taught widely in medical schools, physicians everywhere will honor Dr. Simons, along with his mentor, Dr. Travell, as true medical pioneers.

Into his eighties now, David Simons is still hard at work promoting further research concerning trigger points. His latest book, *Muscle Pain: Understanding Its Nature, Diagnosis, and Treatment* (2001), with coauthor Dr. Siegfried Mense, seeks to impart a better understanding of the neurophysiology of muscles.

The Essentials

Considering the sheer mass of scientific detail that Travell and Simons cover in their first four chapters, it's intimidating for anyone without a scientific education to simply sit and turn the pages. The aim in this chapter is to boil down the essentials of trigger point science and make them accessible to the layman in clear, concise, everyday language. As a consequence, many of Travell and Simons's most carefully reasoned and well-supported assertions can only be summarized here.* If you think you might have the appetite and the capacity to digest the original work of Travell and Simons, by all means go on and do it. You can find their two-volume *Trigger Point Manual* in most university medical libraries. If you're a health care professional, think about buying the books and doing a deeper study than is presented here. A physician should certainly consider his or her personal library incomplete without them.

---

* The pages on which these assertations appear are cited in parenthesis, sometimes accompanied by citations of sources Travell and Simons themselves cited. Due to space considerations, references to Travell and Simons are often listed simply as 1992 or 1999, depending on which volume of the book is cited.

The Price of Ignorance

Travell and Simons believe that trigger points are the primary cause of pain and that the public suffers pain needlessly because too many doctors are still uninformed about them. For that reason, they believe misdiagnosis of pain and ineffective treatments often characterize the practice of medicine, resulting in enormous unnecessary cost, both to the pocketbook and to quality of life (1999, 12, 14, 36). In the *Trigger Point Manual*, they list twenty-four examples of mistaken diagnoses, from angina and appendicitis to tennis elbow and tension headache, that are likely to be made when the physician is unaware that myofascial trigger points may be to blame (1999, 37). Too often, they believe, when pain has a myofascial origin, diagnosis entirely eludes the physician, who then is apt to write the problem off as minor or imaginary and categorize it as untreatable. Too many people grimly live with pain that is very real and that could be very easily treated if their doctor or other health-care practitioner would simply take the time to acquire the appropriate knowledge.

Pills, Pills, Pills

Dr. Sidney Wolfe, in *Worst Pills, Best Pills* (Wolfe et al. 1999), contends that too many physicians resort to prescribing narcotics and other chemical substances for the relief of pain, not necessarily because they don't know what else to offer, but because of the pharmaceutical industry's inordinate influence in the medical community. He believes that the billions of dollars poured into pharmaceutical advertising is one of the biggest causes of the public's almost exclusive dependence on drugs for pain and other conditions.

Wolfe points out that all pain medications have potential adverse effects and that some actually kill thousands of people every year. He believes there are at least twenty commonly prescribed pain medications that are so dangerous they should be taken off the market. He lists thirty-nine others that should have only very limited use. Dr. Wolfe quotes studies suggesting that an appallingly high percentage of physicians are insufficiently aware of just how dangerous some of their favorite drugs can be. He strongly recommends seeking proven nondrug remedies whenever possible before giving in to pharmaceutical solutions. Anyone who regularly takes prescription drugs for any reason should study Dr. Wolfe's book closely. An astounding number of drugs include muscle and joint pain in their list of side effects. Your medicine may be playing a key role in your problem with chronic pain.

Trigger Point Science

Although much of the medical community resists having to learn about what they think are new, untested notions about pain, trigger points aren't really a new concept. Travell and Simons, in an extensive review of the medical literature, found that the knotlike characteristics of trigger points have been written about for over 150 years. Their ability to cause displaced pain was known as early as 1938. Janet Travell first used the term "trigger point" in print in 1942 (1999, 15).

It's a good guess that ancient Chinese systems of therapeutic touch, surviving today as acupressure and related modalities, were probably early attempts to explain and deal with what we now know as trigger points. People have probably been coping with trigger points for many thousands of years in the simple acts of rubbing one another's backs and necks. Massage for the relief of pain by dealing with the "knots" in muscles has been a formal profession in this country for almost a hundred years. People have always known about "knots." It's only that they haven't known about all the ways they connect with pain.

The Prevalence of Trigger Points

Trigger points are remarkably common. Travell and Simons describe them without exaggeration as the "scourge of mankind" (1999, 14). No one escapes trigger points, not even children and babies (1999, 21). Trigger points can develop in any of the two hundred pairs of muscles in the body, which gives them a wide territory for creating mischief (1999, 13). Trigger points can last as long as life and can even survive in muscle tissue after death, detectable until rigor mortis sets in (1999, 68).

The pain inflicted by trigger points may be the biggest cause of disability and loss of time in any workplace or office, in any professional or amateur sport, or simply around home—anywhere people are apt to overdo some activity. Travell and Simons quote studies suggesting that trigger points are a component of up to 93 percent of the pain seen in pain clinics, and the sole cause of such pain as much as 85 percent of the time (1999, 12; Gerwin 1995, 121; Fishbain et al. 1986, 181–197).

An underestimated trait of trigger points is that they can exist indefinitely in a latent state, in which they don't actively refer pain. Travell and Simons believe that the long-term effects of *latent trigger points* may be of even greater concern than the pain caused by active ones. They assert that latent trigger points tend to accumulate over a lifetime and appear to be the main cause for the stiff joints and restricted range of motion of old age. In addition, the constant muscle tension imposed by latent trigger points tends to overstress muscle attachments even in younger people, which can result in irreversible damage to the joints and may be one of the causes of osteoarthritis. You may not suspect that you have latent trigger points, but they're very easy to find. They're exquisitely painful when pressed on. Latent trigger points can be activated by very little stress or strain (1999, 12–21).

Mistaken Identity

Many people have the mistaken impression that trigger points are the same thing as acupressure points. Acupressure points are said to be concentrations of energy or blockages on the meridians, the body's supposed energy pathways. It's difficult to prove that such meridians exist. Trigger points, on the other hand, are demonstrably physical phenomena. Acupressure points don't refer pain as trigger points do and aren't painful to touch unless they happen to coincide with a trigger point. Acupressure and acupuncture both enjoy greater success in relieving pain when a trigger point is present at the same site as an acupressure point (1999, 41–42; Melzack, Fox, and Shilwell 1997, 3–23).

People often say "pressure points" when they mean to say "trigger points," but a pressure point is what you press on to stop the flow of blood from a wound. Pressure is used on a trigger point not to stop blood flow but to increase it. The pressure, of course, is intermittent, in the form of a repeated massage stroke.

Trigger points are also often mixed up with "tender points," one of the official criteria for a diagnosis of fibromyalgia. This is a serious mistake when made by a professional, because it can sentence the person unnecessarily to a life without hope of significant improvement or cure. According to Travell and Simons, many people who have been diagnosed with fibromyalgia are afflicted in reality only with widespread trigger points. Also, a significant part of the pain suffered by someone with genuine fibromyalgia can be due to myofascial trigger points. Massage is widely recognized as an effective way to deal with fibromyalgia when the practitioner has the patience to limit treatment to only what the sufferer can tolerate without adverse reactions (1999, 36–41, 140–142).

There are clear guidelines for distinguishing trigger points from tender points: A trigger point needs firm pressure to elicit pain, while a tender point is so painful it can hardly be touched. In addition, tender points cause only local pain; they don't refer pain to another site as trigger points do. Genuine fibromyalgia sufferers usually have both types of "points." Their states of pain can be improved markedly when they can bear treatment of their trigger points.

Not infrequently, people think that myofascial trigger points cause only pain in the face, teeth, and jaws, getting "fascial" mixed up with "facial." Trigger points certainly can cause face pain, but myofascial pain can occur anywhere in the body. The prefix "myo" in myofascial (MY-oh-FAH-shul) refers to muscle. *Fascia* (FAH-shuh) is the thin, translucent membrane that envelopes and separates muscles like shrink-wrap. (A good place to see fascia is on a chicken leg.) When you have trigger points in a muscle, the fascia covering it typically gets tight and inflexible and becomes part of the problem.

Validation of Trigger Points

There has always been skepticism regarding the reality of trigger points among physicians who have not taken the time to study the subject. Stubborn disbelief remains even today among those who are aware of the evidence unearthed by Dr. Travell in 1957. She discovered that trigger points generate and receive tiny electrical currents and that the activity of a trigger point could be quantified by measuring these tiny signals with electromyographic instruments. She found that the precise location of a trigger point could be determined by this same means. Muscle tissue not in a state of contraction is electrically silent. Electrical activity confined to a very small area shows that only a small part of the muscle is in contracture. Interestingly, pressure on a trigger point increases its electrical activity. Stretching the muscle does the same thing, which explains why stretching so often makes pain worse (1999, 58–69).

The most convincing practical demonstration of the existence of trigger points is to just feel them with the fingers. Active and latent trigger points alike give a distinctively painful response to pressure. If a trigger point is near the surface, sensitive fingers can detect that it's a little warmer than surrounding tissue. This temperature difference, which is due to increased metabolic activity in the trigger point, is measurable (1999, 29–30).

Being soft tissue, trigger points can't be seen on X-ray. They have been viewed, however, with electron microscopy in fresh human cadavers. In the second edition of volume I of the *Trigger Point Manual*, Travell and Simons include a very convincing and elucidating electron microscopic photograph of a trigger point in a dog's leg muscle (1999, 68–69).

A Clear Definition

Travell and Simons define a trigger point as "a highly irritable localized spot of exquisite tenderness in a nodule in a palpable taut band of muscle tissue." The first part of that very exacting definition just means that a trigger point hurts like the devil when you push on it. When a trigger point is active enough, you're likely to startle, wince, and pull away. This is called "giving the jump sign."

The "nodule" in the formal definition is the trigger point itself. To your fingertips, it feels like a knot or a small lump that can range in size from a pinhead to a pea. In the large muscles of the thigh, a trigger point can feel like a lump the size of your thumb. Sometimes a trigger point feels like a short piece of partially cooked macaroni or spaghetti. Your fingers must be sensitive to feel these nodules. Not everyone has that sensitivity. Particularly gifted massage therapists are able to rely entirely on their sense of touch to find trigger points. Luckily, in troubleshooting your own myofascial pain, the trigger point's exquisite tenderness to pressure always gives it away. Trigger points *always* hurt when pressed on—there's never any question.

The "palpable taut band" is a semihard strand of muscle that feels like a cord or cable and is easily mistaken for a tendon. Taut means it's tightly stretched. Palpable means you can feel it with your fingers. Plucking a taut band in some muscles elicits a localized twitch response, which is a brief spontaneous contraction. Taut bands tend to restrict range of motion by limiting a muscle's ability to lengthen. They can exist painlessly in muscles without the presence of trigger points.

A trigger point is not the same thing as a muscle spasm. A spasm involves a violent contraction of the entire muscle. A trigger point is a contraction in only a small part. A spasm can usually be relaxed in a matter of minutes. For physiological reasons, trigger points don't give up that easily.

The Physiology of a Trigger Point

The place where contraction actually occurs in muscle fiber is a microscopic unit called a *sarcomere*. Millions of sarcomeres have to contract in your muscles to make even the smallest movement. A trigger point exists when overstimulated sarcomeres become unable to release their contracted state (1999, 45–47).

Figure 2.1 is a representation of several muscle fibers within a trigger point. It is based on the electron microscope photograph of a trigger point shown on page 69 of the second edition of volume 1 of Travell and Simons's *Trigger Point Manual* (1999), as interpreted by illustrator Barbara Cummings.

Letter A indicates a muscle fiber in a normal resting state, neither stretched nor contracted. The distance between the short crossways lines within the fiber defines the length of the individual sarcomeres. The sarcomeres run lengthwise in the fiber.

Letter B indicates a knot in a muscle fiber consisting of a mass of sarcomeres in the state of maximum continuous contraction that characterizes a trigger point. The bulbous appearance of the contraction knot indicates how that segment of the muscle fiber has drawn up and become shorter and wider.

Letter C indicates the part of the muscle fiber that extends from the contraction knot to the muscle's attachment (to the breastbone in this case). Note the greater distance between the crossways lines, which displays how the sarcomeres in this part of the muscle fiber are being stretched by tension within the contraction knot. These stretched segments of muscle fiber are what give tightness and rigidity to the taut band. Therapy should equalize sarcomere length in the fiber.

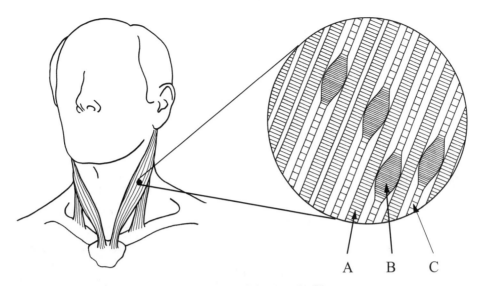

Figure 2.1   Magnified contraction knots (trigger points) in muscle fibers

Normally, sarcomeres act like tiny pumps, contracting and releasing to circulate blood through the capillaries that supply their metabolic needs. When sarcomeres in a trigger point hold their contraction, blood flow essentially stops in the immediate area. The resulting oxygen starvation and accumulation of the waste products of metabolism irritate the trigger point. The trigger point responds to this emergency by sending out pain signals until the brain institutes a policy of rest for the muscle. You stop using the muscle, which then begins to shorten and tighten up (1999, 69–78). To learn more about sarcomeres and the complex chemistry of muscle contraction, consult any good biology or anatomy textbook.

Central Trigger Points

Solving the problem of myofascial pain hinges on locating *central trigger points*, those that occur in the center of a muscle. Trigger points always originate at the midpoint of a muscle's fibers. This is where the motor nerve enters, bringing the signals that tell the muscle to contract. This also happens to be just the place where sarcomeres get into trouble, locking up and forming a trigger point. Knowing how to find the belly (the enlarged, fleshy part) of a muscle often brings you right to the trigger points that are causing the pain (1999, 47–49).

The problem gets more complex when the fibers don't run from end to end in a muscle. The orientation of the fibers in muscles varies, depending on the job they're designed to do (Figure 2.2). In a muscle made for speed, the fibers are parallel (A), running straight from end to end, and its trigger points are easily found, just as expected, halfway along it. However, a muscle made for power will have fibers running diagonally at some angle to its length. A diagram of such fiber arrangements looks like a feather (D) or sometimes a feather bisected down the middle (C). Since trigger points may be found in the center of each individual fiber, they may be situated anywhere along the muscle (1999, 49–53).

Another variation is when a muscle divides into several heads, like the biceps, triceps, or quadriceps. Trigger points may exist in only one head or they may be present in all. In

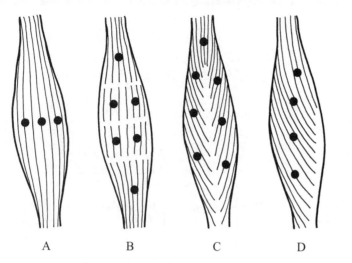

Figure 2.2   Orientation of muscle fibers: (A) parallel; (B) parallel with tendinous inscriptions; (C) bipennate; (D) unipennate

other muscles like the rectus abdominis of the stomach, the muscle may be divided by lateral bands of connective tissue (B), giving several potential sites for trigger points along its length. There are several instances of a muscle being divided lengthwise into two or more bellies. Other examples are the gracilis, sartorius, and semitendinosus muscles of the thigh, all of which, like the rectus abdominis, are long muscles that must exert great power. If you aren't aware that multiple bellies can exist in a muscle, you can easily overlook critical trigger points (1999, 49-53).

Satellite Trigger Points

When a trigger point is created in the pain referral zone of another muscle, it is termed a *satellite trigger point*. (An older term, no long recommended, is *secondary trigger point*.) The trigger point sponsoring the satellite is a *key trigger point* or *primary trigger point*.

Long-term chronic pain is often a compound effect from a chain of satellite trigger points, cascading from muscle to muscle. It's not unusual for one entire side of the body to be involved in this way. Satellite trigger points can sometimes resolve on their own without treatment when the primary trigger point is deactivated. By the same token, satellites can be difficult to deactivate if the primary trigger point is overlooked. Pain referral from diseased internal organs, familiar to physicians for generations, can promote satellite trigger points in chest, back, and abdominal muscles, an effect unfortunately not often recognized (1999, 122–123).

Attachment Trigger Points

Exquisitely painful places are often found at or near where the muscle attaches to bone. Travell and Simons believe these *attachment trigger points* are created secondary to central trigger points in the muscle belly. Rather than being true trigger points, they may be only highly sensitized connective tissue that has been abused by the stress of continuous muscle tension. Attachment trigger points are always under the control of centrally located trigger points, which should be the primary target of treatment. Attachment trigger points generally cease to be tender when central trigger points have been deactivated. In chronic conditions where trigger points have been in place for months or years, stresses at the site of muscle attachment are thought to cause degenerative changes in the joint (1999, 72, 76; Fassbender and Wegner 1973, 355–374).

The Mystery of Referred Pain

The reality of referred pain can be convincingly demonstrated by simply pressing on a trigger point that is bad enough to reproduce its referred pain pattern. It's a little harder to explain why pain is referred at all. Research on pain referral is difficult because the mechanisms of the human nervous system are so unimaginably small. The tiny electrochemical impulses in the nerves can be detected and measured to some extent, but not with accuracy or great discrimination. In addition, there are ethical limits on how far you can go in pain experiments, whether with animals or humans. Nevertheless, scientists have made a number of suppositions about how pain can be displaced from its cause.

The easiest theory to accept regarding referred pain is that the signals simply get mixed in your neurological wiring. Sensory inputs from several sources are known to converge into single nerve cells at the spinal level, where they are integrated and modified before being transmitted to the brain. Under these circumstances, it may be possible for one electrical signal to influence another, resulting in mistaken impressions about where the signals are coming from (1999, 56). On the surface, this looks like bad design, but the displacement of pain seems too consistent to be accidental. Janet Travell's great discovery was that referred pain occurs in very predictable patterns in everyone, with only small variations. This predictability implies that there may be some evolutionary advantage to the referral of pain. It's notable that referred pain occurs very often in or near a joint, where pain is most likely to make you modify the activities or conditions that have created the problem (1999, 96).

Fortunately, it's not necessary to understand why trigger points send their pain elsewhere. All you need to know is that they do. After you've worked with referred pain for a while, you develop an intuition about it. After gaining some experience, people often find that their fingers inexplicably begin going right to the trigger point that's causing the pain, even though it may be some distance away from the pain. It takes time to acquire this facility.

Trigger Point Symptoms

The sensory symptoms created by myofascial trigger points take a variety of forms and they aren't limited to the sense of pain. Symptoms of dysfunction—such as muscle stiffness, weakness, edema, nausea, dizziness, and postural distortions, to name a few—are even more diverse and include a number of surprises.

Referred Pain

The defining symptom of a trigger point is *referred pain*. Characteristically, referred pain is felt most often as an oppressive deep ache, although movement can sharpen the pain. Referred myofascial pain can be as intense and intolerable as pain from any other cause. It should be noted that the pain level depends more on the degree of trigger point irritability than on the size of the muscle. Trigger points in the tiniest muscle can cripple you with pain. Some common examples of referred pain are tension headaches, migraine, sinus pain, and the kind of pain in the neck that won't let you turn your head. Jaw pain, earache, and sore throat can be expressions of referred pain. Another is the incapacitating stitch in the side that comes from running too hard.

Sore legs, sore feet, and painful ankles are examples of referred pain. Stiffness and pain in a joint should always make you think first of possible trigger points in associated muscles. Pain in such joints as the knuckles, wrists, elbows, shoulders, knees, and hips are classic trigger point symptoms. If you don't count headaches and backaches, pain referred to the joints is the most usual manifestation of myofascial pain syndrome.

Back pain always has a myofascial component, no matter the official diagnosis. Although arthritis, bad disks, and displaced vertebrae come quickly to mind when your back hurts, back pain very often is nothing but referred pain from myofascial trigger points. Pain in your low back can come from trigger points in surprising places, such as your buttocks, your stomach muscles, or even knotted-up muscles in your calves. Treatment for back pain often fails when myofascial trigger points are not considered as a possible cause (1999, 804–809; Rosomoff et al. 1990, 114–118).

Unexplained intrapelvic pain and pain connected with sexual function can be referred from trigger points in the inner thighs, the low abdomen, or inside the pelvis itself. It's not unusual for trigger points in these places to refer pain to the ovaries, cervix, uterus, testes, penis, prostate, rectum, or bladder. A woman's vaginal pain during intercourse in the missionary position, with the legs up and spread, can be referred pain from a certain mean-spirited myofascial trigger point high in the overstretched adductor magnus muscle of the inner thigh. Janet Travell believed that even a large part of menstrual pain is due to trigger points in abdominal muscles and could be prevented to a great extent by regular self-applied massage between menstrual periods.

Travell and Simons tell us that many symptoms that seem to be internal may actually be coming from trigger points in external muscles. Stomachaches, heartburn, or pain that feels like an ulcer can be referred from trigger points in the stomach muscles. Referred pain from a trigger point in the rectus abdominis can simulate acute appendicitis. The pain of colic in a baby can have the same source. Other referred symptoms from abdominal trigger points take some interesting forms, like heart arrhythmia, nausea, diarrhea, loss of appetite, projectile vomiting, and urinary incontinence. Older children and adults who wet the bed should know their problem might be only a referred weakening of the urinary sphincters by trigger points in lower abdominal muscles (1999, 941).

Compression of Vessels and Nerves

Muscles that have been shortened and enlarged by trigger points frequently squeeze nearby nerves. Nerves that pass through a muscle are even more vulnerable. Compression of a nerve can distort the electrical signals that travel along it, resulting in abnormal sensations such as numbness, tingling, burning, and hypersensitivity in the areas served by the nerve. This is a very common occurrence in the arms and hands. It's not unusual in the legs and feet. When physicians are unaware that these worrisome symptoms can be coming from myofascial trigger points in muscles, they are apt to label the condition "peripheral neuropathy," which can lead to inappropriate treatment, including unnecessary surgery.

Trigger points can also cause a muscle to clamp down on the blood flow in an artery, making a distant body part feel cold. Trigger points in a calf muscle (soleus) can impede the return of blood in a vein, resulting in a swollen ankle or foot. The same effect in a neck muscle (anterior scalene) can cause a swollen wrist and hand (1999, 509–510).

Autonomic Effects

The autonomic system controls the glands and the smooth muscles of the digestive system, the blood vessels, the heart, the respiratory system, and the skin. Some of the effects of trigger points on these systems may be as yet unknown. Known effects can be quite surprising, verging on the unbelievable. Travell and Simons list some of the known effects as reddening of the eyes, excessive tearing, blurred vision, a droopy eyelid, excessive salivation, persistent nasal secretion, and goose bumps. Trigger points in a pectoral muscle can cause an erect, hypersensitive nipple. Another one on the front of the rib cage can cause an irregular heartbeat.

Problems with Movement

Trigger points can affect movement by keeping muscles short and stiff, which reduces range of motion. They can maintain spasms in other muscles. They prevent muscles from relaxing, causing them to tire quickly, recover slowly from exertion, and contract excessively when they work. They can also keep muscles out of balance to the extent that they partially disarticulate joints, causing them to catch or pop when you move.

Trigger points can distort your perception when gauging the weight of things. They can cause dizziness and imbalance. Their weakening effect on muscles adds to problems with coordination, causing you to stumble, lurch, and unexpectedly drop things, which can provoke needless speculation about neurological problems (1999, 21).

Movement requires some muscles to contract and others to lengthen. Trigger points can make a muscle reluctant to do either. Stretching or contracting irritates trigger points and increases pain, making you less and less inclined to move. If your neck hurts, you stop turning your head. If your back hurts, you stop trying to lean over. If your shoulder hurts, you stop reaching for things. This is called "splinting" or "guarding," a natural protective response that keeps the muscle from suffering further abuse.

Splinting calls other muscles into action to take up the burden. That may sound like a good idea until you realize that the helper muscles are bound to get stressed from doing the awkward, unaccustomed work. Very soon, they develop trigger points too and an entire limb, or one whole side of the body, can become involved. The muscles stiffen and your range of motion becomes progressively limited. Your reluctance to move turns into an inability to move. Depending on the focus of the trouble, you end up unable to bend your knee, raise your arm, turn your head, or reach down to tie your shoelaces.

Unnatural twists or curves in the neck, spine, or hips can also result from this kind of wholesale myofascial trigger point activity. The familiar and much dreaded dowager's hump may begin this way, from the pull of bound-up chest and anterior neck muscles. Trigger points should be one of the first things investigated when scoliosis or any other abnormal spinal curve is being addressed.

Chronically bad posture, especially with the head or hips thrust forward, may not be correctable until certain trigger points are attended to. An apparent short leg is sometimes simply a collection of long-standing trigger points drawing up that side of the body (1992, 32, 42).

Problems with Mood

Untreated myofascial symptoms that go on for months or years can really drag your spirits down. Chronic pain is a well-known cause of depression, especially if you've been told it's untreatable. Therapy for depression should include treatment of trigger points when they're the source of your depressing chronic pain. It can become a deadly cycle when a sense of hopelessness keeps you from taking positive action to combat your trigger points.

Sleeplessness and chronic fatigue are other very common symptoms of myofascial trigger points. As noted above, muscles tend to overcontract and be slow to relax when afflicted with trigger points. The constant tension causes you to tire too easily. Pain from trigger points disturbs your sleep and keeps your muscles from resting. The resulting chronic fatigue should not be a surprise (1999, 110).

Dyslexia, Too?

Travell and Simons don't mention dyslexia in their long list of proven myofascial symptoms. But trigger points provoke such an unbelievable variety of symptoms in the head, neck, and face that it's worth wondering whether dyslexia should be counted among them.

Conventional beliefs about dyslexia blame it on a dysfunction within the brain, but there are other theories. Harold N. Levinson, M.D., in *Smart but Feeling Dumb* (1994), expresses the belief that dyslexia basically stems from an inner ear dysfunction. His reasoning is that the inner ear, mediated by the cerebellum, is vital to the ability of the eyes to track, sort out and make sense of what they see, including the printed word. Dr. Levinson tells of numerous successes in treating dyslexia with finely controlled doses of seasickness medicine and other substances meant for fighting dizziness. Travell and Simons note that trigger points are a known cause of dizziness, indicating that they may affect the inner ear (1999, 314, 334, 383).

In dyslexia, a number of other problems appear to accompany reading difficulty, including headaches, blurred or double vision, balance and coordination problems, speech disorders, poor memory, messy writing, impaired concentration, hyperactivity, and confusion about telling time and direction. Some of these problems are oddly coincident with symptoms of myofascial trigger points. Trigger points in muscles of the neck and jaw can cause discoordination, dizziness, loss of balance, ear pain, and occasionally a unilateral loss of hearing.

We know that children have trigger points, even from birth. Tense, overstressed children, just like adults, are particularly apt to have trigger points in the jaws, neck, and face. Are these kids prone to be dyslexic because of a myofascial effect on the inner ear? It would seem worth checking out. Hopefully, someone in the business of treating dyslexia will be motivated to investigate this question. All the trigger points that might be involved could be treated with the techniques presented in this book.

Trigger Point Causes

Some of the activities and events that create trigger points are obvious, like accidents, falls, strains, and overwork. The onetime episode of overdoing, for example, is notorious for ending in debilitating pain that long outlasts the event. Everyone occasionally lifts or carries unreasonable loads, ambitiously exercises when out of condition, or hammers away too long and too hard at some unaccustomed work. All these things constitute abuse of muscles. It would pay to examine the varieties of abuse more closely.

Avoidable Muscle Abuse

The chronic overloading of muscles in work situations is so common nowadays that it has earned a number of fancy labels. We call it "overuse syndrome," "repetitive motion injury," "repetitive strain," "cumulative trauma disorder," and "occupational myalgia." All these terms look good on an insurance claim, but none of them mean anything other than that you've worked a group of muscles beyond their endurance and now they're making you pay for it.

It's important to look critically at a work situation that causes the overuse of muscles and results in myofascial pain. Trigger points are usually easy enough to deal with, but they tend to come right back if you don't change the conditions that bring them on. On the job, thoughtless positioning of the body is clearly hazardous when it causes strain, inefficient movement, and poor body mechanics. Maintaining an awkward position too long, habitual muscle tension, disregard of efficient methods, and reluctance to take rest breaks are some of the things you need to work on if you hope to end the pain that comes from overwork. Lack of commitment to making improvements may be the biggest obstacle of all.

Along with flagrant, mindless overwork, there are other less obvious ways to abuse muscles and create trigger points. Being overweight and out of shape can set you up for overstressed muscles. Carrying an overloaded purse or backpack just invites trouble. Carrying a fat billfold in the back pocket is famous as a cause of sciatica, which is pain from the sciatic nerve itself and from trigger points in buttock muscles, both created by pressure from the billfold (1999, 139, 147, 175, 182). Muscles of the back, neck, and hips can be severely stressed by the postures dictated by car seats, chairs, and other furniture designed for appearance instead of good support.

Unavoidable Muscle Abuse

Trigger points are created in muscles when they suffer direct impact in accidents such as falls and auto collisions. The sudden wrenching movements that occur during these events, when muscles are either overcontracted or overstretched, can also be expected to result in trigger points. Trigger points are the major source of the pain of whiplash, though they often go unsuspected and unaddressed. They generally accompany fractures, muscle tears, sprains, and dislocations. Failure to recognize and treat trigger points as an inevitable part of any physical injury causes needless pain and can defer complete recovery indefinitely (1999, 437–439).

Unsuspected Muscle Abuse

According to Travell and Simons, many kinds of medical treatment can be unrecognized causes of trigger points and myofascial pain. Trigger points are sure to be provoked by the immobility imposed by braces, slings, and casts. When surgery leaves long-term residual pain, trigger points should be suspected in muscles that have been cut, stretched, or otherwise traumatized. Physicians may persist in trying to treat the site of the pain, not recognizing it as referred myofascial pain, and consequently overlook and fail to attend to the cause.

An ordinary injection in the gluteal muscles can set up trigger points, particularly in the gluteus minimus, leaving a patient with a mysterious agonizing case of sciatica that can last for months.

Steroids injected into painful joints, though seeming to bring relief, may not be an appropriate treatment when the pain is of myofascial origin. The trouble is that the patient, thinking he or she has been cured, goes unmindfully on with the stressful activity that caused the trouble in the first place. The critical trigger points go untreated and continue to pull incessantly on the bones of the joint, ultimately making the problem worse. Steroids themselves, if overused, can seriously degrade the connective tissue of bones, muscles, ligaments, and tendons. Surgery may even be called for to repair the damage.

Pain medications continue to be the treatment of choice because they work so well in reducing the awareness of pain. But pain must always be viewed as a warning that something is wrong and needs attention: it's not enough to murder the messenger and ignore the message. Many people, concerned about unknown side effects, are becoming leery of all medications or foreign substances put into or taken into the body. Medical history is full of tragic examples of the truth about a prescription drug coming out too late. It's not unreasonable to wonder whether your prescription for pain, depression, anxiety, or such conditions as high blood pressure may cause more illness than it cures.

As an example, Travell and Simons tell about research indicating that calcium channel blockers for hypertension appear to irritate and perpetuate trigger points. In other words, your high blood pressure medicine may be worsening your pain (1999, 75). Sidney Wolfe, in *Worst Pills, Best Pills* (Wolfe et al. 1999), lists scores of drugs that are known to have the potential for causing muscle pain as a side effect. If you take prescription drugs for any reason, it would be worth your while to get this valuable book and study it thoroughly.

Fibromyalgia

There's some question as to whether trigger points cause fibromyalgia or whether it's the other way around. Maybe the two conditions aren't connected at all. One thing is certain, however: you can have widespread trigger points (myofascial pain syndrome) and fibromyalgia at the same time. Myofascial pain syndrome and fibromyalgia are both characterized by hypersensitive spots in various parts of the body. With fibromyalgia, these spots are called "tender points" rather than "trigger points." Either condition is easily mistaken for the other if you're unaware of critical differences.

Myofascial pain is usually localized and its cause is very specific in the form of trigger points, whose extreme tenderness always reveals their location. They can often be felt with the fingers. People with fibromyalgia ordinarily hurt all over and often can hardly bear the lightest touch. Tender points are typically present almost everywhere and aren't limited to muscles. Fibromyalgia is believed to have a systemic cause, instead of something specific to the muscles, and the entire body is usually involved.

There are other ways to differentiate between myofascial pain syndrome and fibromyalgia. Muscles with trigger points feel firm; muscles of the fibromyalgia sufferer are soft and doughy. Muscles with trigger points stiffen the joints and inhibit your range of motion. In fibromyalgia, the joints are loose, or even hypermobile, although the person may have an overall subjective sense of stiffness and may be hesitant to move because of ongoing pain. Depression can come with both conditions, but people with myofascial pain can generally go on with life. People with fibromyalgia are frequently overwhelmed by deep fatigue and sometimes can hardly move at all without agonizing pain.

None of the self-treatment techniques in this book will have a direct effect on fibromyalgia itself. However, massage can benefit any myofascial trigger points that may be present among the tender points and significantly reduce the fibromyalgia sufferer's level of pain. (It's wise to carefully avoid overtreatment.) In too many cases, fibromyalgia has been wrongly diagnosed when myofascial trigger points are the true cause of the pain. In such cases, trigger point massage will indeed be helpful for the purported "fibromyalgia" (1999, 36–40).

Trigger Point Persistence

Trigger points can sometimes be very difficult to get rid of. You may find that after you've successfully deactivated them, they seem to come right back. The influence of perpetuating factors on myofascial pain is seriously underestimated, not only by the sufferer, but also by many therapists. Management of perpetuating factors often makes the difference in whether treatment will succeed and whether its benefits will last. A perpetuating factor is sometimes so important that its removal can allow a trigger point to deactivate on its own. Some systemic factors, such as vitamin deficiency, are so strong that they can be the initiating circumstance in the creation of trigger points (1999, 179).

Physical Factors

Congenital irregularities in bone structure, postural stress, poor work habits, repetitive strain, and lack of exercise can all contribute to the difficulty in getting rid of trigger points.

Abnormal Bone Structure

A short leg, an asymmetric pelvis, short upper arms, and a long second metatarsal bone in the foot are conditions that make it necessary for the body to continuously compensate, resulting in perpetual strain on certain groups of muscles. Unequal leg length may create and maintain trigger points in the legs, buttocks, back, and neck. Unless corrected by a heel lift or other means, a short leg may cause persistent or recurrent pain in these areas; a proper heel lift has even been known to stop intractable headaches. Unfortunately, leg length is difficult to measure accurately. Chronically tight muscles can add to the difficulty by drawing up one side of the body and causing the appearance of a short leg.

Sometimes, one entire side of the body is smaller than the other. In such a case, one side of the pelvis is likely to be smaller too, which makes your pelvis tilt while you're sitting. When this happens, the spine curves abnormally, placing an extra load on the quadratus lumborum and other back muscles. The effect can be transmitted as far away as the scalene and sternocleidomastoid muscles of the neck. Crossing your legs with the same leg over all the time may indicate that you're compensating for an asymmetric pelvis. Sitting on a pad or thin cushion under the smaller side of the pelvis can help remedy this condition. Be aware that keeping a thick wallet in your back pocket tilts the pelvis in the same manner and can cause the same kind of perpetual strains.

Short upper arms are more common than you might think and aren't usually recognized as a potential cause for lingering myofascial pain. You should always have elbow support while sitting, and when you have short upper arms, you need higher arms on the chairs you sit in. Lack of support for your elbows causes continual strain on the trapezius and levator scapulae muscles, whose trigger points cause headaches and neck pain (1999, 183).

Morton's foot, an easily corrected disparity in the length of the first and second metatarsal bones of the foot, is known to be the origin of a variety of aches and pains. This condition causes instability in the foot and ankle that can affect virtually the entire body. Morton's foot is discussed in detail in chapter 10 (1999, 179–184).

Postural Stress

Trigger points can be caused and maintained by postural factors such as couches, chairs, and the bucket seats in cars that strain muscles by failing to properly support the body. You may be so accustomed to these strains that you don't notice them. Badly conceived seating is the source of much chronic back and neck pain.

Strained or awkward positions in your work situation can perpetuate trigger points. The apparent comfort and familiarity of a longtime habit can make you unaware of its effects on your muscles. It's wise to examine how you sit, stand, and work to find the ways in which you may be subjecting certain muscles to continuing tension and strain. See if you're keeping an arm or a leg locked in a cramped position while you work. Observe whether you're keeping your head turned or cocked at an angle for long periods of time. Develop an awareness of unusual tightness in muscles that would indicate postural imbalance.

Keeping muscles immobile or inactive encourages them to stiffen and grow weak. A sedentary lifestyle is a great perpetuator of trigger points. Muscles need to work in order to stay healthy (1999, 184–185).

Repetitive Movement

Repetitive movement overloads muscles, even when it requires only minimal effort. Repetitive movement that is strenuous can actually be healthier because you're more apt to be aware when the muscles are growing tired. The seeming effortlessness of office work can have an insidious effect on large and small muscles alike. Working at a computer keyboard is particularly stressful. The small muscles of the forearms and hands have to slave away for hours at a time, contracting hundreds if not thousands of times in a single session. At the same time, larger muscles of the shoulders, upper back, and neck remain static and immobile but under continuous contraction to hold your head and arms in position. The static posture and unrelieved subtle strain of computer work can perpetuate trigger points in any part of the upper body.

Many jobs in industry, because of their repetitious nature, make it impossible to deal effectively with myofascial problems. If the health of the workers is worth anything, it would be much more cost-efficient and productive to allow people to vary their tasks a number of times during the day. Janet Travell's advice to homemakers was always to "scramble" their housework, instead of working all day at one thing. Think of ways to scramble your work, no matter what it is (1999, 185–186).

Vitamins and Minerals

Travell and Simons state that nearly half the patients they treated for chronic pain were found to be lacking certain vitamins or minerals that are necessary for lasting relief. These critical nutrients include vitamins B_1, B_6, and B_{12}, vitamin C, and folic acid. The minerals calcium, iron, magnesium, and potassium are also critically important. Groups of people who are especially likely to be deficient in these are the elderly, pregnant women, dieters, the economically disadvantaged, the emotionally depressed, and people who are seriously ill.

The problem in many cases is not an inadequate ingestion of vitamins and minerals, but the intake of other substances that cause their elimination. Smoking destroys vitamin C. Taking in excessive amounts of water can wash B vitamins out of your system. Alcohol, antacids, and the tannin in tea impair absorption of B_1. Antacids can also affect absorption of folic acid. Oral contraceptives leave you short of B_6, as do antitubercular drugs and corticosteroids. Overdosing on vitamin C or folic acid can deplete your B_{12}.

Levels of the minerals calcium, iron, magnesium, and potassium must be adequate for normal muscle function. The exchange of calcium ions is directly involved in the contraction and relaxation of muscle fibers. Iron enables muscle tissue to use the nutrients and oxygen that are delivered by the blood. Iron also has a role in regulating body temperature. People with inadequate iron feel cold all the time. Too much iron, however, is as bad as too little, sometimes leading to discoloration of the skin, heart disease, and slow recovery from stroke. Potassium deficiency affects heart and other smooth muscle function. Magnesium is needed in conjunction with the body's use of calcium. Low levels of magnesium are associated with muscle hyperexcitability and weakness.

Despite their concern for the balance of the vitamins and minerals in your body and their specific levels, Doctors Travell and Simons find that a good multivitamin with minerals should ordinarily meet your needs. They add the caution not to exceed maximum limits of folic acid, iron, vitamin A, and vitamin B_6 (1999, 186–213).

Metabolic Disorders

You're likely to have trouble getting rid of your trigger points when any chemical or glandular imbalance interferes with metabolism in the muscles. Some conditions to watch out for are thyroid inadequacy, hypoglycemia, anemia, and high levels of uric acid in the blood (uricemia). Nicotine, caffeine, and alcohol cause enough irregularity in the metabolism to make it difficult to keep trigger points deactivated (1999, 213–220).

Low output from the thyroid gland can increase the irritability of muscles, predisposing them to development of trigger points. Thyroid insufficiency is likely to make relief from trigger point therapy very short-lived. Typical signs of hypothyroidism include muscle cramps, weakness, stiffness, and pain. Other symptoms are chronic fatigue, cold intolerance, dry skin, and disturbed menstruation. Some people have trouble losing weight. Thyroid inadequacy may play a role in fibromyalgia. Lithium appears to lower thyroid secretion, while estrogen replacement increases it. Indirectly, lithium may make your trigger points worse; estrogen may make them better (1999, 214–218; Sonkin 1994, 45–60; Bochetta et al. 1991, 193–198).

Recurrent bouts with hypoglycemia (low blood sugar) tend to aggravate your trigger points and decrease the effectiveness of trigger point therapy. Symptoms of hypoglycemia are a fast heartbeat, sweating, shaking, and increased anxiety. A more severe spell can bring visual disturbances, restlessness, trouble with thinking and speaking, and even fainting. Emotional distress makes you more susceptible to hypoglycemia. Caffeine and nicotine both accentuate the secretion of adrenaline, which can worsen this condition. Alcohol should also be avoided (1999, 219–220; Foster and Rubenstein 1980, 1758–1762).

Uricemia can make your trigger points more troublesome. Gout, the deposit of urate crystals in the joints, is the extreme manifestation of this problem. A diet of too much meat and too little water is likely to promote uricemia. Vitamin C helps combat the problem (1999, 220; Kelley 1980, 479–486).

Psychological Factors

Tension, anxiety, and everyday nervousness can make trigger point therapy ineffective. Habitually holding your muscles tight (bracing) never gives them a chance to rest, not even at night when you're sleeping. A tight muscle is working continuously, and the tightness should be considered a form of overuse. You may not be aware of just how much muscle tension you're holding on to. Relaxing your muscles won't get rid of their trigger points, but it will allow therapy to work better.

Cultivate an awareness of when you're holding rigid postures. Going around with hunched shoulders is a classic sign of excessive tension. You may be breathing shallowly when things aren't going well; you may even be holding your breath at times. If you tune in to your body during tense moments, you'll detect the tightness in your chest and stomach. There are several excellent books in the catalog of New Harbinger Publications, the publisher of this book, that can help you learn to deal better with your tensions. Emotional distress can often be relieved by simply relaxing needless or excessive muscle tension. To learn more about dealing effectively with muscle tension, see chapter 12.

Other Factors

A number of other influences may affect your success with trigger point therapy. Chronic lack of sleep can be an important factor. Diseases of internal organs can produce and perpetuate trigger points in muscles. Chronic infections, including sinusitis, can keep trigger points going. An allergy to airborne irritants that causes respiratory distress can make it very difficult to keep up with trigger points in the neck, chest, and abdomen. Food allergies can make all the muscles of the body more vulnerable to stress. Infestation of the intestinal tract can perpetuate trigger points indirectly through depletion of essential nutrients. Infestations can be insidious and are more common than you may think (1999, 220–226).

You can't depend on your control of perpetuating factors alone to get rid of trigger points and myofascial pain. You may even find it hard to judge whether your control of perpetuating factors is having an effect. But keep an open mind and keep exploring. You may happen onto the one factor that makes all the difference.

Therapeutic Methods

Almost any intervention will affect a trigger point, according to Travell and Simons, as long as it's a *physical* intervention. Nothing subtle will do. Trigger points don't respond to positive thinking, biofeedback, meditation, and progressive relaxation. Even physical methods can fail if they're too broadly applied. Conventional stretching exercises, for example, are not sufficiently specific to affect trigger points in a dependable way. When overdone, stretching can actually make trigger points worse. Other therapeutic methods can yield disappointing results. Applications of heat or cold may temporarily reduce pain but they won't deactivate your trigger points. Likewise, electrical stimulation can give temporary relief of pain but not affect a trigger point specifically. Most systems of therapeutic touch, like acupressure, shiatsu, craniosacral therapy, myofascial release, Swedish massage, and even deep tissue bodywork—despite their good uses—are also too nonspecific to guarantee success with trigger points. For dependable results, therapy needs to be applied directly to the trigger point (1999, 126–147).

In *The Trigger Point Manual*, Travell and Simons discuss numerous ways to cope with trigger points, including a few ideas for self-applied massage. They cover only two methods in comprehensive detail: *trigger point injection* and *spray and stretch*. These therapies are designed for use in a doctor's office or a physical therapy clinic.

Trigger points will release when injected with a local anesthetic. They will sometimes do the same when stuck with a dry needle, as in acupuncture. Injection of trigger points requires a high degree of skill. Spray and stretch is safer and easier to use than injection and is the method favored by Travell and Simons for general use in a professional setting. Spray and stretch is fundamentally different from conventional stretching in that it directly addresses the trigger point before the affected muscle is stretched (1999, 126–147).

Trigger Point Injection

The most exacting method of attacking trigger points is to inject them with a mild dose of procaine, a local anesthetic that wears off quickly. The therapeutic effect is in the mechanical disruption of the trigger point's contracted muscle fibers by the needle. The anesthetic keeps it from hurting. The trigger point nodule is hardly ever larger than a pea, and often is no bigger than the head of a pin. It takes exceptional skill to accurately stick one with a hypodermic needle. As Travell and Simons describe it, it's like trying to impale a tiny ball of hard rubber: the needle tends to bounce off the nodule or push it aside rather than penetrate. If you try to hold a trigger point between your fingers, it tends to slip out like a wet noodle. It reacts the same way to a needle.

Trigger point therapy by injection has other drawbacks. The needle usually leaves some postinjection soreness, which can take several days to subside. As with any invasive procedure, injections also risk inadvertent damage to nerves, blood vessels, and vital organs. In addition, your body has to get rid of the anesthetic that has been injected, which limits the number of trigger points that can be injected at any one time. By comparison, a massage therapist in a single session can give attention to every trigger point you may have, with no risk in the worst case beyond low-grade soreness for a day or two.

Trigger points can be difficult to locate precisely enough to inject. They can't always be felt clearly with the fingers, especially if they're buried deep in a muscle. Trigger points are usually quite easy to find on yourself because of the immediate feedback provided by their sensitivity to pressure. It's impossible to have this connection with the trigger points on someone else.

All other considerations aside, injection may be the quickest treatment for myofascial pain if the trigger points haven't been in place too long. Chronic pain from long-standing trigger points may require multiple treatments, as with any other therapy. It's important to accept the fact that trigger points do come back, as life goes on with all its stresses and strains. If you depend on injection therapy, you'll be seeing your doctor a lot (1999, 150–166).

Spray and Stretch

Releasing a trigger point by spraying the skin with a refrigerant, then stretching the affected muscle, is the procedure Travell and Simons call their "workhorse method." Spray and stretch requires less skill than injection does, but there are several stringent requirements to meet so that it can be done safely. First, you must be certain that you're stretching the muscle containing the trigger point that is referring the pain. If you're entirely focused on the place that hurts, you may apply the method to the wrong muscles.

Second, before you even think about stretching, it's imperative that you chill the skin that overlies the trigger point and its area of referred pain with ice or a refrigerant spray. Trigger points are inclined to react to stretching with a defensive tightening. Chilling the skin prevents this by "distracting" the nervous system and temporarily suppressing the pain. In chilling the skin, it's vital to work quickly so that the cooling agent doesn't cool the underlying muscle. Cooling the muscle will inhibit the stretch rather than facilitating it, and more pain will be the likely result. After stretching, a third requirement is that you immediately rewarm the cooled skin with moist hot packs to keep it from drawing heat out of the muscle.

If movement was limited by the trigger point before treatment, a fourth step calls for gentle movement several times through the complete range of motion to let the body know that it is possible to move now.

Even with these safeguards, stretching remains hazardous for many people. Travell and Simons specifically warn that the stretch must not be forced. They advise merely "taking up the slack" and not trying to make the muscle lengthen beyond the onset of resistance. The danger in attempting to stretch a muscle whose trigger points resist release is the chance you may strain the muscle's attachments. This is because the taut bands of muscle on either side of the trigger point are already stretched to their limit. Because of the limits they put on stretching, these taut bands in muscles may be a critical factor in ligament and tendon injuries (1999, 127–135).

Deep Stroking Massage

The safest and most effective method of trigger point therapy, according to Travell and Simons, is deep stroking massage applied directly to the trigger point. It has a more specific effect on the trigger point than spray and stretch and carries much less risk to muscle attachments. Its directness makes deep stroking massage nearly as effective as injection, and actually superior around blood vessels and nerves where injection can be too dangerous to use. Deep stroking massage is also obviously the method most adaptable for self-treatment (1999, 141–142; Danneskiold-Samoe, Christiansen, and Andersen 1986, 174–178).

The next chapter, "Massage Guidelines," will show you how to use deep stroking massage efficiently and effectively.

CHAPTER 3

Massage Guidelines

Although professional massage is unquestionably the best method of trigger point therapy, there are many advantages in doing it yourself. With self-treatment, you don't have to wait for an appointment, you can get help whenever you need it, and you don't pay a cent. Best of all, you don't have to depend on someone else knowing what's causing your pain and knowing what to do about it. You can be the expert.

No one can ever have the connection with your pain that you have. You know exactly where it hurts and how much it hurts. You know better than anyone else when a treatment feels right and when it doesn't. With self-applied trigger point therapy, you'll have direct control over treatment. Most people feel a satisfying sense of empowerment when they discover they know how to get rid of their own pain.

It's important to realize that self-treatment won't all be smooth going. There will be some difficulties to surmount. You can make some kinds of pain go away very quickly but a long-established chronic problem can take a while to clear up. This is because trigger points that have been in place for a long time have made pathways in the nervous system that tend to reinforce and perpetuate them (Travell and Simons 1999, 56–57; Yaksh and Abram 1993, 116–121).

Another reality is that trigger point massage hurts, though if done correctly it will be a pleasant kind of pain, a level of pain you can still relax into. Trigger point massage may not be pleasant at first if you're a person who reactively avoids all pain. If you believe that all pain is bad and that it's a dumb idea to make yourself hurt, you may not be willing to do enough massage on yourself to do any good. On the other hand, if you try too hard to make massage work and do too much of it, your body will react against it and make your pain worse for a day or two. Overenthusiastic use of hard tools for massage can result in bruising not only of the skin, but possibly also of deeper tissues, such as muscles and nerves. When you have a lot of very active trigger points and work too long on yourself, you can come out of it feeling woozy or nauseous. If you have widespread pain, don't try to take care of everything at once. Work on your worst problems first and try to be patient with the method and with yourself.

Also, recognize that some of the trigger points related to your greatest stresses will tend to be recurrent. It's not reasonable to expect that you'll never have pain again. Nevertheless, with your skills at trigger point massage therapy, you'll be better equipped to cope with pain than ever before. Plan to be good at it.

Troubleshooting

Success with trigger point massage depends ultimately on your ability to recognize when your pain is referred pain and to trace it back to the trigger point that is causing it. It's too easy to get caught up in attacking the pain itself and remaining blind to its cause. Although some trigger points cause local pain, myofascial pain will defeat you if you assume that the problem is at the place that hurts. Winning over pain requires giving considerable attention to the referred pain patterns. Only by cultivating a methodical approach to troubleshooting can you become good at finding and deactivating trigger points.

The Trigger Point Guides at the beginning of chapters 4 through 10 give lists of muscles that are known to send pain to particular sites. To find the specific trigger point that is causing pain at a particular location, check the muscles on the appropriate list one at a time. The muscles are listed in order of greatest probability of being involved, the one at the top being the most likely. Always allow for the possibility that a muscle low on the list may be the culprit. It's not unusual for trigger points in several muscles to be contributing to the problem. The page number in parentheses after the muscle name is the beginning of the section where that muscle is discussed. The Trigger Point Guides are adapted from Travell and Simons's *Trigger Point Manual* (1992; 1999).

New Words

It's useful to know the right names for the muscles. Knowing the name of the muscle helps clarify your conception of where it is and makes it easier to find. You certainly have to be able to find the muscle before you can find its trigger points.

There is no other name for most of the muscles except the latinized scientific name. A simplified key to pronunciation is given when the muscle is introduced. With a little practice, you'll find that the words aren't as much a foreign language as they may seem. A great number of the English words you use every day have their roots in Latin and Greek. The classical roots of the English language have enriched it. Knowing the right words for your muscles will enrich you too. When you learn these beautiful new words and start throwing them around, your friends and family will think you're brilliant. The people at work will think you're a snob, but only until you show them how to get rid of that headache or sore back.

Body Mechanics

In the muscle chapters, you'll learn about the job each muscle does. Understanding a muscle's function helps you find the trigger points that are causing your problem. Insight into body mechanics also lets you see what you can do to prevent the problem from recurring. Simply getting rid of the pain is never enough. More than anything else, you need to know how you can keep it from coming back.

Knowledge of body mechanics also fosters an intuition about trigger points. When you know your muscles and have gained some experience finding their trigger points, you'll find your hands going right to them without having to consult the charts. Understanding how the muscles work also increases your awareness of problems when they're just starting up. This helps you nip trigger points in the bud.

Finding Trigger Points

False assumptions about the source of your pain can defeat your every effort to get rid of it. Trigger points are not usually found at the place that hurts. Pain referral is the essential fact about trigger points. Massage in the wrong place can feel good and yet do no good at all for healing your pain. You won't conquer referred pain unless you get good at tracking it to its source.

The illustrations of the referred pain patterns for each muscle are the key to finding trigger points. Go back to these drawings every time you set out to deal with a pain problem. A referred pain pattern can be such a crazy quilt of disconnected locations that if you try to rely on reason or memory, you'll overlook details that may be crucial to a successful search. You'll notice a tendency for trigger points to send their pain away from the center of the body, but the reverse is true too often to infer a perfectly reliable guiding principle. Also, you'll often find that several different muscles send pain to exactly the same spot. Your pain may be coming from only one of them, or each may be contributing. The illustrations are absolutely vital for keeping it all sorted out.

Figure 3.1 shows how muscles, trigger points, and referred pain are indicated in the illustrations. An area of referred pain is portrayed by a group of parallel lines running diagonally from lower left to upper right. Parallel lines also represent a muscle, but the lines are always enclosed within the outline of the muscle. A black dot approximates the location of a trigger point and may stand for several trigger points in the area. To keep the illustrations simple, trigger points are usually shown on only one side of the body, but they can occur on either side or both. Trigger points typically cause pain on their same side of the body. Rarely do they send pain to the opposite side.

Sometimes an illustration will put you exactly on target and sometimes it will only get you in the ballpark. Ultimately you have to zero in on trigger points by feel. The aim is to get to the right area—usually a circle of a couple of inches diameter—then search for that spot of exquisite tenderness. Don't be discouraged if you can't feel the little nodules in the muscles. Some people never acquire that skill. Very experienced massage therapists are able to feel every little bump in muscles. Some can find trigger points with their fingertips without even being told where it hurts, but when you work on yourself you don't have to find them that way. The most reliable criterion for detecting a trigger point is its extreme tenderness. Just seek the spot that hurts the most when you press on it. Obviously, many medical conditions cause tenderness in muscles and other soft tissue. If you're in doubt, check with a physician, preferably one who is informed about trigger points and myofascial pain. It won't hurt to show your physician this book. It may be just the resource he or she has been needing.

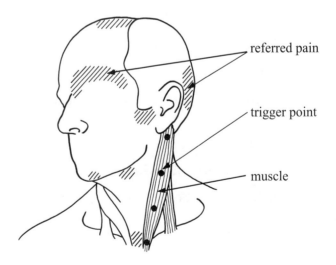

Figure 3.1 Key to pictorial devices. (Throughout the book, trigger points and referred pain are shown on only one side of the body, but they can occur on either side or both.)

Massage Technique

When it comes to doing massage the right way, there are two overriding issues: safety and effectiveness. You have to be able to do massage without straining and exhausting the muscles in your forearms and hands and you have to do it in a way that will actually have an effect on a trigger point.

Table 3.1 lists nine principles of safe, effective, self-applied trigger point massage. These rules define the basic massage stroke that is used everywhere on the body. Massage of a given trigger point should be relatively brief, no more than fifteen or twenty seconds. When you've done that much, stop and move on. That constitutes a treatment. It's not necessary to do more. Doing more may actually be counterproductive. A basic tenet of medicine is that you can only create conditions that promote healing. The body itself is the healer. You must trust your body's natural processes to respond and do their job.

Impatience will tempt you to try to kill the trigger point, to rub it out. That's a normal impulse, but it's not the best therapy. *Never try to force a release.* Trigger points release on their own when they get frequent daily treatment that follows the guidelines given below. You will be surprised at how well this simple routine works. Treatment failures are usually the result of being too aggressive or simply treating the wrong spot.

Table 3.1   Massage Guidelines at a Glance

1. Use a tool if possible and save your hands.

2. Use deep stroking massage, not static pressure.

3. Massage with short, repeated strokes.

4. Do the massage stroke in one direction only.

5. Do the massage stroke slowly.

6. Aim at a pain level of seven on a scale of one to ten.

7. Limit massage to six to twelve strokes per trigger point.

8. Work a trigger point three to six times per day.

9. If you get no relief, you may be working the wrong spot.

Deep Stroking Massage

Established practice in therapeutic massage dictates that you press and hold trigger points for a specified number of seconds, or until they presumably "release." This is known as *ischemic compression*. You literally squeeze the blood out of the tissue. The trouble with pressing and holding a trigger point is that it can become unnecessarily painful if the goal is to make it release. It also requires a sustained contraction of the shoulders, arms, and hands of the person doing the therapy, which can become extremely tiring in a very short time. Massage therapists who use ischemic compression as trigger point therapy very often have constant pain in their arms and hands. This is one of the serious ergonomic hazards causing such a large turnover in the profession. The burnout time for massage therapists averages about three years. As you can see, you must do massage safely or you'll end up with more trouble than you started with. Fortunately, there's a much safer and more effective way to deactivate trigger points.

Instead of the static pressure of ischemic compression, it's altogether better to make a series of strokes across the trigger point nodule. This gets results quicker and with less irritation to the trigger point, less damage to your hands, and less risk of bruising the skin and muscle. In addition, a moving stroke, frequently repeated, elicits a greater change in a trigger point than static compression.

Compressing the trigger point is the right idea, but a repeated "milking" action moves the blood and lymph fluid out more efficiently. The lymph contains the accumulated waste that has been generated by the continuously contracted muscle fibers. Picture how you rinse out a dirty cloth. Wetting and wringing it out only once won't get it clean no matter how long and hard you twist it. You need to run fresh water through it over and over until the water wrings out of it clear. A similar process works best with a trigger point.

Another advantage of using the short, repeated stroke instead of static pressure is that intermittent pain is easier to tolerate than continuous pain. Intermittent moving pressure allows you to go deeper and evoke just a little more pain than you could stand if you just pressed a trigger point and held it. Work deeply and slowly, using very short strokes, and no more than one stroke per second. The massage stroke doesn't need to be more than an inch and a half long. It only needs to move from one side of the trigger point to the other. Rather than sliding your fingers across the skin, move the skin with the fingers. This will help free up the underlying fascia, the thin membrane that envelopes muscles and whose tightness is sometimes part of the problem. Work deeply, pressing the trigger point against the underlying bone. Release at the end of the stroke, then go back to where you started, reset your fingers, and repeat. Each time you release the pressure, fresh blood immediately flows in, bringing a renewing charge of oxygen and nutrients. The trigger point has been deprived of these essential substances because pressure from the knotted-up muscle fibers has been constricting the capillaries that supply them.

Although you'll hear that you should always move the fluid toward the heart, it's not a critical issue here, because so little fluid is being moved. Stroke in whatever direction feels best. If you don't make trigger point therapy as easy as you can, it will wear you out and you won't want to do it.

Another benefit of the deep stroking massage is that it helps get the stretch back into the muscle fibers within the trigger point. Picture what would happen if you applied deep, stroking massage to a ball of modeling clay. It would spread and lengthen in the direction you pushed it. The effect on the muscle fibers is similar, just not as dramatic or as visible. Think of this as a *microstretch*, as opposed to the *macrostretch* of the whole muscle that you do with conventional stretching exercises. The microstretch is applied directly to the trigger point, right where it's needed. Done this way, there's little chance of overstretching the taut bands of muscle fibers that lead from each side of the trigger point to the muscle's attachments at the bone. Abuse of this taut band risks irritating the trigger point and making it hold on tighter.

Hurting Good

Trigger points hurt when compressed, and you may be very reluctant to work them for fear of doing yourself harm or making your pain worse. You have to realize that pain created by massage is beneficial. The electrical impulses of moderate amounts of self-inflicted pain are therapeutic in that they disrupt the neurological feedback loop that maintains the trigger point. Rest assured that self-administered pain is usually self-limiting. Your natural defense mechanisms won't allow you to inflict more pain on yourself than you can stand. It's very unlikely you'll do yourself real harm unless you try to massage too deeply with hard tools (1999, 140–141).

The level of pain caused by massage is useful as a measure of effectiveness. To gain maximum benefits, you should exert enough pressure to make it "hurt good." It should be a pleasant kind of pain. Don't let yourself off too easy, though. Light pressure won't do the job. Aim at a pain level of seven or eight on a scale of one to ten, where number one is no pain and number ten is intolerable.

Another positive effect of pain from massage is that it immediately brings a flood of painkilling endorphins. For this reason, you'll find that the longer you work on yourself, the more pressure you will be able to use. If you have a really bad trigger point that you absolutely hate to work on, try giving it a good initial shot of pain, then back off and wait ten seconds before going on. This gives the endorphins time to kick in and deaden your sensitivity. You'll then be able to work deeper with far less discomfort. Endorphins are related chemically to morphine but have many times the power.

Using the number scale, continue multiple daily treatments of the trigger point until your pressure on it elicits a pain level of only a two or three. Don't expect to reach this goal in a single session. Never try to force the trigger point to release. Normally, you should expect to continue massage for several more sessions after the trigger point has stopped actively referring pain.

Saving Your Hands and Fingers

Considering the risks inherent in overworking your hands and fingers while doing self-applied massage, it's smart to avoid using them if at all possible. You may not have thought of using your knuckles, knees, heels, or elbows as massage tools, but it can be done. See Figures 6.7, 9.21, 10.7, 10.26, and 10.27.

There are also a number of commercially available massage tools ergonomically designed to maximize safety and efficiency. Tools aren't appropriate, however, in sensitive areas such as the face, the front of the neck, the inside of the mouth, or under the arms. When there's no choice but to use your fingers, you must do all you can to avoid injuring them.

The basic principle in using your hands for massage is to apply the most force with the least effort and the least strain. When a thumb is used as a massage tool, back it up with the fingers (Figure 3.2). This is called the *supported thumb*. Don't use the thumb in opposition to the fingers unless there is simply no other way to do it. Gripping or kneading would seem the most natural thing to do, but it is actually quite exhausting. Hands used in this way won't last any time at all. Save the grip for places where absolutely nothing else will do.

When using your hands as massage tools, pair them if you can, using the opposite hand to back up the fingers that are doing the massage (Figure 3.3). This tool is called *supported*

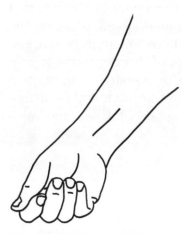

Figure 3.2   Supported thumb

fingers. The single hand shown in the drawing illustrates how the wrist, hand, and fingers are kept straight and yet as relaxed as possible. This takes the hand and forearm muscles largely out of the equation, requiring the force to come from larger muscles of the shoulders, chest, and upper back. The third and fourth fingers are the business end of the tool. The thumb, index finger, and pinky are just along for the ride. This makes a very pointy tool that penetrates with minimal effort. Observe that the supporting hand completely covers the nails. The ulnar side (pinky side) of the hand should make contact with the skin of the place being worked on. Note that the supporting hand helps move the fingertips of the tool hand.

Figure 3.4 illustrates a subtle way to support the fingers back-to-back for self-applied abdominal massage. Other ways to position the hands to give support to the fingers are shown in Figures 7.6, 7.24, and 10.25.

Rather than using the hand to pinch, squeeze, and knead, use the thumb or fingers like the end of a stick to push into the flesh. For the greatest

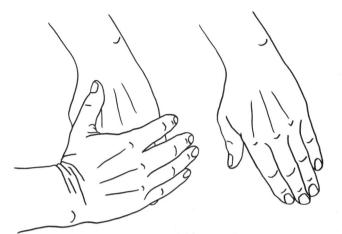

Figure 3.3   Supported fingers (Note that the supporting hand completely covers the nails of the massaging fingers. Both hands work together in making the massage stroke.)

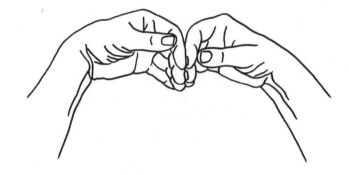

Figure 3.4   Supported fingers back-to-back

mechanical advantage, the fingers or thumbs need to be held nearly perpendicular to the surface of the body (Figure 3.5). This allows the force to be directed in a straight line from the elbow down through the arm, wrist, and hand and out the ends of the fingers or thumbs. You'll see right away that if you have fingernails of even moderate length, you will be prevented from using your hands in this way.

Massage done with the flats or pads of the fingers is ergonomically so poor that you'll find your hands and fingers getting tired before you've gained any benefit. In some lines of work, the inefficiency imposed by long nails contributes significantly to formation of trigger points in the forearms and hands, because the muscles have to work so much harder to overcome the awkwardness. Professional massage therapists keep their nails filed to the quick. You might consider doing the same, at least until your pain is gone.

If you feel that you can't do without your nails, try using *supported knuckles*, as shown in Figure 3.6. Note that

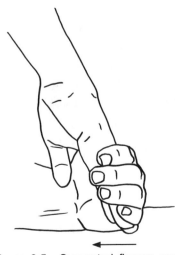

Figure 3.5   Supported fingers nearly vertical to skin

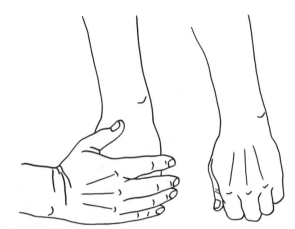

Figure 3.6   Supported knuckles

the "door knocking knuckles" of your third and fourth fingers are the tool. Your wrist and "fighting knuckles" are kept straight to efficiently transfer force from the shoulders. Supported knuckles are in fact a power tool and are rather blunt, as opposed to supported fingers whose best use is very precise massage requiring deep penetration.

A great variety of massage tools are available that will save your hands, amplify your strength, and let you reach difficult places. Three of the most versatile and well-designed tools are the Thera Cane (Figure 3.7), the Backnobber (Figure 3.8), and the Knobble (Figure 3.9). All three items, along with many other useful tools, are available through any massage therapist, massage school, or wellness center. You can also find them online. Addresses and phone numbers of distributors can be found at the end of the book. In most illustrations in this book, you'll see the Thera Cane being applied to bare skin. This was done for the sake of clarity: you won't like it on bare skin. For comfort and to avoid abrasion and bruising, massage tools should always be used through a layer of clothing.

The best massage tool of all for a surprising number of muscles may simply be a ball pressed between the body and a wall. You can use a tennis ball or a hard rubber ball of the same size; smaller rubber balls can be used if you need to go deeper. Putting a tennis ball in a sock lets you hang the ball down behind your back without risk of dropping it and having to chase it all over the room. (See Figure 8.6.) The sock is a convenient handle

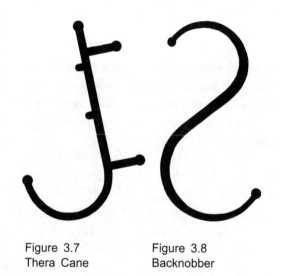

Figure 3.7
Thera Cane

Figure 3.8
Backnobber

that helps you get the ball into position. "High bounce" or "super bounce" rubber balls often come in several sizes in one package and can be found in sports, discount, and variety stores. They're very hard without being too hard, and they make excellent massage tools. Figure 3.10 shows the relative size of balls used for massage of various places. The sixty-four millimeter and fifty-eight millimeter sizes (letters A and B) are meant to be used on the arms, shoulders, hips, back, and buttocks against the wall. The thirty-five millimeter ball (letter C) is for the bottom of the feet against the floor. The twenty-seven millimeter ball (letter D) is for the meaty base of the thumb against a table top.

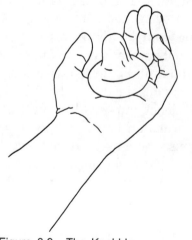

Figure 3.9   The Knobble

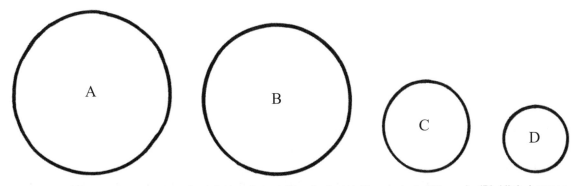

Figure 3.10 Balls for massage against the wall (not life size): (A) Tennis ball (64 mm); (B) High bounce or lacrosse ball (58 mm); (C) High bounce (35 mm); (D) High bounce (27 mm)

A problem with high bounce balls is that they are seasonal toys and often can't be found anywhere in the fall and winter. Another drawback is that the large, fifty-eight millimeter size tends to crack and break down with long-term daily use. A far superior tool for massage against the wall is a lacrosse ball, which is very hard, extremely durable, and can be found in all seasons in large sporting goods stores throughout the country. You may like a lacrosse ball better than a tennis ball because it penetrates with less effort and doesn't slide around as much on the wall.

Making the Method Work

Even though trigger point massage works extremely well for getting rid of trigger points and referred pain, don't be surprised if you encounter some snags.

Worrisome Results

Deep massage may occasionally cause bruising in tender areas. This is usually nothing to worry about, but you might want to let up a little on the pressure you're using. Bruising should be taken as a sign that you're trying too hard. It may also be a sign you're working the wrong place, particularly if you're working a lot and getting little improvement. Trigger points ordinarily respond well to massage and it doesn't take long to feel an improvement. Most treatment failures are the result of working the wrong spot. Always use the Trigger Point Guides at the beginning of the chapters to help find the trigger points you need to treat, and remember that in some areas, such as the hands, shoulders, and low back, pain can be a composite of referral from several muscles.

Half-hearted efforts at self-treatment won't get you very far. Once or twice a week simply won't do it. If you're not getting the results you think you should be getting, consider whether you're doing *enough* massage. Your really bad trigger points should have three to six treatments a day. Remember that treatment should only be 15 or 20 seconds long. Those are only very tiny snippets of time out of your schedule, not enough to slow you down or interfere with your day. You will be disappointed in the outcome if you do less. You only need to do six to twelve strokes per session on any given trigger point to have a beneficial effect. In addition to multiple treatments during the day, be sure to massage your really difficult trigger points just before going to bed and again when you get up in the morning. If pain wakes you up in the night, get up and have a session. As a general rule, massaging *often* is much better than massaging too hard or too long.

Some people have difficulty getting the hang of trigger point massage. You may have trouble finding trigger points, or you may feel clumsy and unsure with the tools and techniques. In such a case, you may benefit from a few sessions with a professional massage therapist who knows trigger points well. Be up-front: tell him or her that you want to learn how to take care of your trigger points yourself. He or she probably already knows about this book and employs its methods. If not, by all means take the book when you go for your appointment.

Trigger point massage works extremely well for myofascial pain. Done correctly, it usually shows clear results well within a week, often in just a day or two. Keep in mind that pain that persists could have an organic or systemic cause. If your pain began with an accident or a fall, you may have bone or tissue injuries that need medical attention. If you hurt all over and massage is doing no good at all or seems to make the pain worse, you may be dealing with fibromyalgia or some other systemic problem and will have to seek other remedies.

Health Factors

If you're successful in deactivating your trigger points but your pain seems to come back after a short time, there may be health factors that are predisposing your muscles to the development and perpetuation of trigger points. These things are discussed in more detail in chapter 2. For an exhaustive discussion of perpetuating factors, chapter 4 in volume 1 of Travell and Simons's *Trigger Point Manual* (1999) is the ultimate resource.

Consider whether you may be lacking B or C vitamins or calcium, magnesium, iron, or potassium. Smoking, excess alcohol, birth control pills, and certain other drugs are all known to deplete these nutrients. You may have a thyroid inadequacy. Hypoglycemia can aggravate trigger points. Question whether you're drinking enough water. Hyperuricemia, a condition where you're not getting enough water or your kidneys aren't doing their job, can keep your trigger points going. Diseased or dysfunctional internal organs can make it difficult to get rid of trigger points in external muscles. Chronic infections or allergies may perpetuate trigger points. Be aware that food allergies can play a role in both myofascial pain syndrome and fibromyalgia.

Expectations

You may wonder what you should expect of trigger point massage. You may want to know how many massage sessions will be needed to make your pain go away. Will your trigger points come back? Can you really expect to be truly pain free? All of these things depend to a great degree on how much intelligence and commitment go into your efforts.

Be realistic regarding expectations of success with trigger point therapy. Although you may occasionally experience the much-desired one-shot fix with trigger point massage, it's wise not to plan on it. Quick fixes are often illusory and can amount to nothing more than having simply swept the problem under the rug. Sometimes, a one-session triumph is genuine. The body can be very good about healing itself with the right stimulus. This happens most often with new pain. Long-standing trigger points require considerable attention; this will be true whether you do the massage yourself or seek help from a professional.

People tend to quit too soon whether they're working on themselves or going to a professional. You will be tempted to stop doing your massage the minute the trigger point stops actively referring pain. Remember that if the trigger point still hurts when you press on it, you've only soothed it into a latent state. Leaving a trigger point in the latent state allows it to be quickly reactivated by almost anything. Massage must continue until the trigger point no longer hurts when you press on it. Massage works miracles with trigger points and their pain, but only when done correctly and completely.

The Learning Curve

You'll be surprised at how quickly you can forget even your most useful discoveries about myofascial pain. It's useful to keep a pain diary about what you learn from day to day, making notes about the tricks and tools that work best. Then, when a problem comes up again, you'll find the solution all worked out in your pain diary and you won't have to reinvent the wheel.

To succeed in making this method work for you, the old rule applies: just keep trying. For difficult problems, read and reread and then read again any passage in this book that may apply. Underline and make notes in the margins. Take time to think. All the anatomical detail and all the ramifications regarding myofascial pain are so new that you're bound to feel mystified and overwhelmed sometimes. However, self-treatment of pain is much simpler than it seems at first and it will eventually all come together. Don't give up! Keep trying!

There's a long learning curve to mastering everything in this book, but you can expect to see positive results from the very beginning. If you study this book on an ongoing basis and keep searching for solutions, you'll learn something useful almost daily. Work on knowing the muscles and bones. It's important that you understand what's beneath the surface of your skin. The muscles and bones in there are part of *you*. To augment what you see in this book, you may want to get Frank Netter's *Atlas of Human Anatomy* and study his magnificent illustrations. If you've got the stomach to learn from dissected bodies, the six-part *Video Atlas of Human Anatomy* by Robert Acland will give you some unique insights. Dr. Acland uses a moving camera technique to create a three-dimensional view, which you can't get from a book, and which can be very revealing of the structure of things. In whatever way you can, keep exploring and keep learning. You deserve to be pain free. Give yourself this gift.

Hidden Benefits

Massage, when done by a professional, can be profoundly relaxing, reducing heart rate, blood pressure, and respiration along with reducing muscle tension. It may not be reasonable to hope for quite as much benefit when you do your own massage, but the relaxing effect can still be considerable. You can use your self-treatment sessions to slow down and calm down. Try consciously relaxing whatever muscle you're working on. When you are able to relax one muscle, your entire body tends to relax too.

The intentional reduction of tension in your muscles can also reduce the pain produced by trigger points. If you're good enough at it, the pain reduction can nearly equal that of a prescribed painkiller. Muscle relaxation won't get rid of trigger points, but it can make the pain more bearable until your self-applied trigger point massage begins to succeed.

CHAPTER 4

Head and Neck Pain

Trigger Point Guide: Head and Neck Pain

Crown Headache
sternocleidomastoid (51)
splenius capitis (64)

Frontal Headache
sternocleidomastoid (51)
semispinalis capitis (65)
zygomaticus (71)
levator labii (71)
frontalis (73)

Temple Headache
trapezius (55)
sternocleidomastoid (51)
temporalis (73)
splenius cervicis (64)
suboccipitals (62)
semispinalis capitis (65)

Eye Pain
sternocleidomastoid (51)
temporalis (73)
splenius cervicis (64)
masseter (67)
suboccipitals (62)
occipitalis (73)
orbicularis oculi (70)
trapezius (55)

Sinus Pain
sternocleidomastoid (51)
masseter (67)
lateral pterygoid (69)
orbicularis oculi (70)
zygomaticus (71)
levator labii (71)

Ear and Jaw Pain
lateral pterygoid (69)
medial pterygoid (68)
masseter (67)
sternocleidomastoid (51)
trapezius (55)

Tongue Pain
sternocleidomastoid (51)
medial pterygoid (68)
mylohyoid (72)

Toothache
temporalis (73)
masseter (67)
digastric (72)
buccinator (70)

Throat Pain
sternocleidomastoid (51)
medial pterygoid (68)
digastric (72)
longus colli (72)
buccinator (70)
platysma (71)

Side of Neck Pain
medial pterygoid (68)
sternocleidomastoid (51)
levator scapulae (60)
digastric (72)

Back of Head Pain
trapezius (55)
sternocleidomastoid (51)
semispinalis capitis (65)
splenius cervicis (64)
suboccipitals (62)
digastric (72)
temporalis (73)

Back of Neck Pain
trapezius (55)
multifidi (66)
rotatores (66)
levator scapulae (60)
splenius cervicis (64)
infraspinatus (90)

Trigger Point Guide: Head and Neck Pain

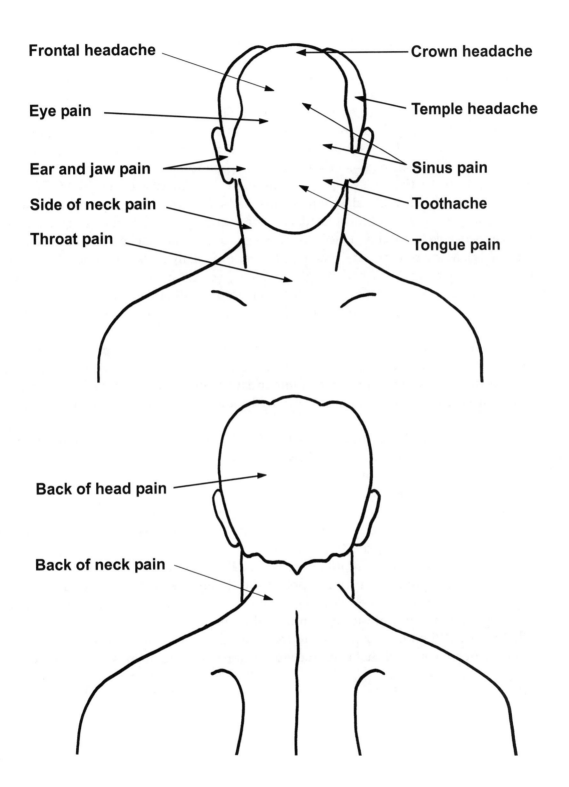

Frontal headache

Eye pain

Ear and jaw pain

Side of neck pain

Throat pain

Crown headache

Temple headache

Sinus pain

Toothache

Tongue pain

Back of head pain

Back of neck pain

Head and Neck Pain

Trigger points cause an astonishing variety of symptoms in the head and neck region. Some of their effects may contradict a lot of what you've always believed. Trigger points are known to cause pain and hypersensitivity in your teeth, pain and stuffiness in your ears, pain and redness in your eyes, sinus pain and drainage, stiff neck, chronic cough, and sore throat. Trigger points can cause dizziness and balance problems. They can blur your vision and make the words dance around on the page when you're trying to read. They can make your lips numb, your tongue hurt, or an eyelid droop (Travell and Simons 1999, 308–316).

Furthermore, trigger points are responsible for much of the pain associated with temporomandibular joint (TMJ) syndrome and are involved in important ways with the other symptoms of this disturbing condition, including popping and clicking in the jaw, dislocation of the jaw, restriction of jaw opening, and faulty closure of the teeth (1999, 379–384).

If this isn't enough, Travell and Simons's work has shown that trigger points are often the hidden and unsuspected cause of most headaches, no matter what name they're given: tension headaches, cervicogenic headaches, cluster headaches, vascular headaches, or migraines (1999, 240–256, 308–314). Many recognized "headache triggers" actually have their effect by cranking up your latent trigger points. A bad cough can do it; so can a viral infection, a hangover, overexertion, analgesic rebound, and too much consumption of sugar. Trigger points are the operational element in headaches set off by allergic reactions, chemical withdrawal, physical trauma, and emotional tension. Even the frustrating, unexplainable headaches that come with fibromyalgia can be shown to be due largely to the presence of trigger points (1999, 242).

The paradox about headaches is that the cause is rarely in the parts of the head that hurt. Most headaches come from trigger points in jaw, neck, and upper back muscles. This physical distance between cause and effect is why headaches can be so mysterious and hard to deal with.

The confusing thing about neck pain is that it is referred most of the time from trigger points in the upper back and shoulders. Few things feel better than a good neck massage, but it's massage of the upper shoulders and upper back that fixes neck pain. Neck massage fixes headaches. Trigger points in posterior neck muscles can participate in producing neck pain, but they are usually only satellites of central trigger points in the trapezius. Because of this satellite phenomenon, the search for the ultimate cause of chronic headaches can lead you down to this very muscle, the trapezius.

Obviously, pain and other symptoms in the head and neck area can have other causes than myofascial trigger points, but trigger points should always be one of the first things to be considered, because they can be so quickly checked out. You only need to know where to look. The Trigger Point Guide at the beginning of this chapter will provide the guidance you need in that regard. When trigger points are the cause of your symptoms, self-applied massage will give a degree of relief that even the strongest narcotic medicines don't provide, and it will last longer. With certain muscles, such as the sternocleidomastoid, relief comes so quickly that the connection between trigger points and your symptoms is hard to deny.

Whiplash

Nicole, a registered nurse, age forty-six, was rear-ended by a semi on the interstate. She wasn't seriously hurt, other than suffering whiplash. But the whiplash left her with pain behind one eye and a constant headache that centered in two places, over her eyebrows and at the base of her skull. A doctor prescribed hydrocodone, which stopped the pain quite well. But as a nurse, Nicole knew the drug was addictive, so she limited herself to using it only when pain kept her from sleeping.

The physician also sent her to a physical therapy clinic where she was given a series of electrical stimulation treatments to her neck and upper back. The electro-stim cut the pain for a day or two, but then it would come right back. Chiropractic treatments delivered similar results. The stretching exercises that everyone gave her made her headaches worse. As a last resort, Nicole decided to try massage.

Pressure on certain spots in her neck and upper back reproduced her various symptoms exactly. The therapist taught her how to massage several of the spots herself. This, along with weekly massage sessions, made her free of symptoms within six weeks. As a health-care professional, Nicole wondered why she had to go outside the health-care system to find something that worked.

Even a minor auto accident can cause whiplash, which typically results from sudden and extreme overstretching of muscles of the chest, upper back, and the front and back of the neck. Whiplash can produce not only widespread pain in the head, neck, chest, and upper back, but also numbness, tingling, and swelling in the hands and fingers. Without appropriate treatment of myofascial trigger points in the injured muscles, the effects of whiplash frequently last for months and can persist literally for years.

Two sets of muscles of the front of the neck, the sternocleidomastoids and the scalenes, can be solely responsible for all of the symptoms of whiplash. Other muscles often involved are the trapezius, levator scapulae, pectoralis major and minor, certain jaw muscles, deep cervical muscles of the anterior spine, and spinal muscles of the posterior neck and upper back.

Three Special Muscles of the Neck

The trapezius, levator scapulae, and sternocleidomastoid muscles are difficult to classify according to location. The trapezius is so large that it covers the upper back, the back of the neck, and part of both shoulders. The levator scapulae starts in the upper back but wraps around to become part of the side of the neck. The sternocleidomastoid also wraps around the neck and could be seen as part of either the side or the front of the neck. Further, the unique multiple functions of these three muscles puts each in a class by itself.

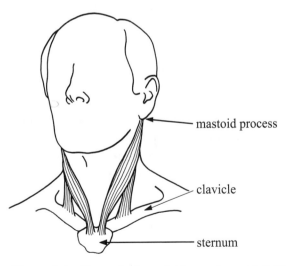

Figure 4.1 Sternocleidomastoid muscles and their attachments

Sternocleidomastoid

The name *sternocleidomastoid* (STUR-no-KLY-do-MAS-toid) is made up of the anatomical names for the bones it attaches to (Figure 4.1). *Sterno* refers to the sternum, or breastbone. *Cleido* refers to the clavicle, or collarbone. *Mastoid* is the mastoid process, the bony knob behind the ear. Don't be intimidated by this long, wonderful word. It has an infectious rhythm that you'll learn to love: say it four times in a row and you'll be on your feet dancing. You'd best make friends with your sternocleidomastoid muscles, because they make more trouble than you can imagine.

Since the sternocleidomastoids are in the front of your neck, you've probably never thought about them or even noticed them. You don't usually get pain in the front of your neck. You get it in the back of your neck. Trigger points in the sternocleidomastoid muscles actually cause an incredible amount of pain, but it's all sent elsewhere. The sternocleido-mastoids themselves rarely hurt, no matter how much trouble they're in or how much trouble they're causing. Tightness or stiffness in these muscles, however, can indicate the presence of trigger points (1999, 308–311).

> *Kate, age fifty-one, was a case that illustrates the unexpected effects that sternocleido-mastoid trigger points can have and the dramatic and swift relief that can occur with appropriate treatment. She'd lived with TMJ pain in both jaws since the age of nine, when she'd had several teeth removed to compensate for a small jaw. She also had frequent headaches and pain deep in her left ear.*
>
> *One day, while reading an article about myofascial pain that suggested neck muscles as the source of many mysterious symptoms, she began feeling her neck muscles with her hand. She was startled to find a big knot in the left side of her neck that she hadn't realized was there—she said it felt just like an egg. While she was massaging the muscle, she experienced a release in her left jaw that was so sudden and intense that it frightened her. The side of her neck felt like it was expanding like a balloon. She ran to look at it in the bathroom mirror but could see no swelling or anything else wrong. Then she noticed the pain in her ear and jaws was gone and her bite felt different. Her jaw felt like it had shifted position. Her dentist, after inspecting the change, told Kate that her TMJ dysfunction had somehow resolved itself and she now had a proper bite.*

From a myofascial viewpoint, massive chronic trigger points in Kate's sternocleido-mastoids were directly to blame for her headaches and ear pain. They had also maintained secondary trigger points in the jaw muscles that were the cause of her jaw pain and the misalignment of her temporomandibular joints. She has learned that a few minutes of massage to her sternocleidomastoid muscles gets rid of her symptoms when she feels them coming back.

Symptoms

People are rarely aware of sternocleidomastoid trigger points, though their effects can be amazingly widespread. Their influence on other muscles extends their effects significantly. Symptoms created by sternocleidomastoid trigger points fall into four groups: referred pain, balance problems, visual disturbances, and systemic symptoms.

Referred pain. Trigger points in the sternocleidomastoid don't cause pain in the muscle itself. They can be so tender to pressure, however, that they can be mistaken for swollen and sensitive lymph nodes ("swollen glands"). They can be the source of a painless neck stiffness that keeps your head tilted to one side. There are important differences in the referred pain patterns for the two branches of the sternocleidomastoid muscle, although both generally send their symptoms upward to the cranium, face, and jaws (Figures 4.2 and 4.3). A frontal headache is practically a signature of sternocleidomastoid trigger points.

Trigger points in the *sternal branch* can cause deep eye pain, tongue pain when swallowing, and headaches over the eye, behind the ear, and in the top of the head. They can contribute to temporomandibular joint pain, their referral pattern tending to promote and perpetuate trigger points in the jaw muscles. Pain is also sometimes sent to the back of the neck. The only referral downward is when pain is sometimes sent to the top of the breastbone. Not shown in Figure 4.2 is an occasional spillover of pain in the side of the face, which mimics *trigeminal neuralgia,* a disorder characterized by brief attacks of pain caused by irritation of the trigeminal nerve. This pain in the cheek can also be mistaken for sinusitis.

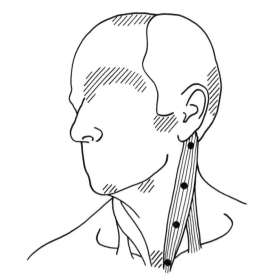

Figure 4.2 Sternocleidomastoid, sternal branch: trigger points and referred pain pattern

Trigger points in the *clavicular branch* can cause a deep earache and a toothache in the back molars. And unusual feature of clavicular trigger points is that the frontal headache can be cross referred to the opposite side of the forehead. (1999: 308–309, 318)

Balance problems. Another unusual trait of trigger points in the clavicular branch is that they are apt to make you dizzy, nauseous, and prone to lurching or falling. Fainting may occur unexpectedly. This dizziness can last for minutes, hours, or days. Often given a diagnosis of vertigo or Ménière's disease, it can become a lifelong recurrent condition, defying all treatments and medical explanations.

The myofascial explanation is that differences in tension in the clavicular branch of the sternocleidomastoid muscles help with your spatial orientation, keeping track of the position of your head. When aberrant tensions in the muscle are caused by trigger points, confusing signals are sent to the brain. Dr. Travell believed that the distorted perception caused by sternocleidomastoid trigger points were a hidden cause of falls and motor vehicle accidents.

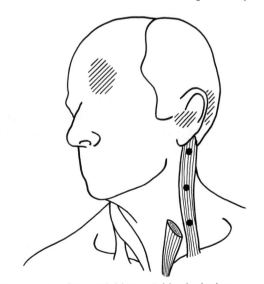

Figure 4.3 Sternocleidomastoid, clavicular branch: trigger points and referred pain pattern

Clavicular trigger points can be a cause of unilateral deafness or hearing loss on the side where these trigger points exist. This is thought to be due to referred tension in the tiny *stapedius* and *tensor tympani* muscles that attach to the equally tiny bones of the middle ear. Tension in these little muscles could inhibit vibration in the inner ear. Massage of the jaw muscles and the sternocleidomastoids has been known to bring back normal hearing when trigger points were to blame for the problem (1999, 314).

Visual disturbances. Sternal branch trigger points can cause dimmed, blurred, or double vision. You may have reddening and excessive tearing of your eyes, along with a runny nose. These trigger points can cause a drooping eyelid from a referred spasm in the orbicularis oculi muscle that surrounds the eye. Referred effects on the orbicularis muscle can also cause twitching of the eye or eyelid. The print on the page may seem to be jumping around when you read.

Systemic symptoms. A fourth group of symptoms from sternocleidomastoid trigger points can include disturbed weight perception, cold sweat on the forehead, and the generation of excess mucus in the sinuses, nasal cavities, and throat. They can be the simple explanation for your sinus congestion, sinus drainage, phlegm in the throat, chronic cough, and continual hay fever or cold symptoms. A persistent dry cough can often be stopped with massage to the sternal branch near its attachment to the breastbone (1999, 308-311).

Causes

A primary function of the sternocleidomastoid is to turn the head to the opposite side. The sternocleidomastoids also help maintain a stable position of the head during movements of the body. Trigger points can therefore be created by postures that keep the sternocleidomastoids contracted to hold the head in position. Holding your head back to work overhead is particularly bad. Keeping your head turned to one side for any reason is sure to cause trouble. Trigger points in the lower half of the body often distort the posture to such an extent that the neck muscles must exhaust themselves in a constant attempt to compensate (1999, 314–316).

A single incident of heavy lifting can strain the sternocleidomastoids. Falls and whiplash accidents cause severe overstretching and overcontraction in all the muscles of the neck, including the sternocleidomastoids. Myofascial symptoms from whiplash in an auto accident can persist for years. Other conditions that encourage trigger points are a tight collar, a short leg, a curvature of the spine, emphysema, asthma, a chronic cough, hyperventilation, emotional stress, and habitual muscle tension. An auxiliary function of the sternocleidomastoids is to raise the breastbone when you inhale. Chest breathing can overwork them.

To avoid unnecessary stress to the sternocleidomastoids, don't sit for long periods with your head turned to one side, don't read in bed, and don't sleep on your stomach. Don't slouch when sitting on a couch or in a chair. Don't hold the telephone to your ear with your shoulder. Learn to breathe with your diaphragm, not with your chest. During normal breathing, your stomach should go in and out; your upper chest should not expand and contract much at all.

Treatment

The good news about the confusing conglomeration of symptoms generated by sternocleidomastoid trigger points is that you can fix them yourself in the simplest way.

To massage the sternocleidomastoid, take all the soft tissue that you can between your fingers and thumb and knead firmly (Figures 4.4, 4.5, and 4.6). Try to discriminate between the two parts of the muscle. One is in front of the other, each about as big around as a finger.

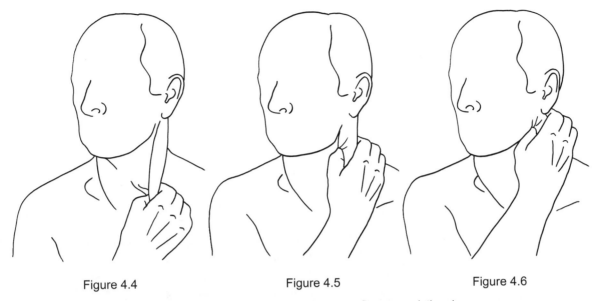

Figure 4.4 Figure 4.5 Figure 4.6

Sternocleidomastoid massage between fingers and thumb

If you pay close attention, you should be able to feel them separately. If you squeeze the inner branch (the clavicular) and then roll off it, you should feel a slight trough between it and the outer branch (the sternal). Search for trigger points in each branch, starting up behind your earlobe, all the way down to your collarbone.

If your sternocleidomastoid muscles hurt when squeezed, they're almost certain to be involved in that chronic headache or whatever other symptom you may be having in your head, face, or jaws. When sternocleidomastoid trigger points are bad enough, a little squeeze will actually reproduce or accentuate a frontal headache, giving you a very convincing demonstration of what trigger points do.

Don't be afraid of these muscles. They may hurt like the devil to massage, but you can't do them any harm. To the contrary, every squeeze you give them will be of benefit. Your symptoms may disappear in a very short time, but continue working the trigger points repeatedly and patiently over several days, until you can no longer find a place that hurts. A single session of sternocleidomastoid massage shouldn't last longer than a minute or two per side. Sternocleidomastoid massage often makes a headache better almost immediately. The same is true for dizziness and many other sternocleidomastoid symptoms.

Some physicians worry that massaging the front of the neck can loosen plaque in the carotid arteries and cause a stroke. These fears are unwarranted if you're mindful of the location of these arteries and simply avoid them. The carotid arteries are vulnerable only where you can feel your carotid pulse, high up under your chin alongside the windpipe. Proper execution of the techniques described here should not endanger the carotids. Don't massage a spot where you can feel a pulse.

Trapezius

The word *trapezius* (truh-PEE-zee-us) comes from the Greek word for a small table, a reflection of the muscle's relative flatness and four-cornered shape. Although the trapezius is

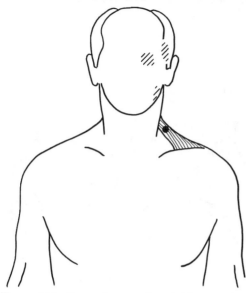

Figure 4.7   Trapezius number 1 trigger point and referred pain pattern: front view

located on the upper back and functions mainly to move the shoulder, it appears in this chapter because its trigger points are a primary source of headaches and neck pains.

A typical case of unsuspected trapezius trouble was Alison, age thirty. Her symptoms didn't seem to have anything to do with her trapezius muscles, although they were the very muscles she had overexercised with her weights. She had awakened the next day with the worst headache she'd ever had. The pain was worst in the back of her head, her forehead, and her right temple. She had a terrible ache behind her right eye. She was also dizzy and nauseous and had been vomiting in the night.

Alison found trigger points in her sternocleidomastoid muscles and the muscles in the back of her neck. Squeezing a trigger point in her right trapezius muscle accentuated the pain in her temple and behind her eye. Several sessions of self-applied massage over the course of a single day got rid of all her symptoms.

Symptoms

The first trapezius trigger point, "trapezius number 1," is located in the very topmost fibers of the thick roll of muscle on top of the shoulder. But it's not in the body of the muscle. You can only find it by pinching a tiny roll of skin right where the shoulder joins the neck (the angle of the neck). The taut band that contains the trigger point feels like a knitting needle between your fingers. It's the primary cause of a temple headache but may also send pain to the masseter muscle at the angle of the jaw, down the side of the neck behind the ear, and deep behind the eye (Figures 4.7 and 4.8). Occasionally, pain occurs in the back of the head (not shown). Most people have trapezius number 1 trigger points at one time or another. Their effects are most often identified as a tension headache (1999, 278–287). Trapezius number 1 trigger point is also a frequent cause of dizziness that is indistinguishable from that caused by a trigger point in the clavicular branch of the sternocleidomastoid. Moreover, it's capable of inducing satellite trigger points in muscles in the temple and jaw, making it an indirect cause of jaw pain and toothache (1999, 279).

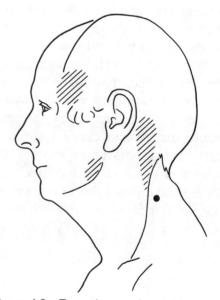

Figure 4.8   Trapezius number 1 trigger point and referred pain pattern: side view

Trapezius number 2 trigger point is actually a pair of trigger points an inch or two apart very deep in the roll of muscle on top of the shoulder. You may have either one or both. It's important to know that they are a major cause of pain at the base of the skull, which may be felt as either a headache or a sore neck (Figure 4.9). This referred pain very often induces satellite trigger points in the muscles of the back of the neck. When neck massage feels good but doesn't get rid of the pain, the problem may be in the trapezius muscles, not the neck.

Trapezius number 3 trigger point can be found in several places along the outer border of the lower trapezius, which crosses the inner edge of the shoulder blade about halfway up (Figure 4.10). This extremely common but easily missed trigger point refers pain to the base of the skull like the trigger points in the upper trapezius. It can also send pain to the upper trapezius itself. Satellite trigger points produced in these two places can in turn be the cause of certain kinds of headache. This cascade or domino effect of myofascial trigger points is one reason why headaches have been so hard to understand and treat effectively.

Trapezius number 3 is also responsible for an oppressive ache or burning pain in the mid back that can come after a long spell at the computer without elbow support. Such aches are very familiar to piano players, who also hold their arms out in front of them unsupported for long periods of time. Although this trigger point is a long way from the neck, it's one of the many causes of a stiff neck. When trigger points weaken the lower trapezius muscles, they may cause the shoulder blades to stick out in back, a condition called "winging" (1999, 280).

Trapezius number 4 trigger point occurs next to the inner border of the shoulder blade in the broad middle part of the trapezius (Figure 4.11). It causes a burning kind of pain nearby, alongside the spine. Superficial trigger points in this area can cause goose bumps on the back of the upper arm and sometimes, oddly, on the thighs (1999, 281–282).

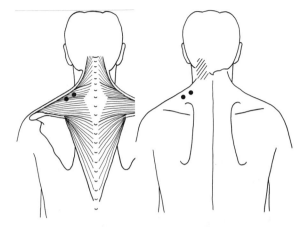

Figure 4.9   Trapezius number 2 trigger points and referred pain pattern

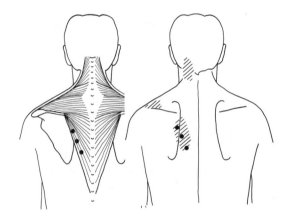

Figure 4.10   Sample trapezius number 3 trigger points and referred pain pattern

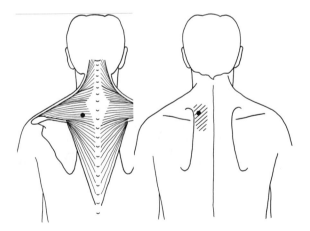

Figure 4.11 Trapezius number 4 trigger point and referred pain pattern

The symptoms generated by trapezius trigger points are widely misinterpreted, producing a whole catalog of misdiagnoses and misdirected treatments. You may be told you have spinal disk compression, spinal stenosis, bursitis of the shoulder, or neuralgia. Headaches caused by trapezius trigger points may be labeled as cervicogenic, vascular, cluster, or migraine when their true cause is not understood. Although there are serious medical causes of headaches, an examination for trigger points should be near the top of any doctor's list (1999, 291–293).

Causes

The trapezius covers most of the upper half of the back, extending upward to cover the central part of the back of the neck. This uppermost part of the trapezius is what gives the back of the neck its shape. The muscle attaches to the base of the skull, the spine, the collarbone, and the shoulder blades. The trapezius supports the weight of the shoulders and must contract strongly to rotate the shoulder blade every time you raise your arm. Another primary function is to hold the shoulder blade solidly in place as a base for the finer operations of the arm and hand.

The uppermost part of the trapezius helps support the weight of the head and neck when you bend your head forward or to the side. Faulty posture, such as slumping while seated or habitually carrying your head forward, places an unnecessary burden on your trapezius muscles, generating trigger points. Shortened pectoral muscles, indicated by a round-shouldered posture, exert a constant pull on the shoulders that the trapezius muscles must constantly counteract.

Another common cause of trapezius trigger points is the emotional tension that keeps your shoulders up. Any work or physical activity that keeps the shoulders raised puts the trapezius muscles at risk of overuse. Trigger points are produced in all parts of the trapezius by a job that requires working with the arms held out in front of the body for extended periods of time. The constant contraction gives them no chance to rest and recover. You subject your trapezius muscles to constant strain when you sit without elbow support. At the computer or any other desk job, use a chair with arms whenever possible. It's not enough to rest your arms on the desk.

Heavy-breasted women may be especially vulnerable to any of the many trapezius symptoms. The strain of supporting heavy breasts can make trapezius trigger points hard to get rid of. Carrying a heavy backpack or a heavy purse hanging from a shoulder strap can be the simple explanation for that chronic "migraine" or stiff neck (1999, 387–388).

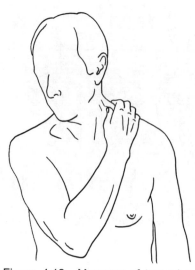

Figure 4.12   Massage of trapezius number 1 with fingers and thumb

Treatment

It's important to understand that trapezius number 1 in the angle of the neck is right under the skin (Figure 4.12). It takes only a shallow pinch to take hold of it. You should feel a firm strand or cord as small as a pencil lead or the tube of a ballpoint refill. It can be as thick as a knitting needle. Massage it by rolling it between your thumb and first two fingers. A good strong squeeze of trapezius number 1 will very often reproduce or accentuate a

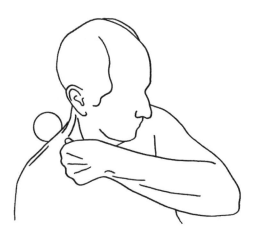

Figure 4.13 Trapezius massage with supported thumb against ball on the wall or bed

temple headache, which verifies it as the cause. If your upper shoulders are very tight or thick with muscle or fat, you may have difficulty grasping it. To make this strand of muscle easier to get ahold of, take some of the strain off the trapezius and loosen it by putting your hand in your pocket. Virtually everyone has this trigger point and it causes an incredible amount of grief.

If massage with fingers and thumb is too tiring for your hand, try pressing a trapezius number 1 trigger point against a ball on the wall with a supported thumb (Figure 4.13). Any of the trapezius trigger points can be massaged with the Thera Cane. Figure 4.14 shows how to hold the Thera Cane for massage of trapezius number 2. Maximum pressure and control is obtained when the hand opposite to the side being massaged is in the crook of the cane. Figure 4.15 shows the crossed position of the hands for reaching over the shoulder to the opposite side of the back to massage trapezius number 4. Figure 4.16 shows the position of the Thera Cane for massage of lower trapezius number 3 trigger point. Although for clarity the Thera Cane is shown being applied to bare skin, always use an intervening layer of cloth. Review the massage guidelines on page 38 to be sure that you clearly understand how to correctly execute the massage stroke.

Leaning against a ball on the wall is especially effective for trigger point number 3 in the lower trapezius where it crosses the shoulder blade (Figure 4.17). Notice that you have a choice of two directions to move the ball: up the back or across it toward the spine. Moving up along the edge of the shoulder blade, you'll feel the ball bump as it goes over the diagonally oriented edge of the muscle. Moving across from the shoulder blade onto the back, it feels like you're pushing the muscle ahead of the ball. There's likely to be more than one trigger point at this site, one on each side of the edge of the shoulder blade. Use a tennis ball if the trigger points are especially tender. A hard rubber ball is better if you have to penetrate a lot of tissue; a very small ball is better yet for penetration. Trapezius trigger points

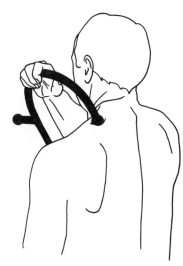

Figure 4.14 Trapezius number 2 massage with Thera Cane

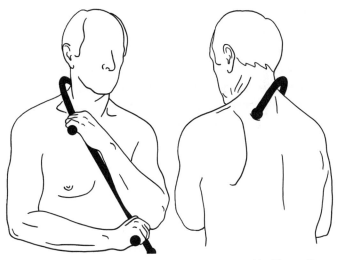

Figure 4.15 Trapezius number 4 massage with Thera Cane over the opposite shoulder

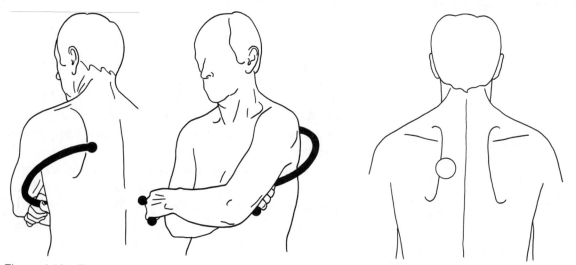

Figure 4.16   Trapezius number 3 massage with
Thera Cane

Figure 4.17   Trapezius number 3 massage
with ball against wall

should be massaged six or more times a day for best results, but limit the session to six to twelve strokes per trigger point. Don't try to kill them. Let your body do the healing.

Levator Scapulae

The *levator scapulae* (luh-VAY-ter SCAP-yuh-lee) is another hardworking muscle that everyone has trouble with. *Levator* is from the same Latin root as "elevator." *Scapula* is Latin for "shoulder blade." The name tells its job: it lifts the shoulder blade. (Note that the word ending "ae" in scapulae is actually a singular form, not the more familiar plural seen in such words as *alumnae*. In common usage, "levator scapulae" is often pronounced as though it were spelled "levator scapula.")

Tony, age thirty-three, had typical levator scapulae trouble. He'd had constant pain and stiffness in the right side of his neck ever since a fender bender three months earlier and couldn't turn his head to the right at all. His insurance was paying for physical therapy, but the stretching and traction only seemed to be making his pain worse. Electrostimulation helped but it didn't last.

Massage to Tony's levator scapulae muscles cut through his pain at once and gave him his first relief. He was shown various ways to do the massage himself, which he was encouraged to do several times a day. Within a week, his pain was gone. In three weeks, he could turn his head again with a full range of motion.

Symptoms

Trigger points in levator scapulae muscles cause pain and stiffness in the angle of the neck (Figure 4.18). When sufficiently active, they also refer a lesser degree of pain along the inner edge of the shoulder blade and to the back of the shoulder (not shown). A levator scapulae trigger point is what keeps you from turning your head to look behind you when you're backing up in your car. You may not be able to turn your head at all toward the side that has the trigger point (1999, 491–492).

Causes

The lower end of each levator scapulae muscle attaches to the inner edge of the top angle of the corresponding shoulder blade. Its upper end attaches to the sides of the top four neck vertebrae. This arrangement allows the levator scapulae to help raise the shoulder blade and thereby raise the shoulder. This function is the very one that gets the muscle into trouble. When stress and bad posture habits keep your shoulders up, you can be sure that the levator scapulae muscles are doing much of the work.

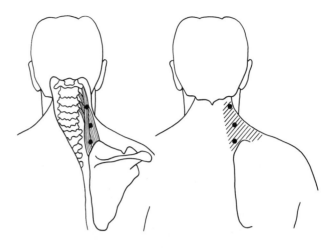

Figure 4.18   Levator scapulae trigger points and referred pain pattern

Because of the attachments to the sides of the neck bones, the levator is also able to help turn your head to the same side. When trigger points disable the muscle, it is reluctant to contract and perform this function. The muscle also resists lengthening, which can keep you from turning your head in the other direction too (1999, 494).

Many things can make trouble for a levator scapulae, including sleeping on your side without support for your head, typing while looking at your copy out to one side, and holding the phone clamped between your head and shoulder. Backpacks and purses suspended from shoulder straps are as bad for levator scapulae muscles as for the trapezius. Both have to stay strongly contracted to counter the downward pull. You'll observe that a woman who carries her purse on a shoulder strap always has her shoulder hiked up to keep the purse from falling off; this causes further strain on the levator scapulae.

Levator muscles are also stressed by overexercise, emotional tension, and armrests that are too high or too low. The levator is one of many muscles that are strained by whiplash. Trigger points set up by an auto accident or a fall can persist undetected for years, the unknown sources of chronic pain and disability (1999, 494–495).

As a pair, the levators serve as a checkrein for the head when it hangs forward. They are consequently severely abused by habitually carrying the head forward. Levator scapulae and trapezius muscles can be strained beyond endurance by habitually reading with your book flat on the desk, since all the muscles of your neck and upper back have to remain contracted all the time your head is hanging forward in that position. Prop your book up when you read so you can keep your head up. Several styles of book stands can be found in any college bookstore.

Treatment

The most accessible levator scapulae trigger point is located just above where the muscle attaches to the upper angle of the shoulder blade. Unfortunately, this isn't the trigger point that causes most of the trouble. It feels good to work this spot but it won't get rid of all your neck pain and stiffness. The middle (central) trigger point is the one to go after. It's buried under the thick upper trapezius, so you'll need to apply strong pressure to get to it. Use a ball against the wall for the lower two trigger points. A Thera Cane or Backnobber also works well (see Figures 4.14 and 4.15). Don't neglect the highest trigger point, high on the side of the neck just behind the top of the sternocleidomastoid muscle. Work it with a supported thumb.

Muscles of the Back of the Neck

Excepting the suboccipital muscles, which constitute a special class, four layers of muscle cover the back of the neck. Picture the plies of a tire: the outer layer is the uppermost part of the upper trapezius; the three deeper layers carry the inevitable Greek-derived and Latinate names that variously describe them or give a clue to their function.

Immediately under the trapezius lie the thin, flat splenius muscles, which cover the others like thin straps. The word *splenius*, in fact, derives from the Greek word for "bandage." Then come the semispinalis muscles, running nearly parallel to the spine as the name suggests. Underneath everything else are the rotatores and multifidi, a multitude of very short muscles that interconnect the neck vertebrae and help rotate the neck and bend it to the side. *Multifidi* literally means "split into many parts."

The massage techniques for all of the muscles of the back of the neck are the same as are shown for the suboccipitals in the following section. The causes of trigger points in the back of the neck are the same kinds of abuse and overuse listed for the trapezius and levator scapulae.

Suboccipital Muscles

The *suboccipital* (sub-ahk-SIH-pih-tul) muscles are located right below the base of the skull; the *occiput* is the back of the head. The suboccipitals consist of four small muscles on each side, each running at a different angle, connecting the top two vertebrae to the skull and to each other (Figure 4.19).

Symptoms

Suboccipital trigger points cause pain that feels like it's inside the head, extending from the back of the head to the eye and forehead (Figure 4.20). It feels like the whole side of the head hurts. This sensation is typical of what you experience with a migraine headache. The treatment of suboccipital trigger points should be part of any approach to dealing with migraine (1999, 472–476).

Oddly enough, suboccipital trigger points don't usually cause neck pain. They can, however, play an important part in neck stiffness. The upper three suboccipitals on each side control nodding and tilting and can inhibit

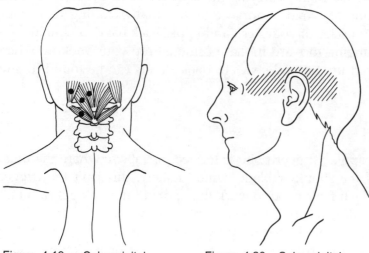

Figure 4.19   Suboccipital muscles trigger points

Figure 4.20   Suboccipitals referred pain pattern

these movements if afflicted with trigger points. The lowest of the suboccipitals, the *obliquus capitis inferior*, connects the top two vertebrae where most of the rotation of the head occurs. This little muscle's trigger points restrict rotation and cause sharp pain high on the side of the neck when you've turned your head as far as it will go. This special muscle can be most effectively worked with supported fingers. The opposite hand crosses over in front so that both hands reach behind from the same side. It's the same tool as illustrated in Figure 4.47, except that the fingers are placed behind the ear just below the base of the skull.

Causes

Suboccipital muscles can be quickly exhausted by frequently moving the head or by any prolonged contraction. Emotional tension tends to keep the suboccipitals contracted, which in some cases may be the physical connection between worry and migraine headaches. Trapezius trigger points contribute to migraine by creating satellite trigger points in the suboccipitals (1999, 241–243).

Treatment

The suboccipitals are the most deeply situated of all the neck muscles. Almost any tool will penetrate to them, however, because the overlying muscles are all relatively thin. Use one of the small nipples on the shaft of the Thera Cane (Figure 4.21). You may also like the Knobble for this, used with both hands either standing or lying down.

A tennis ball or lacrosse ball, held in the palm of the hand, also makes a very good tool (Figure 4.22). Use the other hand to help support the head. This technique is intended for use lying down so you can use the weight of your head for pressure.

The tips of your fingers may be best for massaging the suboccipitals and other posterior neck muscles because they are more sensitive and precise than the hard tools. To massage the back of your neck while standing or sitting, use the fingers of one hand reinforced with the heel of the opposite hand (Figures 4.23 and 4.24). This supporting hand actually does the work. Reverse the hands to massage the other side. Let your head fall back against your hands while doing the supported fingers massage. Letting your head hang forward to any degree contracts the very muscles you're trying to work on. This technique will obviously work best while lying on your back.

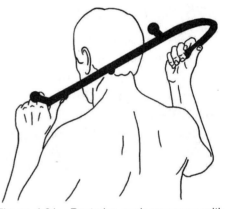

Figure 4.21   Posterior neck massage with Thera Cane

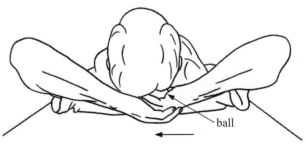

Figure 4.22   Position of hands for posterior neck massage with a ball lying down. Using both hands, stroke toward the center line. Change hands for the other side.

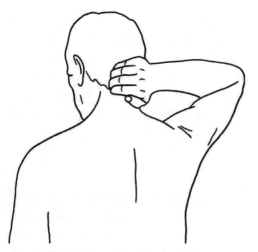

Figure 4.23   First hand in place for massage of opposite side of the posterior neck with supported fingers

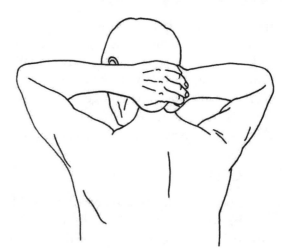

Figure 4.24   Second hand in place for posterior neck massage with supported fingers. Stroke toward the spine; switch hands to work the other side.

Splenius Muscles

Splenius capitis (SPLEE-nee-us CAP-uh-tiss) muscles are broad straps connecting the neck vertebrae to the back of the skull. Their diagonal orientation makes the splenius capitis muscles a major force in turning the head. Splenius capitis trigger points refer pain to the top of the head (Figure 4.25) and are an extremely common cause of headache (1999, 432; Jaeger 1989, 550–607).

Splenius cervicis (SPLEE-nee-us SUR-vuh-sis) muscles connect the vertebrae of the upper back to those of the neck. Their upper trigger points cause pain that begins at the base of the skull and runs forward through the head to the back of the eye (Figure 4.26). It feels like a pulsating ache inside the skull. In addition to pain, this trigger point is capable of blurring your vision. Symptoms emanating from the upper splenius cervicis are an important component of migraine headaches (1999, 432–440).

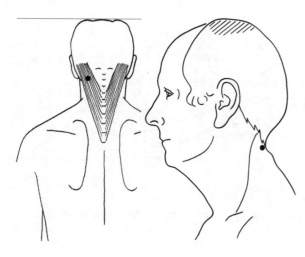

Figure 4.25   Splenius capitis trigger point and referred pain pattern

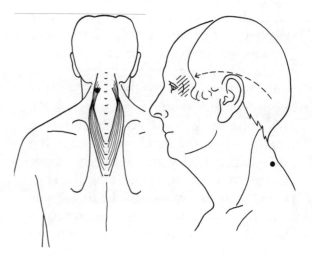

Figure 4.26   Splenius cervicis number 1 trigger point and referred pain pattern: through the head like a spear to the back of the eye

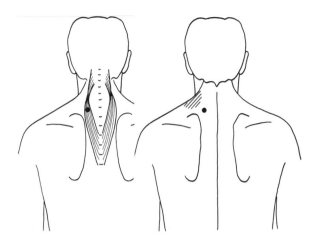

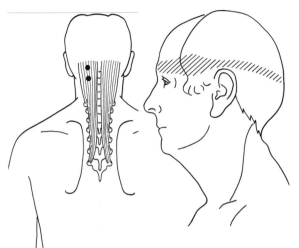

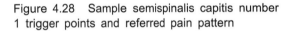

Figure 4.27   Splenius cervicis number 2 trigger point and referred pain pattern

Figure 4.28   Sample semispinalis capitis number 1 trigger points and referred pain pattern

Trigger points in the lower splenius cervicis refer pain to the angle of the neck (Figure 4.27) in a pattern very similar to that referred by the levator scapulae. The upper and lower splenius cervicis trigger points can both cause a sense of numbness or pressure in the back of the head (1999, 434; Graff-Radford, Jaeger, and Reeves 1986, 610–613).

Semispinalis Capitis

Semispinalis capitis (seh-mee-spih-NAH-liss CAP-uh-tiss) muscles connect the vertebrae of the upper back and lower neck to the base of the skull. Because of the segmented construction of this muscle, trigger points may be found anywhere along its length. Semispinalis capitis number 1 trigger points cause a band of pain that encircles half the head just above the ear (Figure 4.28). These trigger points overlie deeper ones in the suboccipitals, which have a similar referral pattern. Semispinalis number 2 trigger points refer pain to the back of the head (Figure 4.29).

Trigger points in semispinalis capitis and trapezius muscles can cause pressure on the greater occipital nerve, which is a sensory nerve for the back of the head. This entrapment of the nerve can be the source of numbness, tingling, and burning pain in the scalp of the back of the head. With this problem, you can't bear the pressure of your head on the pillow (1999, 455).

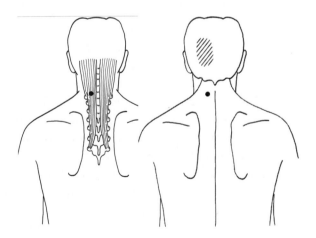

Figure 4.29   Sample semispinalis capitis number 2 trigger point and referred pain pattern

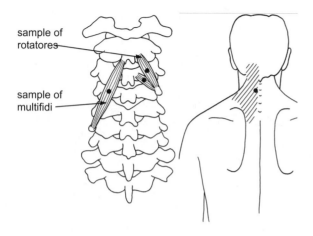

sample of rotatores

sample of multifidi

Figure 4.30   Multifidi and rotatores trigger points and referred pain pattern

Multifidi and Rotatores

The *multifidi* (mul-TIH-fih-dee) and the *rotatores* (ro-tuh-TOR-eez) are the deepest of the neck muscles. Dozens and dozens of these tiny muscles run from vertebra to vertebra at a variety of angles and are important for the finer, more controlled movements of the neck and head.

Multifidi and rotatores trigger points cause intense pain at the site of the trigger point, which usually spreads up or down the spine several vertebrae (Figure 4.30). Pain may be felt as far away as the top of the shoulder and the inner edge of the shoulder blade.

Pain from the multifidi and rotatores feels like it's in the spine itself and is often misinterpreted as resulting from disk compression or disarticulation (subluxation) of the vertebrae. When subluxation, or partial dislocation, does occur, it's caused by extreme tension in one of these small muscles which pulls the vertebra to one side. The vertebra will often pop right back into place when the trigger point is deactivated (1999, 445–459).

Multifidi and rotatores trigger points may occur at any level in the neck. Massage them against the vertebrae with supported fingers (see Figures 4.23 and 4.24). If you can't reach them with your hands, use a ball while lying on your back (see Figure 4.22).

Muscles of the Jaw, Face, and Head

Although there are a great number of muscles in the jaw, face, and head, self-treatment is directed mainly at the two chewing muscles, the masseter and the temporalis. Trigger points in these two muscles, along with those in the trapezius and sternocleidomastoid muscles, account for much of the pain in the jaw, face, and head, including the infamous temporomandibular joint (TMJ). Trigger points in the other muscles of the jaw, face, and head usually exist as satellites to trigger points in these four primary muscles. Symptoms from the smaller muscles may subside spontaneously when the trigger points in the primary muscles are deactivated (1999, 339).

Trigger points in the jaw muscles have a variety of causes, including excessive gum chewing, tooth decay, abscesses, and grinding the teeth at night. Dental work frequently leaves patients with trigger points in the strained or exhausted jaw muscles. Emotional tension, mouth breathing, and the head-forward posture also cause trigger points in the jaw muscles by promoting habitual tension in them. Trigger points in sternocleidomastoid and trapezius muscles resulting from whiplash, falls, and other kinds of physical strain tend to promote trigger points in the muscles of the jaw, face, and head (1999, 335–336; Hong 1994, 29–59).

Masseter

The *masseter* (MASS-uh-ter) muscles are the power muscles of the jaw, exerting the major force in biting and chewing. In the mirror, you can see your masseters contract right in front of your earlobes when you grit your teeth. *Masseter* comes from the Greek word for "to chew." Pain from masseter trigger points can fool even the experts.

> *Mary, age twenty-nine, was a dentist who was frustrated in the treatment of some of her patients who complained of tooth pain but had no problems that she could find. She also had pain in her own jaws and in her own perfectly healthy teeth. She suspected the pain was myofascial but she didn't feel competent to diagnose or treat it. In dental school, they'd been told about trigger points but hadn't spent much time on them.*
>
> *A clue to Mary's own trouble lay in the chronic headaches and neck pain she had suffered since dental school, caused by leaning over all day and twisting to look into mouths.*
>
> *The strain of her work had caused trigger points in her sternocleidomastoid muscles, which in turn were generating secondary trigger points in her masseter muscles. Her headaches were coming from her sternocleidomastoids, the pain in her jaws and teeth from her masseters.*

Trigger points in the masseter muscles cause pain in several places (Figure 4.31). The trigger point in the deep layer right in front of the ear is especially important as a cause of pain in the temporomandibular joint. Masseter trigger points can also increase muscle tension to such an extent that it restricts opening of the jaw. This jaw tightness encourages tightness in the vocal mechanism. Singers have reported hitting their high notes with greater ease after they've worked on their masseters and other jaw muscles (1999, 334–335).

Masseter trigger points cause pain in both upper and lower teeth. They are also a common source of tooth hypersensitivity to heat, cold, and touch. Misinterpretation of these symptoms can result in unnecessary dental work, including needless tooth extraction. Masseter trigger points may cause you to neglect to brush and floss sensitive teeth, which can lead to their deterioration (1999, 329–339).

Trigger points in the masseter muscles also cause pain in the front of the face, under the eyes, and over the eyebrows, symptoms often mistaken for sinusitis. They can even cause sinus drainage. When sinus medicine doesn't help your sinus pain, masseter trigger points may be the problem (1999, 330).

Bags under the eyes can be caused by trigger points in masseter muscles. They can also cause pain deep in the ear, accompanied by a sense of stuffiness or the sound of low roaring. They're often responsible for that maddening itch inside your ear that you can't quite seem to reach (1999: 338).

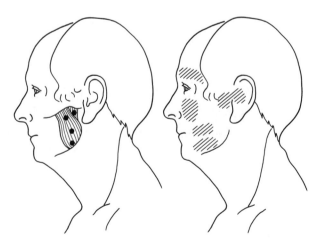

Figure 4.31 Masseter trigger points and referred pain pattern

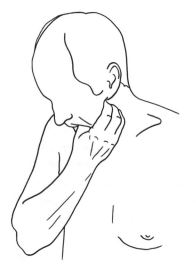

Figure 4.32   Masseter massage with thumb and fingers (thumb inside the mouth)

Trigger points can be found at any place in the masseter, from the cheekbone to the bottom edge of the jaw. Massaging the masseter from outside the mouth with supported fingers is good therapy (see Figure 4.47). To work the masseter most effectively, however, it's necessary to put your thumb inside your mouth and knead the muscle between thumb and fingers (Figure 4.32). The masseter feels very firm, thick, and rubbery. If you're working the right place, you'll feel the tip of your thumb touching the coronoid process, the sharp-edged, fin-shaped piece of bone rising from near the back of the jawbone.

Seek out each exquisitely tender knot, from the cheekbone to the bottom of the jaw, and massage it as strongly as you can bear. Massaging the masseters is extremely painful when they're afflicted with trigger points, and you should expect to experience soreness afterward for a day or two. This residual soreness only indicates how badly the muscles need the attention. Don't let the discomfort make you give up. Work on them every day until squeezing the muscle no longer hurts.

You can go a long way toward preventing trouble with the jaw muscles by giving up chewing gum. In addition, avoid biting your nails, don't chew on ice, and don't open things with your teeth. Find out what you can do to stop grinding your teeth in your sleep. Train yourself not to clench your jaws when you're tense and under pressure. See chapter 12 to learn more about reducing habitual muscle tensions.

Pterygoid Muscles

The *pterygoid* (TEHR-uh-goyd) muscles are well hidden by the lower jawbone, which is very inconvenient, since their trigger points are a frequent cause of pain in temporomandibular joints of the jaw. The word *pterygoid* comes from the Greek for "winglike," a reflection of their shape. The root word is similar to that of "pterodactyl," the name of the winged dinosaur.

The *medial pterygoid* muscle causes pain in the temporomandibular joint and the ear, which increases when you bite down on something (Figure 4.33). It can also refer pain to the back of the mouth, hard palate, and tongue and can make it hurt to swallow. Medial pterygoid trigger points make it difficult to open the mouth wide. A sense of stuffiness in the ear can come from a tight medial pterygoid when it prevents the eustachian tube (in the middle ear) from opening. This may occur because of referred effects on the *tensor veli*

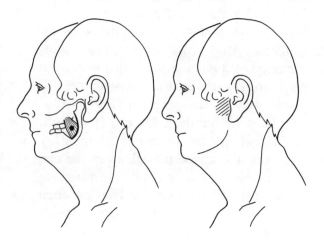

Figure 4.33   Medial pterygoid trigger point and referred pain pattern

palatini and *salpingopharyngeus* muscles in the back of the throat, which have more direct control over the eustachian tube. The medial pterygoid muscle helps close the jaw. Its problems are therefore strongly associated with those in the masseter (1999, 365–366; Bell 1969, 154–160).

You can massage the medial pterygoid by pressing up with your thumb inside the inner edge of the back of your lower jaw (Figure 4.34). This can be an exceedingly painful spot. As with the masseter, massage of the pterygoids can leave you sore, so go easy at first.

The other pterygoid muscle, the *lateral pterygoid*, is the number one myofascial source of pain and temporomandibular joint (TMJ) dysfunction (Figure 4.35). Constant trigger point–generated tension in the lateral pterygoids tends to pull the lower jaw forward and disarticulate, or partially dislocate, the joint. Popping or clicking

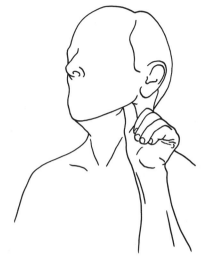

Figure 4.34   Medial pterygoid massage with thumb

in the jaw is the result of this displacement (1999, 383; Reynolds 1981, 111–114; Marbach 1972, 601–605).

As with the masseter, trigger points in the lateral pterygoid refer pain to the cheek, mimicking sinus pain. They can also stimulate sinus secretions. Many "sinus attacks" are simply the effects of lateral pterygoid trigger points (1999: 383).

Travell and Simons link tinnitus (ringing in the ears) to trigger points in the sternocleidomastoid, masseter, and lateral pterygoid muscles. They quote studies showing that trigger point injection can completely relieve the condition.

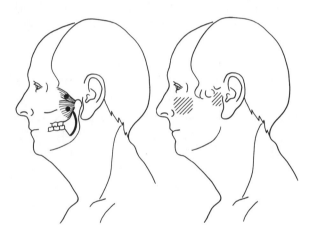

Figure 4.35   Lateral pterygoid trigger points and referred pain pattern

This author, who suffers from tinnitus, has not found that massage of these muscles has any ameliorating effect on tinnitus. The key muscle may be the lateral pterygoid, which is very well hidden by the jawbone, making it much less accessible to the finger than to the needle. The function of the lateral pterygoid muscles is to help the digastric muscles open the jaw. As a consequence, trigger points are created in the lateral pterygoids when you have trouble breathing through your nose and must keep your mouth open in order to breathe. Satellite trigger points set up in the front of the face by the lateral pterygoids may account for much of the face pain that comes with allergies. Major dental work that stresses jaw muscles by requiring you to hold your mouth open for long periods of time can be the unsuspected cause of long-term chronic pain in the face and jaws. Trigger points in masseter and temporalis

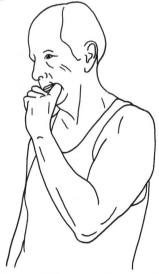

Figure 4.36   Lateral pterygoid massage with index finger in mouth

muscles can cause trigger points to develop in the lateral pterygoids by making them work harder to open the mouth (1999, 379–384).

Massage the lateral pterygoid with the index finger of either hand inside the mouth (Figure 4.36). The fingertip should seek the deep pocket back beyond your upper molars—the place you have to dig peanut butter out of. Push back as far as you can, then push both inward and upward using tiny, short strokes. If trigger points are present, this can be excruciatingly painful. You won't be able to do this massage unless your fingernail is very short. If you have chronic jaw or face pain, cut your nails to the quick so you can do this work. It's well worth it.

Buccinator

The *buccinator* (BUCK-sih-nay-tur) is a cheek muscle and is located between the masseter and the mouth. The buccinator draws the corners of the mouth back for facial expressions. It also helps move food around in the mouth and tightens the cheeks for blowing.

Buccinator trigger points cause pain in the upper gum that can be misinterpreted as evidence of tooth decay or an abscess (Figure 4.37). They also cause diffuse pain on chewing and swallowing (1999, 416–422; Curl 1989, 339–345). Massage the buccinator between the fingers and thumb with the thumb inside the mouth, the same way you massage the masseter muscles (see Figure 4.32).

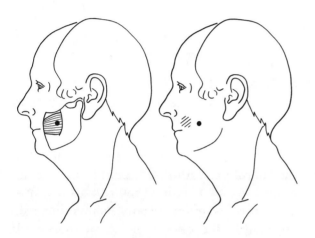

Figure 4.37   Buccinator trigger point and referred pain pattern

Orbicularis oculi

The *orbicularis oculi* (or-bic-yu-LAIR-iss AHK-you-lye) surrounds the eye and is responsible for closing the eye and for squinting. The word *oculi* refers to the eye. *Orbicularis* refers to the circle the muscle makes around it.

Nervous tension, eyestrain, and poor eyesight can keep this muscle constantly contracted and set up trigger points. Orbicularis oculi trigger points cause pain immediately above the eye and to the bridge and side of the nose (Figure 4.38). They also cause the print to jump around on the page when you try to read. They can also be responsible for twitching of the eye or

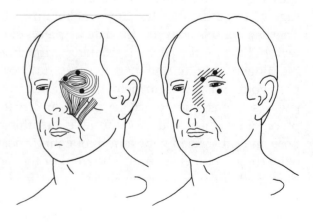

Figure 4.38 Obicularis oculi trigger points and referred pain pattern

drooping of the upper eyelid. Sternocleidomastoid trigger points may be at the heart of these problems, because of their referred influence on the orbicularis oculi. To treat the orbicularis muscles, massage around the eyes carefully with the fingertips. It may do more good, however, to massage the sternocleidomastoid (1999, 416–422).

Zygomaticus and Levator Labii Muscles

The *zygomaticus* (zi-go-MAT-uh-cus) and *levator labii* (luh-VAY-ter LAY-bee-aye) are cheek muscles that lie between the buccinator and the nose. They attach to the cheekbone and the rim of the eye socket. These small muscles function primarily as muscles of facial expression, functioning to pull the upper lip up and back.

Trigger points in zygomaticus and levator labii muscles cause pain in the face below the eye, along the side of the nose, and over the bridge of the nose as far as the middle of the forehead (Figure 4.39). They can cause allergy symptoms such as runny nose, sneezing, and itchy eyes and may contribute a significant part of your "sinus" pain or tension headaches (1999, 422). Massage the entire area below the eye down to the upper lip with the tips of the fingers, using short, deep strokes (Figure 4.40). Knead the area just below your cheekbone between your fingers and thumb (Figure 4.41).

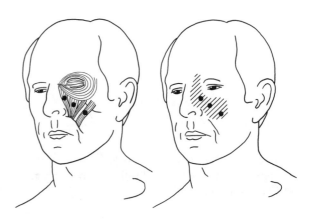

Figure 4.39 Zygomaticus and levator labii trigger points and referred pain pattern

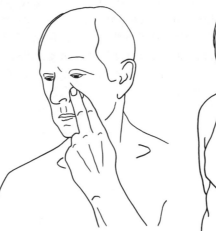

Figure 4.40 Zygomaticus and levator labii massage with fingertips

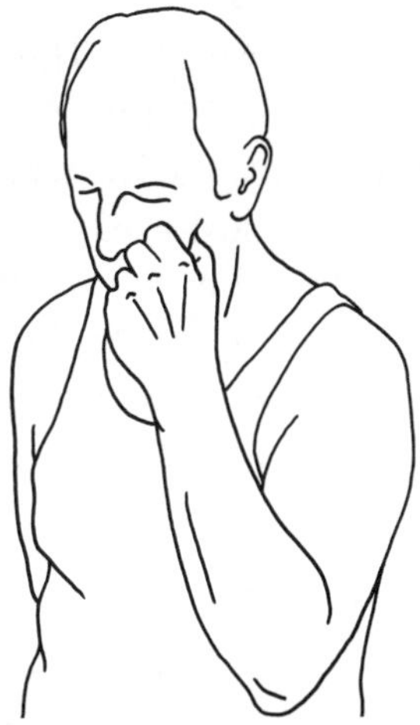

Figure 4.41 Kneading the zygomaticus between fingers and thumb

Throat Muscles

The *platysma* (pluh-TIZ-muh) is a very thin sheet of muscle lying right under the skin and covering the entire throat area from the chin to the collarbones (not illustrated). The word *platysma* is derived from two Greek words meaning "broad muscle." Platysma trigger points can cause a prickling sensation over the lower part of the cheeks, and the chin, throat, and upper chest (not shown). Trigger points in the scalenes and sternocleidomastoid muscles activate platysma trigger points. They may also arise from habitual overuse of the platysma in certain emphatic facial expressions (1999, 421). Massage all of the throat area with kneading strokes of the fingers and thumb.

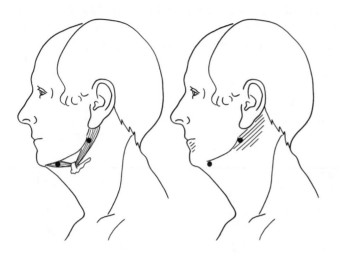

Figure 4.42   Digastric trigger points and referred pain pattern. Pain shown below the lower lip is actually felt in the lower teeth.

Trigger points in the *digastric* muscle are under the chin behind and below the corner of the jaw, immediately in front of the top of the sternocleidomastoid. The word *digastric* comes from Greek words meaning "two bellies." The posterior digastric trigger point, lying just behind the corner of the jaw, refers pain to the top end of the sternocleidomastoid muscle and the mastoid bone (Figure 4.42). The anterior trigger point, which is under the chin, sends pain to the lower front teeth. The *mylohyoid* muscles, also under the chin, refer pain to the tongue (not shown). Digastric and mylohyoid trigger points are also one of the many causes of pain when you swallow. Trigger point tenderness under the chin is often mistaken for swollen lymph nodes (1999, 397–404).

Since the function of the digastric muscles is to open the mouth, habitual mouth breathing promotes the development of trigger points in them. The problems of allergy sufferers are frequently made worse by the effects of trigger points in the digastric and lateral pterygoid muscles. These muscles have to stay contracted to keep your mouth open when you have difficulty breathing through your nose (1999, 404–405). Massage both bellies of the digastric muscle by deep stroking with the fingertips (Figures 4.43 and 4.44). Use the fingertips in the soft area under the chin to massage mylohyoid muscles. Massaging the muscles under the chin can help free up a tight voice and make it more resonant.

The *longus colli* (CO-lye) muscles lie alongside the windpipe on either side, attaching to the front side of the neck vertebrae. Their trigger points are thought to cause sore throat and to make it hurt to talk or sing. To massage the longus colli, insert the fingertips between the

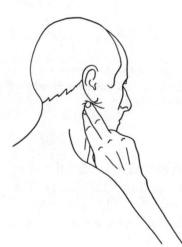

Figure 4.43   Posterior digastric massage with fingertips

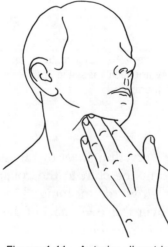

Figure 4.44   Anterior digastric massage with fingertips

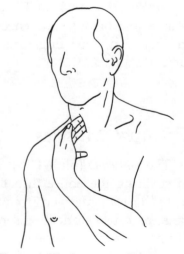

Figure 4.45   Longus colli massage with fingertips. Avoid pressure on the carotid arteries where you feel your pulse.

windpipe and the sternocleidomastoid and push back against the vertebrae (Figure 4.45). If you feel the carotid artery pulsing under your fingers on either side of your windpipe, just move them slightly to the outside.

It's important to know that trigger points in the longus colli, digastric, mylohyoid, and other muscles of the front of the neck can be created in whiplash-type accidents (1999, 404).

Scalp Muscles

The *temporalis* (tem-por-AL-iss) is a large, flat muscle covering the temple above and in front of the ear (Figure 4.46). The attachment of the temporalis to the coronoid process of the lower jaw allows it to assist the masseter in bringing the jaws together. Like the masseter, the temporalis is a chewing muscle.

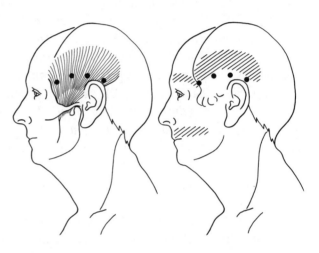

Temporalis trigger points contribute to headaches in the front and sides of the head. They're also a very common, though usually unsuspected, cause of pain and hypersensitivity in the upper teeth, along with pain and minor inflammation in the upper gums. Your teeth may be bothered more by hot and cold than by pain. Diffuse pain in the upper teeth or jaw when you chew or bite down is apt to be coming from the temporalis muscles. Your teeth may feel like they don't fit together right (1999, 349–357).

Figure 4.46 Temporalis trigger points and referred pain pattern

Trigger points in the masseter and sternocleidomastoid muscles sponsor trigger points in the temporalis and can quickly reactivate them after you've gone to the trouble of subduing them. Muscles have this kind of effect on one another. It's important to track down and treat all the muscles that are interrelated by proximity or function—in this case, the masseter, sternocleidomastoid, and temporalis (1999, 345–355). Massage the temporalis with supported fingers (Figure 4.47). In the illustration, observe that the weight of the head exerts the pressure.

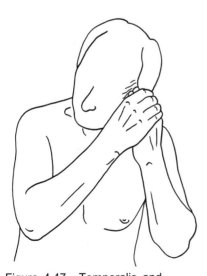

Figure 4.47 Temporalis and masseter massage with supported fingers

A large, thin muscle with two bellies covers the front, top, and back of the head. The front half of this muscle is called the *frontalis* (frun-TAL-iss). The back half is called the *occipitalis* (ahk-sih-pih-TAL-iss). Trigger points in the frontalis refer pain to the forehead (not shown). Trigger points in the occipitalis refer pain to the side and back of the head and through the head to the eye (not shown) (1999, 427).

The occipitalis is the muscle that lets you wiggle your ears. It also establishes a base for contraction of the frontalis, which raises the eyebrows and wrinkles the forehead. Anxiety and excitement overwork these muscles. You can exhaust them with by habitually contracting your face and forehead in an expression of rapt attention. Massage the frontalis and occipitalis muscles with your fingertips (not shown).

The following case history demonstrates the complex interrelationships that exist between the muscles of the head, neck, and upper back. When a myofascial problem presents itself, there are usually multiple symptoms. Trigger points are typically found in all the muscles in the area and all the connections and relationships may not be immediately apparent.

Richard, age fifty-one, had constant pain in the right side of his tongue. His right cheek and his lower teeth on the right side sometimes hurt too. His right upper lip was hypersensitive and often tingled. His right shoulder also hurt most of the time and he had difficulty lifting his arm. Richard didn't know what was wrong with his face, but he was pretty sure that his shoulder trouble came from lifting fifty-pound bags of chemicals at work to dump them into a hopper. His doctor mistakenly concluded that all his symptoms stemmed from one cause: a malfunctioning shoulder joint. He suggested that Richard get a shoulder operation and then change jobs.

Trigger points were found in all the muscles of Richard's right shoulder, the right side of his neck, and his right jaw and cheek. Particularly bad were the sternocleidomastoid, masseter, pterygoid, buccinator, and zygomaticus muscles of his neck, face, and jaw. His sternocleidomastoids had been strained by the lifting, along with his shoulder muscles. The afflicted neck muscles had then created secondary trigger points in his jaw and face.

With trigger point therapy to the muscles in his neck, jaws, and face, much of which he could do himself, all the symptoms in Richard's face soon went away. Self-treatment of his shoulder muscles also enabled him to be without shoulder pain for three or four weeks at a time, before the heavy lifting started it up again. It was clear that a shoulder operation wouldn't be needed. He took the rest of his doctor's advice seriously, however. His retirement plan would allow him to quit his factory job in two years. He was looking forward to it.

CHAPTER 5

Shoulder, Upper Back, and Upper Arm Pain

Trigger Point Guide:
Shoulder, Upper Back, and Upper Arm Pain

Front of Shoulder Pain

infraspinatus (90)

anterior deltoid (96)

scalenes (78)

supraspinatus (88)

pectoralis major (134)

pectoralis minor (139)

biceps (100)

latissimus dorsi (98)

coracobrachialis (99)

Back of Shoulder Pain

scalenes (78)

levator scapulae (60)

posterior deltoid (96)

supraspinatus (88)

teres major (98)

teres minor (92)

subscapularis (93)

serratus posterior superior (86)

latissimus dorsi (98)

triceps (101)

trapezius (55)

superficial spinal muscles (165)

Side of Shoulder Pain

infraspinatus (90)

scalenes (78)

lateral deltoid (96)

supraspinatus (88)

Front of Arm Pain

scalenes (78)

infraspinatus (90)

biceps (100)

brachialis (113)

triceps (101)

supraspinatus (88)

anterior deltoid (96)

subclavius (137)

Back of Arm Pain

scalenes (78)

triceps (101)

posterior deltoid (96)

subscapularis (93)

supraspinatus (88)

teres major (98)

teres minor (92)

latissimus dorsi (98)

serratus posterior superior (86)

coracobrachialis (99)

Upper Back Pain

scalenes (78)

levator scapulae (60)

supraspinatus (88)

trapezius (55)

rhomboids (84)

latissimus dorsi (98)

deep spinal muscles (162)

superficial spinal muscles (165)

serratus posterior superior (86)

infraspinatus (90)

serratus anterior (141)

Trigger Point Guide:
Shoulder, Upper Back, and Upper Arm Pain

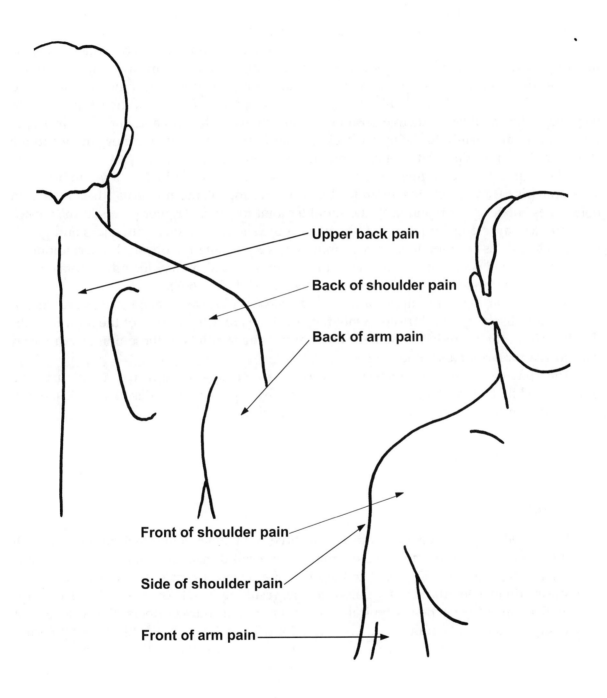

Upper back pain

Back of shoulder pain

Back of arm pain

Front of shoulder pain

Side of shoulder pain

Front of arm pain

Shoulder, Upper Back, and Upper Arm Pain

Muscles whose trigger points cause shoulder, upper arm, and upper back pain can be divided into five groups: scalenes, shoulder blade suspension muscles, rotator cuff muscles, upper arm muscles, and spinal muscles.

Although the scalenes are neck muscles, their trigger points cause a surprising amount of pain in the upper back, shoulder, and upper arm. Scalene trigger points also contribute significantly to pain and other symptoms in the forearm and hand. The scalenes are so important that they should always come first in troubleshooting pain in all these areas.

The shoulder blade suspension muscles are the rhomboids, levator scapulae, and trapezius. They suspend the shoulder blade from the spinal column and their function is to help move the shoulder blade into position for all actions of the arm and hand. Their trigger points send pain mainly to the upper back and neck, referring only a minor amount to the shoulder. The trapezius and levator scapulae are discussed in chapter 4.

The four rotator cuff muscles are the supraspinatus, infraspinatus, teres minor, and subscapularis. They attach the shoulder blade to the top of the humerus, the upper arm bone. They rotate the arm and keep the shoulder joint together. Trigger points in the rotator cuff muscles cause a major portion of the pain in the shoulder, along with clicks and grinding noises and loss of mobility. They're indirectly responsible for physical deterioration of the shoulder joint and can predispose it to serious physical injury, including rotator cuff tears and dislocation (Travell and Simons 1999, 538–571, 596–607).

Muscles that move the upper arm include the deltoids, teres major, latissimus dorsi, coracobrachialis, biceps, and triceps. Only the last three are actually part of the arm. In addition to pain in the shoulder, back, and upper arm, trigger points in these muscles can send pain to the forearm, hand, and fingers.

The spinal muscles interconnect the vertebrae and have no direct connection to the shoulder. While they're a common source of upper back pain, they're discussed in chapter 8 along with similar muscles of the mid and low back.

Scalenes

The *scalenes* (SKAY-leenz) are a group of three, sometimes four, small muscles in each side of the neck. The word *scalene* comes from a Greek word meaning "uneven." The scalene muscles are all of different lengths, like the sides of a scalene triangle. In addition, each scalene muscle divides to attach to several vertebrae, resulting in sets of muscle fibers of varying lengths. Since trigger points typically occur midway in muscle fibers, the scalenes can have many trigger points in many different locations. The following case histories are a sampling of the broad diversity of problems that can originate in the scalene muscles. In each case, self-applied trigger point massage solved the problem.

Betsy, age thirty-two, had worked for the post office until someone rear-ended the vehicle she was driving. It was only a minor accident, but it left her with periodic disabling spasms in the right side of her neck. Almost any little strain would set it off. When she had a flare-up, she typically needed several days to recover. In the meantime, she was unable to work.

Hong Sun, age thirty-one, a ballet dancer, complained of a constant ache in his upper back at the inner edge of his left shoulder blade. It felt good to reach over his shoulder and massage the place with his fingers, but it didn't stop the pain. He had had the pain for several years.

Amy, age seventeen, had been a serious student of the cello but she'd had to quit playing because of weakness and numbness in her shoulders, arms, and hands. Her parents believed the problem might be related to an accident in the swimming pool that had strained her neck. Thousands of dollars worth of medical tests had turned up nothing.

Gerhardt, age fifty-six, had suffered shooting pains in his left shoulder and upper arm ever since taking a fall on the ice a year and a half earlier. The pain increased when he carried or tried to lift anything. Physical therapy made the pain worse.

Connie, forty-nine, a potter, had pain in her shoulder and all down her right arm. It was always worse in the morning and often awakened her in the night. Her forearm and hand were vaguely numb most of the time and the hand often felt swollen. She was concerned that she wasn't going to be able to continue her work and support herself if the trouble got any worse.

Symptoms

Trigger points in the scalenes cause an impressively wide distribution of pain, numbness, and other abnormal sensations in the chest, upper back, shoulder, arm, and hand (Figures 5.1, 5.2, and 5.3). Pain may occasionally occur in the back of the neck (not shown). Any of the trigger points in the scalene muscles can cause symptoms in any part of the referral areas, though certain trigger points may favor certain areas. Trigger points low in the middle and posterior scalenes, for instance, are more often the ones that cause chest pain. Trigger points high in the middle and anterior scalenes are more often the cause of pain in the upper arm and shoulder.

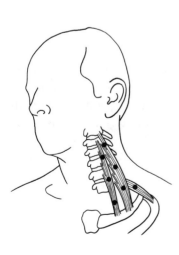

Figure 5.1 Scalene trigger points

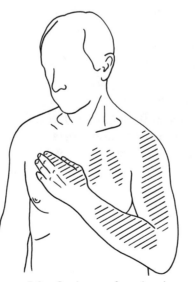

Figure 5.2 Scalene referred pain pattern, front view

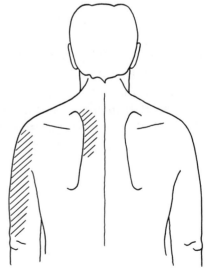

Figure 5.3 Scalene referred pain pattern, back view

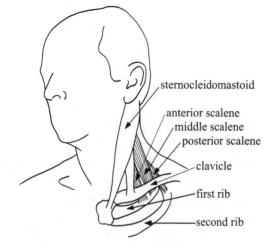

Figure 5.4   Location of anterior, middle, and posterior scalene muscles behind the sternocleidomastoid

The scalenes are rarely suspected as the source of the trouble because they're almost entirely hidden by the sternocleidomastoid muscles (Figure 5.4). Pain is hardly ever felt in the scalenes themselves, but scalene trigger points can be the primary source of pain in their referral areas. Unsuspected scalene trigger points are often the critical element in the failure of conventional therapies. Satellite trigger points are likely to be created in scalene referral areas, which make scalene trigger points quite frequently the ultimate source of pain in the chest, upper back, shoulder, arm, and hand (1999, 514–525; Lindgren, Manninen, and Rytkonen 1996, 254–256).

Symptoms created by the scalenes are easily misdiagnosed. Upper back pain evoked by scalene trigger points is almost always wrongly blamed on the rhomboid muscles. Restlessness in the neck and shoulder, a classic sign of scalene trigger points, is written off as a nervous tic. Pain referred from the scalenes to the chest is mistaken for angina. Pain sent to the shoulder by the scalenes is almost universally mislabeled bursitis or tendinitis. Scalene-referred pain down the front and back of the upper arm is mistakenly treated as muscle strain. The pattern of scalene referral in the shoulder, arm, and hand may make a neurologist infer that a degenerated vertebra or collapsed disk is causing compression of a cervical nerve root (1999, 509–511; Long 1956, 22–28).

When trigger points shorten the scalene muscles, they tend to keep the first rib pulled up against the collarbone, squeezing the blood vessels and nerves that pass through the area on their way to the arm. Termed *neurovascular entrapment,* this impeded blood flow and disturbance of nerve impulses causes pain, swelling, numbness, tingling, and burning in the arm and hand. The collection of symptoms caused by this compression of the nerves and vessels is properly termed *thoracic outlet syndrome,* although it is very often incorrectly diagnosed as carpal tunnel syndrome. Scalene-induced weakness in the forearms and hands that makes you unexpectedly drop things is likely to be ascribed to a neurological defect. Unexplained "phantom pain" in an amputated arm or hand can actually be coming from scalene trigger points (1999, 505; Sherman 1980, 232–244).

When treatment fails to affect symptoms created by scalene trigger points, you may be told it's all in your head. This "diagnosis" is especially apt to be given when the unremitting discomfort from the scalenes makes you sleepless, irritable, and depressed. Given that all these effects occur so far from their source and are so variable, it's no wonder that their cause is misunderstood. Fortunately, once you do understand that all these things can be coming from the scalene muscles in your neck, the solution is remarkably simple and quick (1999, 504–525).

Causes

The scalene muscles attach to the sides of your neck vertebrae and to your top two ribs. Although the scalenes help stabilize and flex the neck, their main job is to raise the upper two ribs on each side when you inhale. They're active to some degree in every inhalation and they work extremely hard when your breathing is labored during vigorous activity.

Habitually breathing with the chest instead of with the diaphragm severely taxes the scalene muscles. Simple nervous hyperventilation stresses them too. People who are prone to emotional tension should expect to find terrible trigger points in their scalene muscles. The struggle for breath in people who suffer from asthma or emphysema can promote scalene trigger points, as can a bad cough from pneumonia, bronchitis, allergies or a common cold. Playing a wind instrument commonly fosters scalene trouble (1999, 510–511).

Many ordinary activities cause scalene trouble when overdone to the point of strain. Working for long hours with the arms out in front of the body can be very stressful for them. Pulling, lifting, and carrying heavy loads can be bad. Carrying a heavy backpack is especially rough for the scalenes and for several other muscles not designed for mule duty, such as the trapezius, pectoralis minor, and sternocleidomastoid. The scalenes are among the muscles most abused in sports activities. They are also very likely to initiate and perpetuate secondary trigger points in other muscles (1999, 510–511).

You can expect the violent movement of the head during a fall or an auto accident to bring about trigger points in the scalenes. Both the scalenes and the sternocleidomastoids are severely affected by whiplash and are easily overlooked in the treatment of pain from this type of injury. Apparent neurological symptoms in the upper back, shoulders, arms, and hands that mysteriously persist after an auto accident can often be traced to the scalenes (1999, 511).

Scalene muscles help manage the weight of the head. Anything that creates an imbalance puts an additional burden on them. For this reason, it's wise to be aware of posture that may be holding the head off center. Slouching or habitually carrying your head forward is sure to keep trigger points going in these muscles (1999, 510–511).

Treatment

Success in finding and dealing with the scalenes depends on your understanding of their relationship to the sternocleidomastoid muscle (Figure 5.4). The *anterior scalene*, the front-most scalene muscle, lies between the sternocleidomastoid and the neck vertebrae and is almost completely hidden. The *middle scalene* is behind the anterior scalene, more on the side of the neck, with its lower half free of the sternocleidomastoid. The *posterior scalene* lies almost horizontally behind the middle scalene in the soft triangular depression just above the collarbone and below the front edge of the trapezius. A fourth scalene muscle, the vertically oriented *scalenus minimus*, is found behind the anterior scalene. Not everyone has a scalenus minimus; it's a normal human variation.

The scalenes cling closely to the neck and feel much firmer than the soft, loose sternocleidomastoids. When massaging the scalenes, you will be pressing them against the bony vertebrae underneath.

To massage the anterior scalene, which is the chief troublemaker, you have to get your fingers between the neck vertebrae and the sternocleidomastoid. To do this, first grip the sternocleidomastoid between your fingers and thumb as if you were going to massage it. Then let go with your thumb and with your fingers pull the entire sternocleidomastoid toward the windpipe. The idea is to get your fingertips as far around in front of the vertebral column as you can, with the sternocleidomastoid pulled out of the way. In this position, you

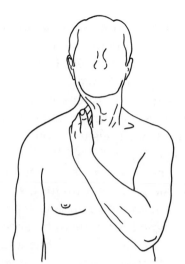

Figure 5.5   Anterior scalene massage. Pull the sterno-cleidomastoid out of the way, firmly toward the windpipe.

can press the anterior scalene against the vertebral column with the tips of your fingers (Figure 5.5).

This will not hurt unless you encounter a trigger point, in which case it will be extremely painful. Pressure on a scalene trigger point evokes a spooky kind of pain that will make you duck and cringe: it can feel like you're pressing on a nerve. At the same time, you may feel the referred pain or other symptom being reproduced or accentuated. This can be a very convincing demonstration of the reality of referred myofascial pain.

The massage stroke is executed by pressing with your fingertips as you push them across the muscle toward the side of the neck. The skin of the neck should move with the fingers. At the end of the stroke, which will be only an inch long, release the pressure, reset your fingers where you began the stroke and repeat. This procedure should be carried out all along the back edge of the sternocleidomastoid, from up under your ear clear down to the collarbone. You'll find some of your worst scalene trigger points behind the sternocleidomastoid where it attaches to the collarbone (Figure 5.6). You may even find a trigger point hiding down behind the collarbone at that spot.

To massage the middle scalene, use this same stroke on the side of the neck. Six strokes on each scalene trigger point are enough for one session. Come back to them six or eight times during the day. You may find as many as five spots of exquisite tenderness in your scalenes.

To massage the posterior scalene, push your middle finger under the front edge of the trapezius muscle near where it attaches to the collarbone (Figure 5.7). Exert downward pressure and drag your finger toward your throat parallel to the collarbone. This stroke is also about an inch long and should move the skin with it. The boniness you feel under your finger as you do this stroke is the top surface of your first rib. Don't neglect the posterior scalene. It can have trigger points when the other scalene muscles don't.

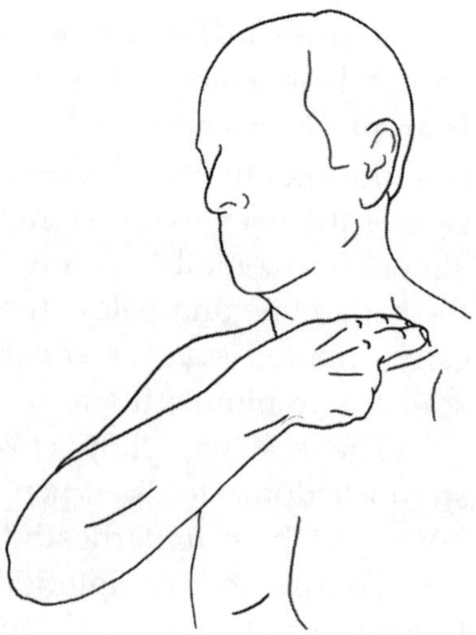

To massage the scalenes effectively and without damaging the skin, the fingernails must be cut and filed to the quick. Your scalenes will be among the most difficult muscles to understand, locate, and treat, but any success you have with them will be well worth the effort. The scalenes are likely to be involved in any myofascial pain problem in the upper body.

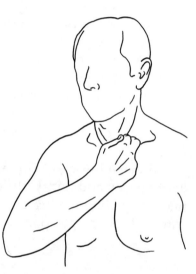

Figure 5.6   Scalene massage behind the sternocleidomastoid attachment to the collarbone

Figure 5.7   Posterior scalene massage pressing down where the trapezius attaches to the collarbone

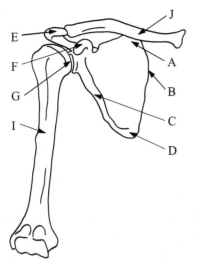

Figure 5.8   Anatomy of the right shoulder (front)

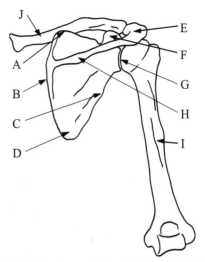

Figure 5.9   Anatomy of the right shoulder (back)

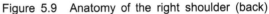

The Shoulder Blade

Seventeen muscles attach to each of your shoulder blades. Finding these muscles for massage is made much easier if you have a clear idea of what a shoulder blade looks like and can find its bony landmarks (Figures 5.8 and 5.9). The following is the key to both illustrations:

A. Superior angle of the shoulder blade

B. Medial border of the shoulder blade

C. Lateral border of the shoulder blade

D. Inferior angle of the shoulder blade

E. Acromion

F. Coracoid process

G. Head of the humerus and the glenoid cavity (the ball and socket)

H. Scapular spine (the spine of the shoulder blade)

I. Humerus (upper arm bone)

J. Clavicle (collarbone)

The *acromion* (E) is the flat shelf of bone at the point of the shoulder. The word *acromion* is a combination of two Greek roots that literally means "tip of shoulder." The *coracoid process* (F) is like a bony bent finger that sticks through the shoulder and comes out in front just below the collarbone. The end of it feels like a marble nestled in the front of the shoulder beside the head of the humerus. *Coracoid* means "curved like a raven's beak."

The most touchable part of the shoulder blade is the *scapular spine* (H). Looking over one shoulder in the mirror, you'll be able to see the scapular spine behind each shoulder if you're slender. Even if you're heavy, you should still see an angular bulge behind the

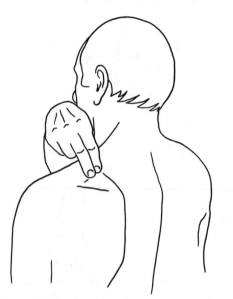

Figure 5.10 Locating the superior angle of the shoulder blade

shoulder that suggests the presence of this bony ridge beneath the skin. See if you can find and trace it with your fingers.

Just above the scapular spine, feel for the bony *superior angle* (A) of the shoulder blade (Figure 5.10). This is an important landmark for locating the supraspinatus, one of the rotator cuff muscles. Under your arm at the edge of your back, you should be able to feel the *lateral border* (C) of the shoulder blade. Trace it down to the lowest point of the shoulder blade, the *inferior angle* (D). If your range of motion isn't hampered by shoulder pain, try reaching all the way across to touch the inner edge of the shoulder blade, the *medial border* (B). Otherwise, try to touch the upper part of the medial border by reaching over your shoulder.

Take some time to learn the terms for the different parts of the shoulder blade. It will aid your comprehension of the discussion of the individual muscles and, ultimately, your ability to successfully treat your trigger points. Sooner or later, you will want to talk to other people about these things, and it helps to know the right words instead of having to point and grunt.

Upper Back Muscles

Putting muscles into logical groups is easy if you're viewing the question anatomically. All you have to do is decide the physical boundaries. When you try to group muscles according to the pain caused by their trigger points, it's like shuffling a deck of cards. Everything changes. This is why certain upper back muscles have ended up in other chapters in this book.

The trapezius and levator scapulae, though located in the upper back, are discussed in chapter 4 because their trigger points send pain mainly to the head and neck. The rotator cuff muscles are located in the upper back, covering both sides of the shoulder blade, but are considered as shoulder muscles because their trigger points send pain mainly to the shoulder. The upper spinal muscles, which do cause pain in the upper back, have been left to the chapter on the lower back and buttocks, because they're simply a continuation of the muscles in those parts of the body. Only three muscles fall into no other group but the upper back. They are the major and minor rhomboids and the serratus posterior superior.

Rhomboids

The *rhomboid* (RAHM-boid) muscles attach to several vertebrae of the upper back and to the inner edge of the shoulder blade. The minor rhomboid is higher and somewhat separate from the major rhomboid, but the two are indistinguishable by touch. The function of the rhomboids is to move the shoulder blade toward the spine, to help raise the shoulder blade, and to hold the shoulder blade still when needed, as a solid support for the operations of the arm and hand.

Trigger points in the rhomboids cause an aching kind of pain along the inner edge of the shoulder blade, which becomes more noticeable at rest (Figure 5.11). A significant amount of pain at this site may also be coming from the serratus posterior superior muscle, which lies beneath the rhomboids, and from the middle trapezius covering them. There may be trigger points in all three layers. Other muscles that send pain to the inner edge of the shoulder blade include the scalenes, infraspinatus, latissimus dorsi, serratus anterior, and levator scapulae. The spinal muscles (discussed in chapter 8) cause pain at this same level but nearer the spine.

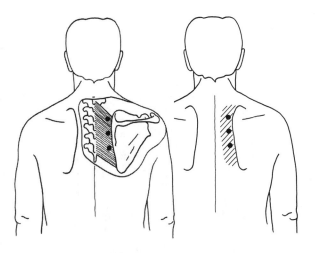

Figure 5.11   Rhomboid trigger points and referred pain pattern

It's important to check for trigger points in your scalenes before going to the trouble of treating all these other muscles. The scalenes are among the most common sources of pain along the inner edge of the shoulder blade. Without first taking care of the scalenes, massage applied to the rhomboids or to any of the others listed here, though it may feel good, can be a complete waste of time. A symptom that may help verify rhomboid involvement in your pain is the sound of snapping or crunching in them during shoulder movement (1999, 616).

To avoid overusing the rhomboids, it's wise to moderate any activity that requires continuously or repeatedly raising the shoulders. The unnatural military posture of keeping the shoulders pulled back requires that the rhomboids remain continuously contracted. Throwing a ball or rowing a boat can exhaust the rhomboids. Habitual tension that keeps the shoulders up stimulates formation of trigger points in many muscles, including the rhomboids. If you would like to learn how to deal more effectively with habitual muscle tension, see chapter 12.

A cause of trouble in the rhomboids that might never occur to you is tight pectoral muscles. Trigger points keep the pectoral muscles shortened, which causes them to pull the shoulder blade forward. The rhomboids must then tighten in response to try to keep the shoulder blade in place. The rhomboids are easily stretched to their maximum length while contracting to counter the pull of the pectoral muscles. This is an exhausting kind of muscle work called *eccentric contraction*, which is guaranteed to set up trigger points (1999, 613, 616).

The pull of tight pectorals causes your shoulder blades to stick out in back and gives you a round-shouldered, flat-chested posture. It's very difficult to correct your posture or to give relief to the rhomboids without first deactivating trigger points in the pectoral muscles. Attempts to stretch the rhomboids for the purpose of therapy when they're already stretched to maximum length by the pectoral muscles can strain them even further, irritating their trigger points and making the pain worse (1999, 618; Kendall, McCreary, and Provance 1993, 282–283).

Rhomboid massage can be applied easily and efficiently with the Thera Cane, although a tennis ball against a wall is a friendlier tool. Use a lacrosse ball for greater pressure and even more control. Long-term, chronic knots in the rhomboids will give the ball a bumpy ride.

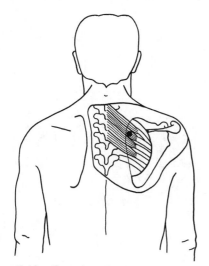

Figure 5.12   Sample serratus posterior superior trigger point

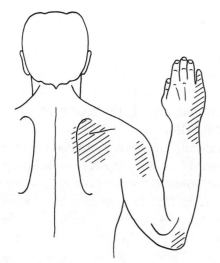

Figure 5.13   Serratus posterior superior referred pain pattern

Serratus Posterior Superior

Although the *serratus* (seh-RAY-tus) *posterior superior* muscles attach to the spine like the rhomboids and run in the same direction, they don't attach to the shoulder blade. Instead, they go underneath the shoulder blade to connect with several upper ribs (Figure 5.12). The serratus posterior superior muscles raise the ribs during inhalation to help fill the lungs. The word *serratus* means "saw-toothed," which relates to its appearance, sequentially attached to several ribs. The word *superior* means that it is the highest of the serratus muscles.

The pain pattern of the serratus posterior superior is very broad (Figure 5.13) and overlaps the patterns of a great number of other muscles. (See the Trigger Point Guides in chapters 5 and 6.) A deep ache under the shoulder blade is the most characteristic symptom. Pain may also be felt in the back of the shoulder, the point of the elbow, and the little finger side of the wrist and hand. Pain in the little finger is a signature of serratus posterior superior trigger points. The referral pattern in the hand is sometimes experienced as numbness. Occasionally, pain may occur over the back of the upper arm and forearm and even in the pectoral area (not shown) (1999, 900–901).

Strenuous breathing during sports activity has the potential for creating trigger points in the serratus posterior superior muscles. Nervous hyper- ventilation or habitual chest breathing can overwork them. Especially taxing for them is the struggle for breath in respiratory illnesses such as asthma, bronchitis, pneumonia, emphysema, and smoker's cough (1999, 902).

Because the serratus posterior superior is largely hidden by the shoulder blade, its trigger points are normally inaccessible. The big bite taken out of the shoulder blade in Figure 5.12 illustrates this. Luckily, the shoulder blade can be moved out of the way by simply reaching the hand across to the opposite shoulder while applying massage. This is accomplished by working with the Thera Cane or Backnobber over the opposite shoulder with the hand in the bow (Figure 5.14). The ball on the wall works well, provided the arm is held across the body to move the shoulder blade aside.

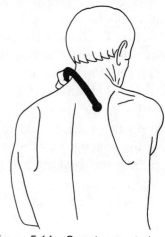

Figure 5.14   Serratus posterior superior and rhomboid massage with Thera Cane or Backnobber (hand at opposite shoulder)

Shoulder Muscles

Up to twenty muscles are involved in operating the shoulder and all of them are vulnerable to strain, because the shoulder is such a hardworking part of the body. Shoulder trouble takes a predictable course. When a shoulder muscle is weakened and made dysfunctional by trigger points, associated muscles have to take up the slack. Under the extra burden, they fall like dominoes, each acquiring trigger points in turn, until every muscle in the region has joined the party.

Simple chores become impossible. You can no longer scratch your back, comb your hair, or reach up to get the cereal off the shelf. If you need two hands for something, you have to use your good arm to lift your bad one. You may not even be able to reach across your body to fasten your seat belt. Constant pain disturbs your sleep and makes your job miserable. In its fully developed state, shoulder trouble can persist for months, and sometimes for years (1999, 604–606; Bonica and Sola 1990, 951).

Diagnosis for this condition usually focuses on the joint: arthritis, bursitis, tendinitis, rotator cuff injury, adhesive capsulitis, and so on. Another rationale for shoulder pain is the presumed deterioration of joint cartilage, which X-rays often seem to confirm. Even with such "proof," it can be a mistake to automatically assume that the trouble is in the shoulder joint. Trigger points in nearby muscles are often the real source of pain. When trigger point therapy takes the pain away, this can be hard to dispute (1999, 544–546, 604–605).

Shoulder trouble can be extremely frustrating when therapists don't understand shoulders.

Jeanie, age forty-five, had pain in both shoulders after trying to catch herself during a fall on the stairs where she worked. Doctors had offered only two options: cortisone shots or exploratory surgery, both of which she declined. She went through two ineffective courses of physical therapy and then settled into getting professional massage once a month. The "feel good" massage was relaxing but did little to relieve her chronic shoulder pain. She lived with her shoulder trouble for the next fifteen years.

In a class on the self-treatment of pain, Jeanie discovered trigger points in all of her rotator cuff muscles. The massage techniques she learned the first night in class brought more relief of her shoulder pain than she'd had from any previous treatment. She had spent thousands of dollars on therapy. She wondered why these trigger points had never been found.

Trigger points in the four rotator cuff muscles are the most frequent cause of shoulder pain, loss of upper arm motion, and clicking or catching in the joint. When you're able to manage these trigger points yourself, you may be able to avoid forced manipulation of the shoulder, steroid injections, and harsh physical therapy. Exercise and stretch, the most common form of physical therapy for shoulder problems, often yields disappointing results when the rotator cuff muscles are stiff and resistant. The safest and most direct and effective therapy for shoulder pain is specific trigger point massage of these muscles. Even when surgery must be done to correct a genuine structural problem, massage of the trigger points in the rotator cuff muscles is vital for eliminating residual pain (1999, 141–142, 542, 556, 599; Danneskiold-Samoe, Christiansen, and Andersen 1983, 17–20).

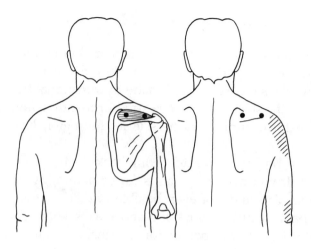

Figure 5.15   Supraspinatus trigger points and referred pain pattern

Supraspinatus

The *supraspinatus* (soo-prah-spih-NAH-tus) is buried in a pocket in the top of the shoulder blade above the scapular spine (Figure 5.15). The word *supraspinatus* means "above the spine." At its outer end, the muscle passes under the acromion and crosses over to attach to the outer side of the top of the head of the humerus. This attachment gives the supraspinatus great leverage for helping raise the arm. It also allows the muscle to help the other rotators hold the joint together.

The supraspinatus is not the easiest muscle to massage and it's not the easiest to find. Many massage therapists, even quite good ones, don't even try. Nevertheless, this muscle is too important a part of common shoulder problems to ignore. The supraspinatus can be self-treated if you understand it well enough and are determined to take it on.

Supraspinatus trigger points can be at the heart of an otherwise unexplainable problem.

Erik, age fifty-five, had had a bad fall while skiing. Eighteen months later, he still felt the effects in the outside of his left shoulder and in his left elbow. He couldn't raise his arm without the most excruciating pain. Sometimes it hurt just to walk across the room with his arm hanging at his side. Playing the piano, something he had always done on weekends for extra income, had become an unpleasant ordeal. After many tests, Erik's doctor still wasn't sure what was wrong.

Pressure applied to an extremely tender spot in the supraspinatus muscle of Erik's left shoulder blade reproduced the pain in his elbow and shoulder. He was shown how to massage the muscle himself. Within three weeks, by his own efforts—after a year and a half of misery—his pain was finally gone.

Symptoms

Pain from supraspinatus trigger points is felt primarily as a deep ache in the outer side of the shoulder (Figure 5.15). Occasionally, pain spreads to the outer side of the upper arm and forearm and into the wrist (not shown). It's exceedingly painful even to start to raise your arm. Putting your arm overhead is next to impossible. It becomes a problem to wash or comb your hair. These difficulties and the pain causing them are frequently misdiagnosed as bursitis (1999, 538; Bonica and Sola 1990, 947–958).

Supraspinatus trigger points are to blame for the clicking or popping that is sometimes felt or heard in the shoulder joint. The muscle is kept so tight that the head of the humerus is prevented from gliding smoothly in its socket. The popping stops when the trigger points are deactivated (1999, 542-543).

The supraspinatus is also one of many sources of the pain in the outer elbow known as "tennis elbow." Although commonly given such catchall diagnoses as arthritis, tendinitis, or inflammation, tennis elbow is often just referred pain from myofascial trigger points that can be treated very effectively with massage. Trigger points in the triceps or one of the forearm muscles are the most usual cause of tennis elbow. Supraspinatus trigger points, being so far away and a less frequent cause, are generally overlooked as a source of this common pain (1999, 538–546).

Causes

The supraspinatus is commonly overloaded during a onetime incident of extreme exertion, such as moving a large couch or carrying heavy weight like boxes or suitcases. The supraspinatus muscles have to work extraordinarily hard to keep the shoulder joints from pulling apart, especially when you carry something like a suitcase with your arm hanging straight down. Repetitive strain such as working with the arms overhead for long periods of time or typing at a computer keyboard with no elbow support can also exhaust supraspinatus muscles. The simple act of swinging your arms while walking can add an intolerable degree of strain on the supraspinatus when it's already in trouble. A fall can also initiate supraspinatus trigger points. So can a large, strong, eager dog who can't be broken of pulling on the leash (1999, 542; Hagberg 1981, 111–121).

Treatment

You will find the supraspinatus muscle at the top of the shoulder blade, immediately behind the thick roll of the trapezius muscle that lies on top of the shoulder. Place your fingers between the scapular spine and the superior angle of the shoulder blade (Figure 5.10 shows how to find the superior angle). If your hand is in the right place, the blunt ends of your fingers will be contacting the top edge of the scapular spine and the heel of your hand will be resting on your collarbone. To verify that you're touching the supraspinatus, begin to raise your arm forward and a little to the side. Just as your arm starts to move, you should feel the muscle contract and bulge up under your fingers.

Trigger points occur in two places in the supraspinatus (Figure 5.15). One is in the belly of the muscle, just below the superior angle of the shoulder blade. The other is an inch or two further out, near where the muscle dives under the acromion, the bony point of the shoulder. The trigger point is right in the bony V formed by the scapular spine and the collarbone that come together at this spot.

The sensitivity of the fingers is helpful for locating trigger points in the supraspinatus, but massage with the fingers is very hard to sustain. It's also difficult to get the pressure needed to go deep enough, because the supraspinatus can be quite thick. The Thera Cane is a better tool, at least as a finger saver, though the knob may be a little large for use in this narrow spot on children and smaller adults (Figure 5.16). It helps to first guide the knob carefully into place with your fingers, feeling for the superior angle of the shoulder blade and the scapular spine. The smaller knob on one end of the Backnobber probably makes it the better tool for this job. With either tool, the opposite hand in the bow gives you the greatest leverage for digging into this deeply situated muscle.

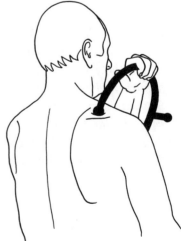

Figure 5.16 Supraspinatus massage with the Thera Cane (opposite hand in the bow)

It's conceivable that you'll need some help in dealing with the supraspinatus. If so, a partner standing behind you (with you seated) can get to the supraspinatus with paired thumbs, supported fingers, or a Knobble. If you go to a massage therapist, you might ask him or her to try standing at the head of the table and using paired thumbs, with you facedown. In this position, it's very easy to use deep stroking massage on the entire length of the supraspinatus along the scapular spine. The trick is to use the body weight to lean in and bury the thumbs in the muscle. This technique is illustrated in Figure 11.12.

Pain in the outer shoulder will tempt you to expend energy massaging the deltoid muscle. Deltoid massage is easy, feels great, and may even do some good, but it won't fix your shoulder pain if it's coming from the supraspinatus.

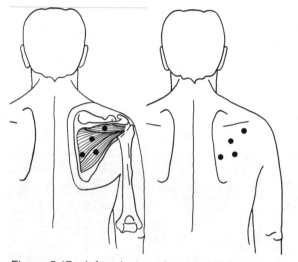

Figure 5.17   Infraspinatus trigger points

Infraspinatus

The *infraspinatus* (in-frah-spih-NAH-tus) covers almost all of the shoulder blade below the scapular spine (Figure 5.17). The word *infraspinatus* means "below the spine." At its outer end, the infraspinatus attaches to the back of the head of the humerus, giving it the ability to rotate the arm outward, as when you pull your arm back to throw a ball or prepare to make a forehand stroke with a tennis racket. Without outward rotation, the arm can't be raised above the level of the shoulder. The infraspinatus is also a strong participant in keeping the head of the humerus in its socket.

The infraspinatus is one of the most frequently afflicted muscles of the body. It's capable of ending an athletic career, as illustrated by Kim's story.

She was a thirty-two-year-old professional tennis coach who had lived with pain in both shoulders ever since she began playing tennis as a child. Diagnosed with rotator cuff tendinitis, Kim had had numerous steroid injections and was going for physical therapy almost weekly. Despite the treatments, pain kept her from playing much of the time. She was very concerned that several of her young players were developing shoulder pain very similar to her own. "I make them play through the pain just like we were told to do at their age," she said. "I'm afraid they'll end up as tennis cripples like me, but I don't know what else to do. They want to play so badly."

After a massage therapist showed Kim how to self-treat her shoulder with a tennis ball against a wall, she became free of shoulder pain for the first time since the age of fourteen. She felt that the best part about the new trick was that she could pass it on to her students.

Symptoms

Paradoxically, though located *behind* the shoulder, infraspinatus trigger points are the most common source of pain in the *front* of the shoulder (Figure 5.18). This pain usually feels like it's deep in the joint and may travel some distance down the biceps. Extreme tenderness in the anterior deltoid and the bicipital groove in the head of the humerus can lead to an erroneous diagnosis of bicipital tendinitis. Pain can also shoot down the outer side of the shoulder. Occasionally, pain is referred to the back of the neck, the inner border of the shoulder blade, all the way down the upper arm and forearm, and into the entire thumb side of the hand. When pain is referred to the forearm, it tends to promote formation of satellite trigger points in the hand and finger extensors, compounding pain and other

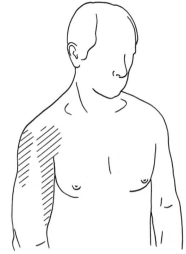

Figure 5.18   Infraspinatus referred pain pattern

symptoms in the hand. Many hours can be wasted rubbing all these places when you don't realize that the problem may be in the infraspinatus (1999, 552–554; Pace 1975, 107–113).

Other symptoms of infraspinatus trigger points include weakness and stiffness in the shoulder and arm, which can cause your shoulder and arm to tire easily. Both inward and outward rotation of the arm is restricted, making it difficult to move the arm in any direction. Since arm rotation is necessary for reaching behind you, it becomes impossible to reach up behind your back. A woman can't fasten or unfasten her brassiere. You struggle getting your jacket on or off. Lying on the afflicted shoulder is painful. Lying on the opposite side is painful as well, because the weight of the afflicted arm pulls on the infraspinatus (1999, 556; Sola and Williams 1956, 91–95).

Dysfunction of the infraspinatus typically causes the other rotators to tighten up in an effort to compensate, which tends to overload them too. All four rotators end up with trigger points and soon you're unable to move the arm at all. The rigidity of the shoulder imposed by the stiffness of the muscles can give your doctor the idea that you have adhesions in the joint, or adhesive capsulitis, which can lead to a recommendation for forced manipulation under anesthesia. Nevertheless, this condition, commonly called a "frozen shoulder," can often be treated very successfully with trigger point massage of the rotator cuff muscles (1999, 552–558).

Causes

Working at a job that requires keeping the arms overhead or out in front for long hours is abusive to the infraspinatus muscles, since they have to stay contracted to keep the arms up. Repeatedly reaching back in work or play can leave the infraspinatus in a shortened state and full of trigger points. Accidents, falls, and many kinds of sports activity can overload the infraspinatus. Driving a car with the hands on the top of the wheel puts continuous strain on both the infraspinatus and the supraspinatus, since they work together to keep the arms up (1999, 556; Baker 1986, 35–44).

For the same reason, working at a computer keyboard without elbow support easily exhausts both muscles. Keeping your hand on the mouse out to one side can be the cause of your chronic shoulder pain on that side, since this position requires nearly maximum outward rotation of the arm and continuous contraction of the infraspinatus. Study your activities to

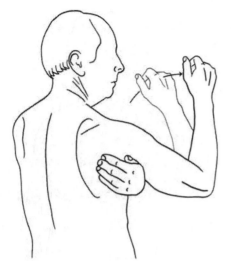

Figure 5.19 Arrow shows outward rotation for locating infraspinatus with isolated contraction

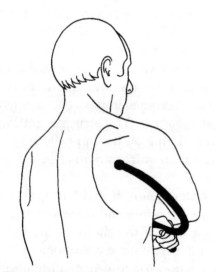

Figure 5.20 Infraspinatus massage with Thera Cane. Place a ball on the same spot for massage against wall.

discover other ways an infraspinatus muscle may be involved in a habitual overload or repetitive strain, related to its function in outward rotation of the arm. As an example, it might be worth the trouble to learn to use the mouse with your left hand. The right infraspinatus is subject to more strain than the left since the right hand has to reach farther to the side because the right side of the conventional keyboard has so many extra keys.

Treatment

The infraspinatus, being on the outside of the shoulder blade, is an easy muscle to treat with self-applied massage. Confirm its location by feeling it contract and bulge as you put the arm into outward rotation (Figure 5.19). The Thera Cane works well for infraspinatus massage , as does the Backnobber (Figure 5.20). You may like a ball against the wall even better. When you exert pressure on infraspinatus trigger points, the pain reaction takes awhile to wake up, so don't conclude too quickly that you have no problem there. It may take several seconds of deep massage before you feel the characteristic exquisite tenderness. Six to twelve massage strokes constitute a treatment, but come back to it several times a day.

The infraspinatus is an especially sneaky muscle. You'll rarely experience pain in the infraspinatus itself. You'll find yourself rubbing away at the front or outer side of your shoulder, forgetting that infraspinatus trigger points are almost always the cause of pain felt there. You won't know the infraspinatus is the culprit until you press on it.

Be wary of exercising and stretching the infraspinatus or any of the other shoulder muscles until the trigger points have been taken care of. Trigger points in the infraspinatus are unusually irritable, making stretching counterproductive as therapy. A therapist may insist on the need for exercising the shoulder, but the weakness and stiffness that seem to be the problem are actually part of the protection the trigger points are trying to provide. Muscle strength comes back quickly when trigger points are deactivated. Exercise and stretching are helpful for getting your range of motion back, but not until the trigger points are gone.

Teres Minor

The *teres* (TEH-reez) *minor* muscle lies right below the infraspinatus on the shoulder blade and has a similar attachment to the back of the head of the humerus (Figure 5.21). The teres minor helps the infraspinatus rotate the arm outward.

The pain pattern for the teres minor is very different from that of the infraspinatus; it refers primarily to a very confined spot on the back of the shoulder in the area of its attachment to the humerus. Pain from trigger points in the teres minor may not be noticed until after more oppressive problems with other shoulder muscles are dealt with.

Teres minor trigger points can also be the cause of a worrisome numbness or tingling in the fourth and fifth fingers, which occurs nearly as often as the pain at the back of the shoulder. Note that a comparable pattern of finger numbness can also come from trigger points in the pectoralis minor. Pain instead of numbness in these two fingers suggests latissimus dorsi trigger points (1999, 564, 572).

The place to find teres minor trigger points is right at the upper outer edge of the shoulder blade. Feel the

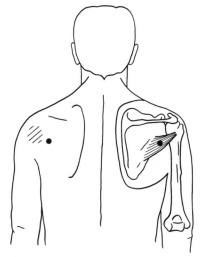

Figure 5.21 Sample teres minor trigger point and referred pain pattern

muscle bulge up at this spot as you rotate your arm outward, as you did with the infraspinatus (see Figure 5.19). Teres minor trigger points are only an inch or so away from those in the infraspinatus and can be massaged at the same time with the same techniques. A tennis ball against the wall is the perfect tool: roll it slowly back and forth across the teres minor against the wall.

If pain persists in the back of the shoulder after teres minor trigger points have been deactivated, consult this chapter's Trigger Point Guide for the many other muscles that refer pain to this same place. The subscapularis is a good bet, especially if you've already found trigger points in the other rotator cuff muscles.

Subscapularis

The *subscapularis* (sub-scap-yu-LEHR-us) is an exceptionally powerful muscle lining the underside of the shoulder blade (Figure 5.22). Visualize it sandwiched between the shoulder blade and the ribs. (In the illustration, the ribs have been removed and you're looking through the body to the back.) The muscle's attachment to the head of the humerus allows it to rotate the arm inward. This attachment also enables the subscapularis to help keep the joint together and the head of the humerus centered in its socket.

You'd think that the subscapularis muscle would be unreachable and untreatable, buried as it is on the underside of the shoulder blade. Actually, it's surprisingly accessible if you go about it in the right way. This

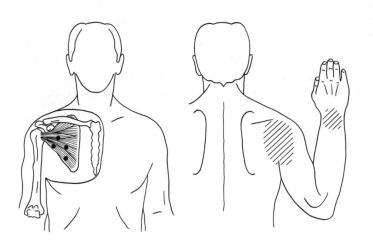

Figure 5.22 Subscapularis trigger points and referred pain pattern

is good news, because the subscapularis is often at the very heart of the problem with shoulder pain. With a frozen shoulder in particular, knowing how to treat subscapularis trigger points can be the key to recovery; without this knowledge, recovery can be a very long time in coming (1999, 599, 603–607; Cantu and Grodin 1992, 154–155; Voss, Ionta, and Myers 1985).

Bernie, age forty-eight, had endured pain in his left shoulder for several months. The problem had begun when he tripped and fell while picking up broken branches after a storm. The shoulder ached all the time and woke him repeatedly in the night. He'd stopped even trying to raise his arm and dreaded putting on his shirt in the morning. He hated the idea of going to the doctor, but the problem wasn't getting any better.

Bernie's wife gave him a gift certificate for a massage and to her great surprise he went. The therapist worked on an extremely painful place under his arm and then showed him how to massage the spot himself. His shoulder was better right away, which encouraged him to continue working on it on his own. When asked at work three months later how his shoulder was doing, he realized he'd had no pain in quite a while. To test it, he raised his arm all the way up. "I'd forgotten about it," he said. "I don't even think about it anymore."

Ruth's shoulder trouble came about in a very different way. At age sixty-seven, she had decided to pursue her lifelong dream of learning to play the banjo. But soon after her first lessons, she began having pain behind her left shoulder whenever she sat down to practice. It hurt just to stick her arm out to hold the neck of the instrument. Luckily, her teacher knew something about trigger points, having had problems of his own.

He explained that the position of the left hand when playing a banjo, guitar, or even a violin requires maximum outward rotation of the left arm. To permit this, the subscapularis muscle has to lengthen all the way, which can be a terrific strain if you try to practice too long and the muscle isn't strong and resilient. "And then you get trigger points," he told her. After he showed her how to do self-applied subscapularis massage, Ruth was able to continue playing her banjo, pain free, as long as she didn't overdo it.

Symptoms

The main symptom of subscapularis trigger points is severe pain deep in the back of the shoulder (Figure 5.22). An ache in the back of the wrist is almost always present and should be seen as a virtual signature of subscapularis trigger points. Sometimes the shoulder pain extends down the back of the upper arm (not shown). You may also have an extremely tender spot on the front of your shoulder where the troubled subscapularis has been continuously pulling and jerking on its attachment to the humerus (1999, 556, 600).

The pull of the four rotators must be in balance in order for the shoulder joint to operate smoothly and freely. A subscapularis muscle weakened by trigger points allows the supraspinatus to pull up on the head of the humerus unopposed, jamming it against the acromion. A clicking or popping noise when you move your shoulder indicates probable trigger points in the subscapularis or the supraspinatus, or both (1999, 545–546; Lippitt and Matsen 1998, 20–28).

Subscapularis trigger points also keep the muscle from lengthening, reducing the shoulder's range of motion and restricting rotation of the arm in either direction. This makes it difficult to reach above your head, across your body, or up behind your back. The disabling pain and stiffness caused by subscapularis trigger points are commonly mistaken for bursitis, arthritis, bicipital tendinitis, rotator cuff injury, and adhesive capsulitis (1999, 596–607).

Causes

A sudden unprepared overloading of the shoulder muscles, such as might occur during a fall, is especially likely to make trouble for the subscapularis. Your shoulders are more vulnerable to this kind of accident when you're an older person, overweight, or simply out of shape. Another common cause for the development of subscapularis trigger points is prolonged immobilization of the shoulder for healing of a broken arm. Stroke victims who have lost the use of an arm often develop subscapularis trigger points because of inactivity (1999, 599–600, 606).

Trigger points commonly develop in the subscapularis when you overexert yourself during exercise or sports activity without proper conditioning. Fitness enthusiasts, swimmers, tennis players, and ball throwers of all kinds are in special danger of abusing their subscapularis muscles. Pitchers who have to retire prematurely because of chronic shoulder pain might well be able to return to the mound if their subscapularis and other rotator muscles were given some trigger point therapy (1999, 599–600).

Treatment

Luckily, the most troublesome subscapularis trigger points occur near its accessible outer edge. They can be easily reached for massage if you position your arm in a way that will move the shoulder blade forward and around the side of the body. Figures 5.23 and 5.24 show how the fingers or thumb should be placed inside the edge of the shoulder blade. The raised arm in these two drawings is only for clarity in showing how to get to the muscle. For the actual work, the arm doesn't need to be raised this far, but it does need to be across the body as far as you can get it (Figure 5.25). Put your hand on your opposite shoulder if possible. This pulls the shoulder blade around the side of the body and exposes a good bit of its underside. With the arm across the body, you can massage the subscapularis muscle while sitting, standing, or lying down. You'll quickly discover that long fingernails will keep you from effectively self-treating your subscapularis muscles. Fingernails grow back. Make the sacrifice.

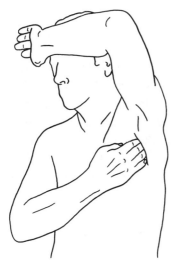

Figure 5.23 Position of the fingers for subscapularis massage. (The arm is up for clarity. Keep the arm down for massage.)

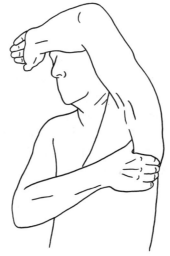

Figure 5.24 Position of the thumb for subscapularis massage. (The arm is up for clarity. Keep the arm down for massage.)

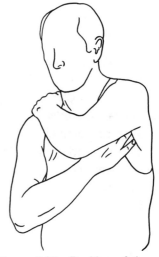

Figure 5.25 Position of the arms for subscapularis massage

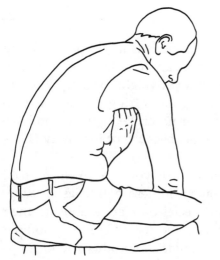

Figure 5.26 Subscapularis massage with arm hanging down between legs

Another technique for gaining maximum access to the subscapularis is to sit with the bad arm hanging down between your legs (Figure 5.26). This position relaxes the shoulder muscles and brings even more of the shoulder blade around the body. With the flats of your fingers firmly against your ribs, push deep into the slot between the ribs and the roll of muscle that defines the back of the armpit. If your hand and fingers are tight against your ribs, the blunt ends of the fingers will bump right into the subscapularis. Try your thumb for this technique; you may like it better. This technique was the primary therapy the author used to treat his own frozen shoulder, as described in chapter 1. Although many other muscles were involved, the subscapularis was the heart of the problem.

If massage in this position is too tiring for your neck, rest your forehead on a table with a folded towel as a pad. If you're unsure whether you're touching the subscapularis, contract it by strongly rotating your arm inward. Inward rotation is when your elbow is turned outward.

Search for exquisitely tender spots all along the outer edge of the shoulder blade. For the uppermost ones you will be poking very high in the armpit and aiming at the joint itself. Don't overlook trigger points near the bottom end of the shoulder blade as you approach its inferior angle. When you find a trigger point, treat it with slow, short strokes from the ribs outward. Give subscapularis trigger points six to twelve strokes several times a day. If pain wakes you up in the night, have another massage session; it should cut the pain enough to let you get back to sleep.

Continue daily massage until you can no longer find trigger points. Significant relief can come right away, but complete deactivation may take as long as six weeks. Trigger points that have been in place for months or years will require a great deal of attention.

Deltoid

The *deltoid* muscle, if flattened out on a table, would resemble the Greek letter delta, which has the shape of a triangle. On the body, the deltoid muscle completely surrounds the shoulder like a cap. Although the deltoid is technically a single muscle, it has three fairly distinct parts, the *anterior, posterior,* and *lateral deltoid,* on the front, back, and outer side of the shoulder, respectively. Because of this, the deltoid muscle is often spoken of as "the deltoids."

The deltoids attach to the collarbone, scapular spine, and acromion, the bony point of the shoulder. Their lower attachment is to a slight bump about halfway down the outer side of the humerus. In conjunction with the supraspinatus muscle, the function of the deltoids is to raise the arm in any direction—front, back, and sideways.

Symptoms

Pain from deltoid trigger points is unusual in that it is not referred to distant places, but is felt at the site of the trigger point or nearby (Figures 5.27, 5.28, 5.29, and 5.30). Pain originating in the deltoids is felt mainly when you move the arm, and less often when the arm is

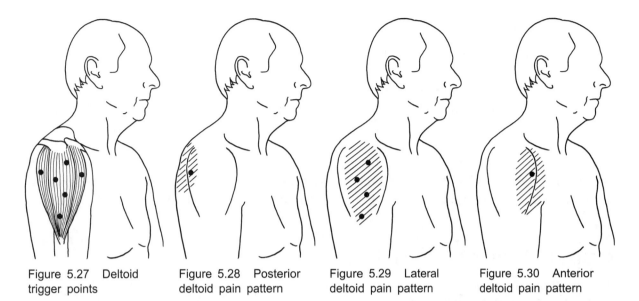

Figure 5.27 Deltoid trigger points

Figure 5.28 Posterior deltoid pain pattern

Figure 5.29 Lateral deltoid pain pattern

Figure 5.30 Anterior deltoid pain pattern

at rest. In contrast, pain referred to the deltoids from elsewhere is felt continuously, or in relation to activity in other muscles (1999, 623–624, 628–629).

Trigger points in any part of the deltoid weaken the shoulder and impair its efforts to raise the arm. Performance in sports or on the job can be seriously degraded. When health-care practitioners are unaware of myofascial causes, pain caused by trigger points in the deltoid muscles is apt to be blamed on arthritis, bursitis, or rotator cuff tendinitis (1999, 628–631; Reynolds 1981, 111–114).

Deltoid trigger points never exist by themselves and are almost never the primary cause of shoulder pain. They're very often created as satellites of trigger points in the scalenes, pectoralis major, or rotator cuff muscles, all of which send pain to the deltoid area—the front, back, and side of the shoulder. See this chapter's Trigger Point Guide for the extensive list of muscles that send pain to the deltoid region.

Causes

The deltoids are frequently overloaded in athletic activities that require forceful flexion of the shoulder, particularly swimming, skiing, weight lifting, and ball playing. In the workplace, the deltoid is overused by having to hold heavy tools up to do a job, or by repeatedly reaching up, out, or back, hour after hour. Picking up and carrying a baby or small child is a very common way to abuse the deltoids and other shoulder muscles (1999, 628–629; Cailliet 1966, 81–85; Jonsson and Hagberg 1974, 26–32).

To reduce repetitive strain to the deltoids, look for ways to change the job that will help keep the elbows down. Typing taxes the deltoids when the keyboard is too high. Good ergonomics dictates keeping the elbows tucked in and the keyboard level with them. Support the elbows whenever possible and try not to sit in chairs that don't have arms.

Keep in mind that the deltoid muscles must work hard to keep the arms from being pulled from their sockets when you carry or lift heavy weights. They also are likely to suffer during any accident or fall that wrenches, jams, or pulls on the arms. An impact injury to the shoulder can be expected to set up trigger points in the deltoids (1999, 628–629).

Treatment

Using your hands to massage the deltoids will needlessly exhaust them. Use a tennis or lacrosse ball against the wall instead. Turning at an angle to the wall will allow you to roll the ball over any of the three parts of the muscle.

Note that trigger points will be found only at midmuscle in the anterior and posterior deltoids. In the lateral deltoid, because of its bipennate fiber arrangement (see Figure 2.2), trigger points can occur anywhere from the point of the shoulder to the attachment in the middle of the upper arm. Most of the knots will actually be found in the lateral deltoid, because it's the largest part of the muscle and works the hardest. Lean into the wall and roll the ball from top to bottom and back again, ironing every inch of the muscle's area.

Upper Arm Muscles

Body builders have an intense appreciation of their upper arm muscles. Everybody else is inclined to forget them. When the upper arm muscles are out of condition, your job or recreational activities can put demands on them that easily exceed their strength and endurance. The upper arm muscles have to support the weight of whatever is in your hand, whether it's a baby, a bag of groceries, or a heavy tool. Sometimes the upper arm muscles are called on to support the weight of the entire body. Simply getting in and out of chairs or in and out of your car can sponsor trigger points in the upper arm muscles, especially if you're carrying a few extra pounds of body weight.

Teres Major and Latissimus Dorsi

The *teres* (TEH-reez) *major* and *latissimus dorsi* (luh-TISS-uh-mus DOR-sye) come together at the back of the armpit and then go around to attach to the front of the upper arm bone near its top (Figures 5.31 and 5.32). Their action is to bring the arm down and in toward the chest. With the help of the posterior deltoid, they also extend the arm backward. *Teres major* means "big round muscle." *Latissimus dorsi* means "wide back muscle." Although the *latissimus dorsi* is a muscle of the lower back, it's included in this chapter because it moves the upper arm and causes pain in the mid and upper back.

Trigger points in the teres major produce sharp pain in the posterior deltoid (Figure 5.31) when you rest your elbows on a table or desk, or reach up and forward to get something from a shelf. When a nearby latissimus trigger point is active, this same motion causes pain in the mid back centered on the inferior angle of the shoulder blade

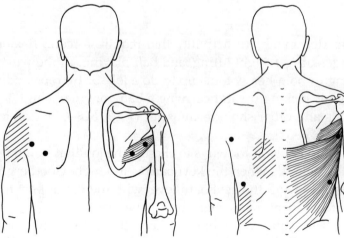
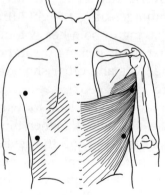

Figure 5.31   Teres major trigger points and referred pain pattern

Figure 5.32   Latissimus dorsi trigger points and referred pain pattern

(Figure 5.32). A trigger point lower in the latissimus causes pain low on the side of the abdomen. When latissimus trigger points are unusually active, pain may extend to the inner side of the arm all the way down to the ulnar or pinky side of the hand and the fourth and fifth fingers (not shown). Trigger points in either the teres major or latissimus dorsi can also inhibit the full stretch that is necessary to reach up and forward. They keep you from fully lifting your arm (1999, 572–578).

When you consider the importance of the teres major and latissimus dorsi for strongly pulling the arm downward, it's easy to imagine the kinds of strains and overuse that can affect them. For the causes of trouble, look at activities such as gymnastics, tennis, swimming, rowing, chopping wood, pitching, or throwing a ball. Go easy with any exercise that involves pulling yourself up or pushing down

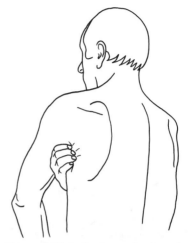

Figure 5.33 Latissimus dorsi and teres major massage between fingers and thumb

with your arms. Be cautious with work that makes you overstretch or repeatedly strain these muscles by reaching forward or overhead.

Pinching the wad of muscle behind the armpit with the fingers and thumb is very effective for locating teres major and latissimus dorsi trigger points (Figure 5.33), but massaging them with the hand tires it very quickly. Luckily, these trigger points can be massaged almost without effort with the Thera Cane or a lacrosse ball against the wall. You may encounter an extremely tender area on the ribs just in front of the edge of the latissimus dorsi. This is a serratus anterior trigger point, which can make horrible pain in the side (see chapter 7).

Coracobrachialis

The *coracobrachialis* (COR-ah-co-bray-kee-AH-liss) lies between the biceps and the triceps on the inner side of the upper arm. The muscle is a little larger than an index finger and about twice as long. At its lower end, it attaches about halfway down the upper arm bone. At its upper end, it attaches to the coracoid process, the little piece of the shoulder blade that sticks through to the front of the shoulder (see Figure 5.8). The action of the coracobrachialis pulls the arm tight against the side.

Pain from coracobrachialis trigger points is felt in the anterior deltoid, triceps, back of the forearm, and back of the hand (Figures 5.34 and 5.35). The more active the trigger points are, the more extensive the pain

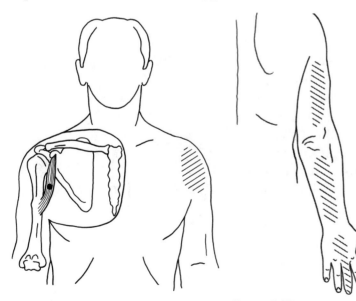

Figure 5.34 Sample coracobrachialis trigger point and anterior referred pain pattern

Figure 5.35 Coracobrachialis posterior referred pain pattern

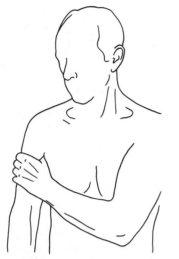

Figure 5.36   Coracobrachialis massage with thumb

pattern becomes. Under extreme conditions, pain may reach as far as the end of the middle finger. You may not become aware of the involvement of the coracobrachialis in this pattern until more obvious trigger points in the shoulder and upper arm have been deactivated. Trigger points in this muscle can make it difficult to put the arm behind your back or raise it up overhead. A coracobrachialis shortened by trigger points can also squeeze the nerves that supply the arm, causing numbness in the biceps, forearm, and hand (1999, 638–644).

Examples of activities that can strain this muscle are push-ups, rock climbing, rope climbing, swimming, throwing a ball, and playing golf and tennis. Any job that requires repeatedly pulling something downward can stress the coracobrachialis. Be careful about lifting heavy weight with the arms stretched out in front and the palms up.

To locate the coracobrachialis, press your thumb against the inner side of the humerus as high up as you can (Figure 5.36). You can feel the muscle contract at this location when you clamp your elbow tight against your side. This is also the place where you will find coracobrachialis trigger points. Massage them with gentle upward and downward strokes of the thumb, taking care to stay on the muscle. Major nerves to the arm run alongside the coracobrachialis in this area, so be conservative with your pressure.

Biceps

The *biceps* has two heads, one head attaching to the coracoid process alongside the coracobrachialis, the other head attaching to the shoulder blade just above the socket (Figure 5.37). This attachment to the shoulder blade lets the biceps help raise the arm. The lower end of the biceps attaches to the bones of the forearm, which allows it to bend the elbow and help turn the hand over palm side up.

Another extremely important function of the biceps is to participate in keeping the arm firmly in its socket. Many muscles work to maintain the shoulder joint, but without the biceps it would be impossible to carry any weight at all without pulling the joint apart.

Trigger points in the biceps cause pain or aching primarily in the front of the shoulder itself and in the crease of the elbow (Figure 5.37). They cause little pain in the biceps itself. You may also experience weakness in the arm and difficulty in completely straightening the arm with the palm facing down. A vague ache may sometimes be felt in the supraspinatus area behind the shoulder (not shown). Pain referred to the shoulder from the biceps may be mistaken for tendinitis or bursitis (1999, 654).

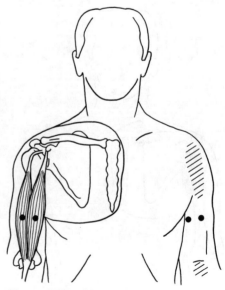

Figure 5.37   Biceps trigger points and referred pain pattern

Trigger points can be started in the biceps by pain referred to it from the infraspinatus or subclavius muscles (1999, 652). Other common causes of trigger points are overexertion in sports activities, lifting heavy weights with the palm up, and exercises that strongly flex the elbow, such as pulling up to a chinning bar. Repetitive strain in the workplace—for example, continuously turning a screwdriver—will exhaust the biceps. Be mindful of any activity that necessitates maintaining a contracted biceps. An example of this is violin playing, which requires the left biceps to be in maximum contraction to keep the hand in position on the fingerboard. Violinists' right biceps often develop trigger points from the continual contracting and lengthening during bowing.

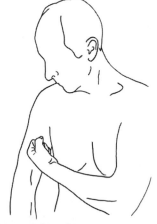

Figure 5.38   Biceps massage with knuckles

Trigger points may be found in either head of the biceps at the midpoint of the muscle. Massage the muscle with the supported thumb or rake it deeply with the knuckles (Figure 5.38). Don't get caught up in massaging the tender referral area on the front of the shoulder. Consult this chapter's Trigger Point Guide for all the muscles that refer pain to this area: note that the biceps is low on the list.

Triceps

The *triceps* is a long, broad muscle with three branches or heads. The attachment of the muscle to the ulna, one of the two bones of the forearm, gives it great leverage for straightening the elbow: the triceps is solely responsible for this function. The attachment of the long head of the triceps to the shoulder blade helps keep the arm in its socket. Triceps trigger points occur at five different sites and evoke five distinct pain patterns.

Triceps number 1 trigger point sends pain to the back of the shoulder and the outer elbow (Figure 5.39). When bad enough, it can refer pain into the upper trapezius and the base of the neck (not shown). Although this is the most common triceps trigger point, its location at the inner edge of the triceps makes it easy to miss (1999, 667–668).

Triceps number 2 trigger point, being very close to the elbow where the muscle is relatively thin, is also easy to miss. It's one of many sources of the pain in the outer elbow known as "tennis elbow" (Figure 5.40). Pain may extend some distance down the back of the forearm (1999, 668–669).

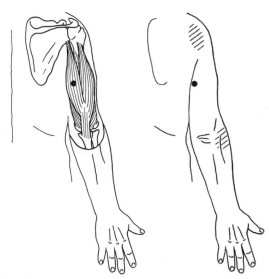

Figure 5.39   Triceps number 1 trigger point and referred pain pattern

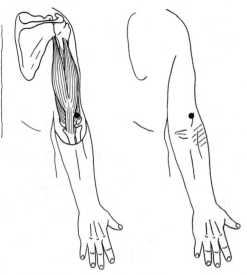

Figure 5.40   Triceps number 2 trigger point and referred pain pattern

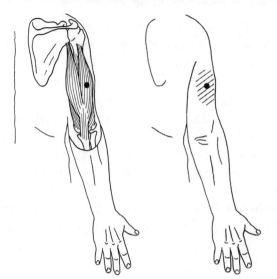

Figure 5.41   Triceps number 3 trigger point and referred pain pattern

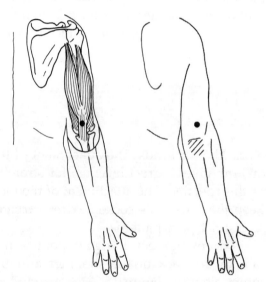

Figure 5.42   Triceps number 4 trigger point and referred pain pattern

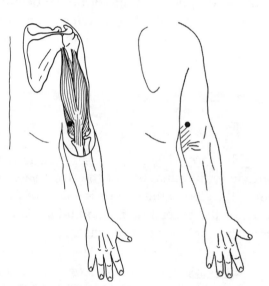

Figure 5.43   Triceps number 5 trigger point and referred pain pattern

Triceps number 3 trigger point in the lateral head causes local pain in the back of the upper arm (Figure 5.41). It has special importance because it can keep the lateral head tight enough to compress the radial nerve, causing numbness in the thumb side of the forearm and hand (1999, 668–669).

Triceps number 4 makes your elbow hypersensitive to touch (Figure 5.42), making it unbearable to rest it on a tabletop or the arm of a chair (1999, 668–669).

Triceps number 5 refers pain to the inner elbow and sometimes to the inner forearm (Figure 5.43). Pain at this site is sometimes called "golfer's elbow" (1999, 668–669).

When active enough, any of these trigger points can cause pain in the fourth and fifth fingers. Any of them can also create an oppressive sense of achiness in the back of the forearm and in the triceps itself. Triceps trigger points can be expected to weaken the elbow and limit both its bending and straightening. Arthritis, tendinitis, and bursitis are common explanations for pain referred to the elbow by the triceps when the effects of trigger points haven't been considered.

Overexertion in sports or the workplace can create trigger points in the triceps, particularly any strong, repetitive pushing action. Simply holding something down for a long, unrelieved period can make the triceps knot up. Sometimes trigger points in the triceps are satellites of unsuspected trigger points in the latissimus dorsi or the serratus posterior superior.

A convenient and effective way to massage the triceps is with your knuckles, using a tennis ball to give support to your hand (Figure 5.44). This technique works best on a desktop, a tabletop, a filing cabinet, or even the top of an old-fashioned upright piano. You can also use the ball-and-knuckles trick against your chest or on your knee. Another good idea, especially for the outer edge of the triceps, is to use a ball against the wall (Figure 5.45).

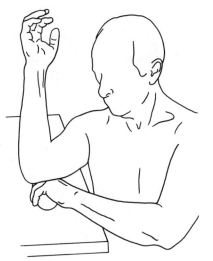

Figure 5.44   Triceps massage with knuckles and ball

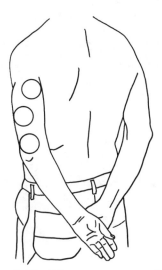

Figure 5.45   Triceps massage with a ball against the wall

CHAPTER 6

Elbow, Forearm, and Hand Pain

Trigger Point Guide: Elbow, Forearm, and Hand Pain

Outer Elbow Pain

extensors (114–121)

triceps (101)

brachioradialis (116)

supinator (116)

supraspinatus (88)

anconeus (119)

Outer Forearm Pain

triceps (101)

scalenes (78)

extensors (114–121)

brachioradialis (116)

brachialis (113)

flexors (121–126)

infraspinatus (90)

teres major (98)

coracobrachialis (99)

supraspinatus (88)

Outer Wrist and Hand Pain

subscapularis (93)

extensors (114–121)

scalenes (78)

serratus posterior superior (86)

first dorsal interosseous (128)

latissimus dorsi (98)

coracobrachialis (99)

Thumb and Web Pain

brachialis (113)

scalenes (78)

supinator (116)

infraspinatus (90)

extensor carpi radialis longus (115)

brachioradialis (116)

opponens pollicis (126)

adductor pollicis (127)

first dorsal interosseous (128)

flexor pollicis longus (125)

Inner Elbow Pain

triceps (101)

flexor carpi ulnaris (122)

pectoralis major (134)

pectoralis minor (139)

serratus anterior (141)

serratus posterior superior (86)

Inner Forearm Pain

palmaris longus (123)

pronators (124)

serratus anterior (141)

triceps (101)

latissimus dorsi (98)

pectoralis major (134)

pectoralis minor (139)

serratus posterior superior (86)

Inner Wrist and Palm Pain

opponens pollicis (120)

flexors (121–126)

palmaris longus (123)

pronators (124)

pectoralis major (134)

pectoralis minor (139)

latissimus dorsi (98)

serratus anterior (141)

Inner Finger Pain

flexor digitorum (124)

interosseous (128)

triceps (101)

latissimus dorsi (98)

serratus anterior (141)

Outer Finger Pain

extensor digitorum (119)

scalenes (78)

triceps (101)

interosseous (128)

pectoralis minor (139)

latissimus dorsi (98)

Hand and Finger Numbness

scalenes (78)

serratus posterior superior (86)

teres minor (92)

pectoralis minor (139)

triceps (101)

coracobrachialis (99)

brachialis (113)

supinator (116)

extensor carpi radialis brevis (117)

flexor carpi ulnaris (122)

flexor digitorum (124)

pronator teres (124)

Trigger Point Guide:
Elbow, Forearm, and Hand Pain

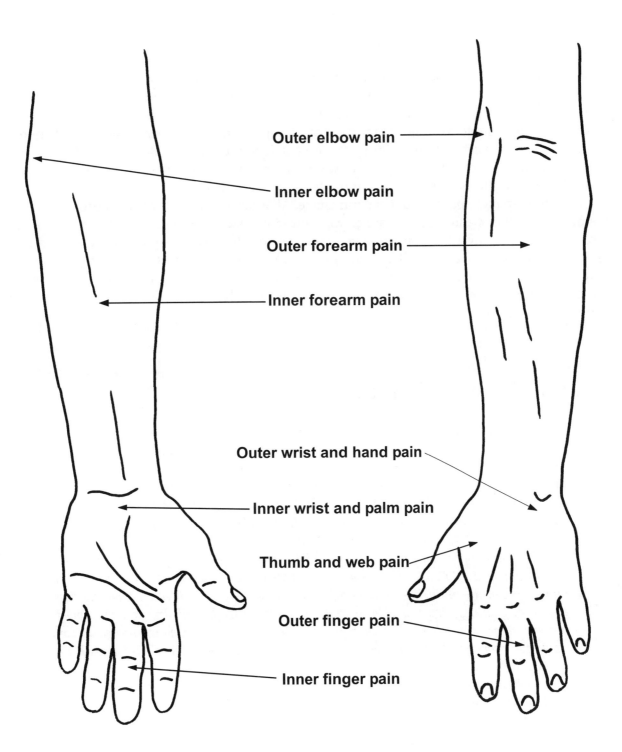

Outer elbow pain

Inner elbow pain

Outer forearm pain

Inner forearm pain

Outer wrist and hand pain

Inner wrist and palm pain

Thumb and web pain

Outer finger pain

Inner finger pain

Elbow, Forearm, and Hand Pain

Myofascial symptoms in the elbows, forearms, wrists, hands, fingers, and thumbs are extremely common. In addition to pain and aching, trigger points can cause numbness, tingling, burning, swelling, hypersensitivity, weakness, and joint stiffness. The combined effects of several of these things can cause you to unexpectedly drop things.

When the practitioner is uninformed about trigger points, these symptoms are likely to be mistakenly interpreted as indicating epicondylitis, arthritis, bursitis, tendinitis, tennis elbow, carpal tunnel syndrome, or a neurological defect. Conventional treatment of symptoms in the forearms and hands is usually local, despite the fact that many of these problems originate with trigger points in the neck, chest, upper back, or shoulders. Because of the displacement of symptoms, relief obtained from local treatments with magnets, wrist splints, pressure straps, electro-stimulation, ultrasound, and acupuncture is likely to be temporary at best. Similarly, since drugs don't affect trigger points and may only mask their symptoms, any beneficial effects of pain medication can only be transitory.

Two extremely popular but often mistaken diagnoses, carpal tunnel syndrome and lateral epicondylitis (tennis elbow), are of particular interest. When your symptoms receive one of these labels, conventional treatments may cause needless suffering and expense and give far less than satisfactory results. Even after surgery, cortisone shots, and physical therapy, symptoms often remain unchanged and sometimes are made worse. When trigger point therapy is tried first, more extreme measures can usually be avoided (Travell and Simons 1999, 685–799).

Carpal Tunnel Syndrome

Libby, age forty, suffered with chronic pain in her shoulders, arms, and hands. In addition, her fingers felt numb, stiff, and swollen. When she went out walking on her lunch hour, the swelling in her hands became so uncomfortable that she often held them up in the air for relief. Her doctor had urgently recommended carpal tunnel surgery to arrest the condition before it got worse. He didn't know whether it would help her shoulder pain but said it was worth a try. She felt like she was in a corner and didn't know what else to do but go through with it.

On the recommendation of a friend, Libby decided to try trigger point therapy before committing to surgery. Massage immediately decreased the pain in her shoulders and arms and the numbness and swelling in her hands. After three massage sessions and some coaching, she was able to continue the massage herself. In six weeks, most of her symptoms were gone. Some of the pain in her forearms and hands tended to come back after working all day at the computer, but she was able to minimize it with the massage techniques she had learned.

Libby was able to determine that although her job with an insurance company had made all her symptoms worse, her problems actually had started with whiplash she'd suffered in an auto accident three years earlier. Trigger points created in her scalenes by the accident accounted directly for many of her symptoms and had predisposed muscles in her forearms and hands to trigger points of their own.

When confronted with pain, numbness, tingling, stiffness, burning, or swelling in the hands and fingers, the universal tendency nowadays is to immediately apply the label "carpal tunnel syndrome" or "peripheral neuropathy" and do no further thinking about it. Very often, myofascial trigger points are the sole cause of all of these symptoms. Typically, trigger points in the scalenes, brachialis, and muscles of the forearms are found to be causing most of the trouble. With severe symptoms, all the muscles of the neck, upper back, shoulder, arm, and hand may be involved (1999, 688).

The carpal tunnel is formed in the wrist by the carpal bones and the ligaments and other fibrous tissues that keep them together. The median nerve and several tendons pass through the carpal tunnel on their way to the fingers and hand. The nerve and tendons can be compressed when this passageway is swollen or otherwise restricted.

Although numbness and tingling in the hands, the most easily recognized signs of carpal tunnel syndrome, are clearly the effects of nerve compression, these symptoms may not be coming from the carpal tunnel. The critical impingement frequently occurs in the thoracic outlet, the opening behind your collarbone through which the nerves and blood vessels pass on their way to and from the arm. The impeded return of blood and lymph from the arm is often the cause of the swelling in the wrist and hand that in turn may cause the restriction in the carpal tunnel. When this happens, carpal tunnel surgery may release the constriction in the wrist and relieve the symptoms in the hand to a degree, but it doesn't treat the real cause. It's the thoracic outlet that needs attention, not the carpal tunnel (1999, 514–516).

The size of the thoracic outlet is reduced when trigger points shorten the scalene muscles in the front of the neck. Tight scalenes pull the first rib up against the collarbone, squeezing the blood vessels and nerves that pass between them. Pressure on these nerves is often the cause of numbness and tingling in the hands and fingers. The pectoralis minor, triceps, brachialis, and certain forearm muscles are also capable of compressing the nerves of the arm and causing numbness in the forearms and hands. It's not helpful when a physician labels your problem "peripheral neuropathy." This needlessly frightening term is only a fancy way of saying that something is pressing on a nerve and making your hands or feet numb (1999, 459, 514–525, 688).

Use the Trigger Point Guide at the beginning of this chapter to help track down the likely sources of numbness in your elbows, forearms, and hands as well as the various origins of pain, burning, or other sensations in those areas. For each area that has such symptoms, start at the top of the list and check the listed muscles one at a time for trigger points. Keep in mind that a good rule in troubleshooting your "carpal tunnel" symptoms is to always start with the scalenes. They're often at the very root of the trouble, setting up a chain of effects all the way down the line. A little attention to your scalenes can make an immediate improvement in many of your shoulder, arm, and hand symptoms. Note that numbness in the hands and fingers can also be caused by trigger points in the serratus posterior, teres minor, pectoralis minor, triceps, coracobrachialis, brachialis, supinator, extensor carpi radialis brevis, flexor carpi ulnaris, flexor digitorum, and pronator teres.

Tennis Elbow

Martha, age forty-eight, had been told she had epicondylitis in both elbows from repetitive strain. The pain had become so bad that she was unable to work and had to quit her job. Worry about the future kept her from sleeping. She felt worn out and tense all the time. She'd gotten many conflicting recommendations regarding treatment, ranging from extended rest to various types of reconstructive surgery. Workman's compensation would pay for almost anything she needed. She'd gone to physical therapy for months and she wore braces on her elbows most of the time, but progress had been negligible. Now her doctor wanted to put her arms in casts to immobilize them. After being shown how to massage her forearm and triceps muscles with a ball against a wall, Martha was able to get rid of most of her pain in just three weeks.

The traditional explanation for epicondylitis, or tennis elbow, is that you have tendinitis, in other words, that the tendons around your elbow have suffered microscopic tears through injury or overuse. A diagnosis of tendinitis is an easy one to make, but it may be the wrong one unless you've had an obvious physical injury. Travell and Simmons believe that trigger points in the forearm muscles, not tendinitis, are the most common cause of pain and weakness in the elbow. Other muscles sometimes contribute to the problem, as can be seen in the Trigger Point Guide for this chapter. When relief is obtained by trigger point massage, tendinitis can be quickly ruled out (1999, 736).

Rest is always recommended for tennis elbow, but it's not the best therapy when trigger points are the cause of the pain. Rest may lull trigger points into a quiet, latent state, but it doesn't get rid of them. When you resume whatever activity caused the tennis elbow in the first place, the pain comes right back, rarely diminished in the least. Inactivity tends to promote atrophy and stiffness in the muscles of the forearm, which perpetuates their trigger points, often making them worse and increasing your pain.

On the other hand, activity can be just as bad for tennis elbow if it takes the form of a program of exercise and stretch. Muscles afflicted with trigger points actively resist stretching because of the risk of overstretching the taut bands of muscle fibers. Also, a painful elbow can appear weak, but exercise for the purpose of strengthening it is not only ineffective but unnecessary. Myofascial trigger points weaken muscles associated with the elbow as a means of protection from further overuse or abuse. Full strength ordinarily returns within a short time after trigger points are deactivated.

Pain in the inner elbow, which is less common than pain in the outer elbow, is called "golfer's elbow," though it probably results less frequently from playing golf than from overexercise or overuse in the workplace. Observe that the list of muscles potentially involved in inner elbow pain is quite different from the list for outer elbow pain. In troubleshooting either condition, remember that two or more muscles may be referring pain to the same place.

Organize your search with the help of the Trigger Point Guide for this chapter. If you find your efforts have been only somewhat effective in that some level of pain is still present, you've probably missed a trigger point somewhere. If massage doesn't seem to be helping at all, you're very likely working the wrong muscle. Tennis elbow can be quickly gotten rid of when you take the time to troubleshoot it in a thorough manner.

Safe Massage of the Forearms and Hands

It's easier than you might think to get rid of the pain and other symptoms in your forearms and hands. You can make things worse, however, if you don't use your hands intelligently when applying trigger point massage. You need to give scrupulous attention to ergonomics, or the safe, effective use of your hands as tools.

Also, massage of the forearms and hands becomes easier and more efficient when you have a good understanding of the function and location of the individual muscles. It helps to be familiar with the bones of the forearm and hand so that you can make use of their *bony landmarks* in locating muscles.

Ergonomics

You won't get much massage done before com-pletely trashing your forearms and hands if you go about it in unintelligent ways. You may not realize how tiring it is for the hands and forearms, for instance, to do massage with your thumb working in opposition to the fingers (Figure 6.1). The reason for this is that all the muscles in the forearm participate in the grasping function, and the harder you grip something, the harder they all contract. The forearm muscles, whose function is to operate the hands and fingers, work harder than any other muscles in the body, pound for pound.

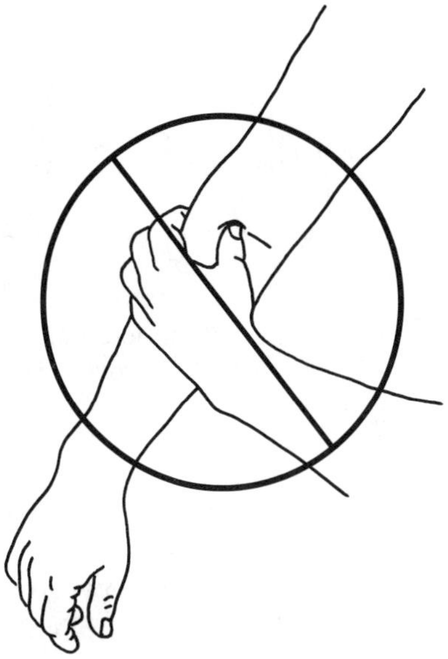

Figure 6.1   Avoid grasping with thumb and fingers

Unfortunately, it's so natural to grasp with the hand that people do it without thinking. If you do massage without thinking, you're guaranteed to end up with more trigger points—and more pain—than you started with. It's best to avoid using your hands at all in massage if you can find any other way. (Note that some muscles, such as the masseters and the sternocleidomastoids, can only be massaged by kneading them between the thumb and fingers: save your hands for them.)

You'll observe that many massage techniques in this book employ straight fingers or a straight thumb reinforced by the opposite hand. Supported fingers or the supported thumb largely eliminate the use of the forearm muscles (see Figures 3.2 and 3.3). The fingers or thumb are held as nearly perpendicular to the skin as possible so that the force is applied through their very tips. With this technique, the supported fingers or supported thumb func-tion as the end of a very long prod that has a straight line to the elbow. When this is done correctly, the shoulder muscles and the weight of the body do most of the work and the muscles of the forearm and hand can remain relatively relaxed. People who try to do mas-sage with long nails find that their hands tire quickly and that they are unable to use some of the most useful techniques.

A tennis ball or a lacrosse ball against the wall is a useful tool for massage of your fore-arms and hands, although they can never have the sensitivity of your fingers and thumbs. The ball on the wall technique, however, does give you the advantage of using your whole body to apply the pressure. While the Knobble can be a hard and insensitive tool, it can also be used on the thicker forearm muscles instead of supported fingers or supported thumb. Though less than perfect, it may make a serviceable compromise for those who can't bear to sacrifice their nails. Hold the Knobble loosely; don't grip it hard. You should sense that the

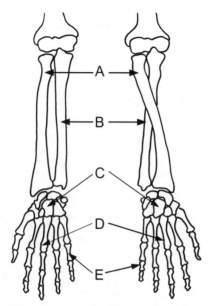

Figure 6.2   Bones of the forearm and hand:
(A) radius; (B) ulna; (C) carpals; (D) metacarpals;
(E) phalanges

force behind the Knobble is coming from the shoulder, not from the forearm or hand. Remember also to use the Knobble through a layer of cloth, not on bare skin.

Bony Landmarks

The ability to find and massage specific muscles depends on being able to find nearby bones. The knobby ends of bones, in particular, serve as valuable landmarks. The better you are at locating these landmarks, the better you'll be at locating trigger points.

There are only two bones in the forearm: the *radius* and the *ulna* (UL-nah). Figure 6.2 shows them in the right arm in two different positions. The upper end of the ulna is familiar to you as the point of your elbow. The sharp bony ridge all along the underside of your forearm is the shaft of the ulna. The knob on the little finger or pinky side of your wrist is the ulna's lower end: this is called the *styloid process*. The thick bone in the thumb side of the wrist is the lower end of the radius. When you turn your hand over, the lower end of the radius moves the entire hand around the lower end of the ulna a full 180 degrees. Try this and observe that the ulna itself doesn't turn. With the radius and ulna parallel, the hand is supinated. When the radius crosses the ulna, the hand is pronated.

The upper end, or head, of the radius is at the elbow. It rotates in its socket when the hand turns over, and this movement can be felt. Feel for two knobs on your outer elbow, about an inch apart. Place a finger on each knob. The one further toward the hand is the head of the radius. Feel it turn as you turn your hand over and back several times. Notice that the knob touched by your other finger doesn't move. It's the *lateral epicondyle*. The bone that sticks out on the inner side of the elbow is the *medial epicondyle*. The epicondyles are parts of the enlarged lower end of the humerus or upper arm bone.

The eight small wrist bones are called the *carpals*. The carpal bones give the hand mobility, enabling it to move in any direction. Because of this great flexibility, the carpals also serve as shock absorbers, protecting the wrist by spreading stresses over a greater total surface area.

The four bones in the hand and the bone that forms the base of the thumb are called the *metacarpals*, meta meaning "after." The metacarpals "come after" the carpals. There are small muscles between the metacarpal bones called the *interosseous muscles*. Trigger points in the interosseous muscles are the source of some kinds of finger and knuckle pain.

The bones of the fingers are called *phalanges* (fuh-LAN-jeez). The thumb has only two phalanges; each finger has three. There are no muscles in the fingers, just lots and lots of tendons, through which the fingers are moved by remote control by the muscles in the forearm and hand.

Explore your forearms and hands, feeling for these various bones. Try to visualize how things are arranged under the skin. The better mental picture you have of the bones, the better you'll be at picturing the muscles in there too.

Brachialis Muscle

The *brachialis* (brah-kee-AH-liss) muscle is the workhorse of the elbow. Lifting by bending the elbow requires contraction of the brachialis. It does much of the work normally credited to the biceps. Although it's an upper arm muscle, the muscle is included in this chapter because the trouble it causes is felt in the hand.

The brachialis lies under the biceps, covering the front of the lower half of the humerus (Figure 6.3). Its upper end attaches to a bony mound on the outer surface of the humerus about halfway down, just below the attachment of the deltoid muscles. The other end of the brachialis attaches to the ulna.

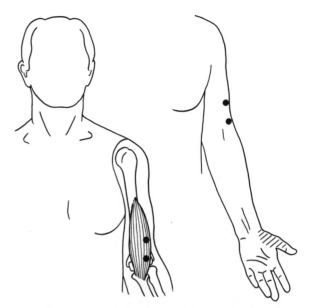

Figure 6.3   Brachialis trigger points and referred pain pattern

Symptoms

Trigger points in a brachialis muscle make it difficult to straighten the elbow, but they cause pain primarily at the base of the thumb. You may also feel some degree of pain in the front of the shoulder and just below the crease in the elbow (not shown). There may be an oppressive ache or tightness on the outside of the upper arm near the elbow. Compression of the radial nerve that passes through the brachialis can make the thumb and the back of the forearm tingle or feel numb (1999, 662).

As can be seen in the Trigger Point Guide for this chapter, many muscles are capable of referring pain to the area of the thumb, but the brachialis and scalene muscles are always the prime suspects. It's natural to massage the thumb when it hurts, but remember that it's a waste of time when the pain is being sent from somewhere else.

Causes

The brachialis can be overworked by carrying heavy bags of groceries, carrying a baby around, picking up growing children, or carrying a purse hanging on the forearm. Brachialis muscles are stressed by holding up heavy tools for long hours and by any repetitive action of the elbow on the job. You can foster trigger points in your brachialis muscles by pulling yourself up too many times to the chinning bar or by any other strained flexion of the elbow in exercise or sports activity.

Working all day at a computer keyboard with your arms held out in front necessitates continuous contraction of the brachialis muscles of both arms. For this reason, computer users nearly always have brachialis trigger points.

Oboe, clarinet, and some saxophone players often suffer from chronic pain and numbness in the thumb of their right hand, which has to continuously support the weight of the instrument. Though the thumb itself may seem to be the trouble because that's where the pain is felt, the real problem is in the brachialis muscle, which has to stay contracted all the time the instrument is being played. In addition to frequent trigger point massage, a wind

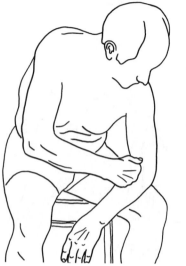

Figure 6.4   Brachialis massage with supported thumb, just above the inner elbow crease

player should put the instrument down at every opportunity and let the arm hang at the side, allowing the brachialis to lengthen and relax.

Treatment

Brachialis trigger points are found under the outer edge of the biceps, just above the crease of the elbow (Figure 6.3). Push the biceps aside to access the trigger points and massage them against the bone with a supported thumb (Figure 6.4). Notice that the arm getting the work is braced against the thigh. The trigger point that causes entrapment of the radial nerve lurks in a sort of lump in the muscle a short way above the elbow on the outside of the arm—it's the upper of the two shown in Figure 6.3. This lump tends to slip out from under the supported thumb, but it's less elusive when worked with a ball against a wall. Occasionally, trigger points occur under the inner edge of the biceps (not shown).

Hand and Finger Extensor Muscles

The *extensor* muscles are on the outer or hairy side of the forearm. Their upper attachments are to the lateral epicondyle, which is the uppermost bony protuberance on the outer elbow. They then attach by long tendons to various bones of the hand and fingers. The extensors bend the hand back and straighten or raise the fingers. When you're gripping with the hand, the extensors must contract to keep the finger flexors from bending the wrist inward. (The flexors are on the inner or hairless side of the forearm.) A strong grip requires strong action in both the flexors and the extensors. The extensor muscles are constantly working in almost everything you do. They're extremely prone to repetitive strain among musicians, who use their fingers intensely for hours on end.

> *Perry, age twenty-three, a graduate student in the saxophone, had excruciating pain in his hands and wrists when he practiced or performed. He'd been working hard preparing for an upcoming recital, but his fingers felt slow and sluggish and his playing was getting worse, not better. After being shown how to massage the backs of his forearms, Perry was able to play without pain for the first time in a year. Working on his forearms before and after practicing helped keep the pain from coming back.*

Trigger points in the extensor muscles cause pain in the outer elbow and in the back of the forearm, wrist, hand, and fingers. They also cause hand weakness, finger stiffness, and knuckle tenderness. Other effects in the hands and fingers are numbness, tingling, and discoordination. When your hand and finger extensors are in trouble, you're apt to drop things unexpectedly.

When the extensors have been abused for a long period of time, your first attempts at therapeutic massage can be extremely painful. Just begin with whatever pressure you can bear, don't expect too much progress too soon, and keep at it. Success in managing trigger points in the extensors can be one of your most important victories.

Extensor Carpi Radialis Longus

The *extensor carpi radialis longus* (ex-TEN-sur CAR-pee ray-dee-AH-liss LONG-gus) attaches to the lateral epicondyle of the humerus and to the base of the metacarpal bone of the index finger (Figure 6.5). The muscle and its tendon are aligned along the full length of the radius. Its job is to bend the wrist toward the thumb side of the hand. The wrist action in throwing a Frisbee is a perfect example of this motion. This long extensor of the hand also helps bend the wrist back and participates in bending the elbow. These two actions keep the hand in position for such activities as typing or playing the piano. Without this muscle and the other two hand extensors, the hand would hang limp at the wrist when you hold your arm out in front of you.

Trigger points in the extensor carpi radialis longus are a common cause of tennis elbow. They also send a kind of burning pain to the outer side

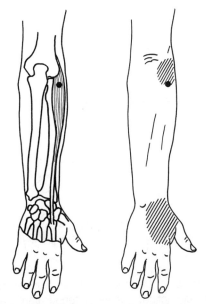

Figure 6.5 Extensor carpi radialis longus trigger point and referred pain pattern. (The drawings show the outer side of the forearm and hand.)

of the forearm and the back of the wrist and hand. A tight elastic brace is sometimes worn at the elbow to subdue such pain. Pressure from the elastic is believed to interfere with transmission of pain signals. This is a stopgap remedy at best, although it's useful on a job where you simply must keep going. A better therapy is to work on deactivating the trigger points.

The extensor carpi radialis longus muscles are stressed by repetitive activity involving the hands, such as tennis, golf, typing, playing a musical instrument, or stirring cookie dough. When you play the violin, you can get tennis elbow by overworking the extensors in your bowing arm. Orchestra conductors often get pain in their elbows from the continual flexing of the wrist of the baton hand. Diehard Frisbee players get it too. Any intensive wrist action tends to exhaust all the muscles of the forearm.

In the workplace, study how you might be overusing the extensor carpi radialis longus muscles. Suspect any position that requires their constant contraction to keep the hands in position, such as when you work long hours at the computer keyboard.

Extensor carpi radialis longus trigger points are found in the thick roll of muscle at the outer elbow. They're at the outer end of the elbow crease. To locate the muscle by isolated contraction, place your fingers on this area and feel the muscle bulge when you cock your wrist hard in the direction shown in Figure 6.6. Your "fighting knuckles" are good tools for massaging this muscle (Figure 6.7). A tennis ball or a lacrosse ball on the wall with the arm oriented straight down may be even better

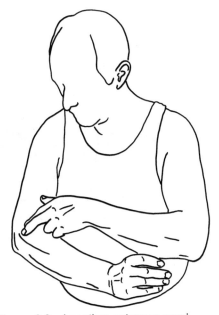

Figure 6.6 Locating extensor carpi radialis longus by isolated contraction

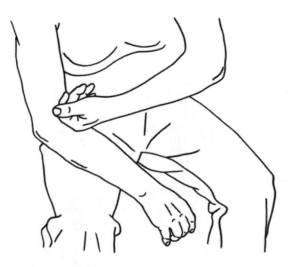

Figure 6.7   Massage of three muscles around the head of the radius (extensor carpi radialis longus, supinator, and brachioradialis) using knuckles and loose fist

(Figure 6.8). Keep the thumb side of the hand toward the wall and exert pressure by leaning the body against the arm. Roll the ball slowly and repeatedly over the trigger points with short deep strokes.

Deep massage all around the head of the radius with the ball will incidentally deactivate trigger points in two less frequently involved muscles: the *brachioradialis* (brah-kee-oh-ray-dee-AH-liss), which lies alongside the extensor carpi radialis longus (Figure 6.9); and the *supinator* (SOO-pih-nay-tur), which lies under both (Figure 6.10). Trigger points in these three muscles are hard to differentiate from one another, and they all have similar pain patterns. The brachioradialis helps bend the elbow. The supinator turns the hand palm side up. Under the influence of trigger points, the supinator can squeeze the radial nerve, which may result in numbness in the thumb side of the hand (1999, 734).

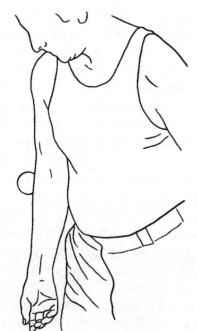

Figure 6.8   Extensor carpi radialis longus massage with ball against a wall

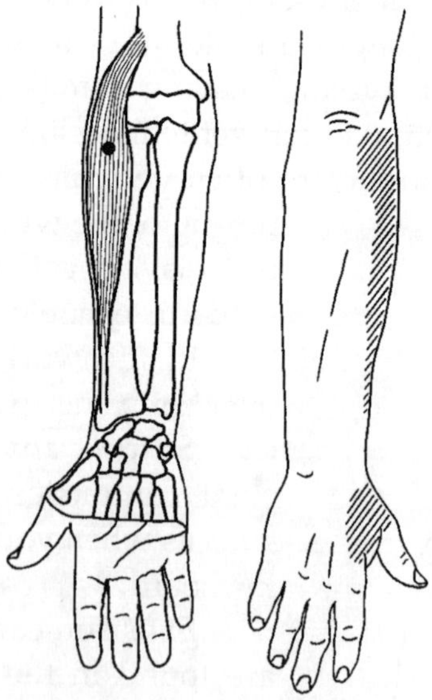

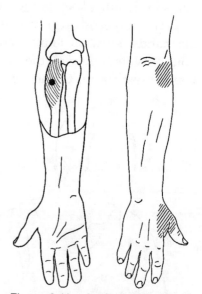

Figure 6.9   Brachioradialis trigger point and referred pain pattern

Figure 6.10   Supinator trigger point and referred pain pattern

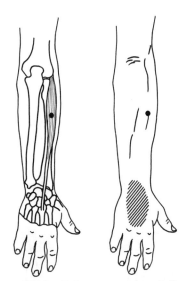

Figure 6.11 Extensor carpi radialis brevis trigger point and referred pain pattern

Extensor Carpi Radialis Brevis

The *extensor carpi radialis brevis* (ex-TEN-sur CAR-pee ray-dee-AH-liss BREH-vis) attaches to the lateral epicondyle and to the base of the metacarpal bone of the middle finger (Figure 6.11). Although it's called the "short extensor," it can be a surprisingly big muscle, lying all along the length of the back of the radius.

Trigger points in the extensor carpi radialis brevis send pain to the back of the wrist and hand. A sense of tightness, burning, or aching in the back of the forearm can be coming from this muscle (not shown). Sometimes an extensor carpi radialis brevis staying tight from the influence of trigger points can compress the radial nerve and cause numbness and tingling in the hand.

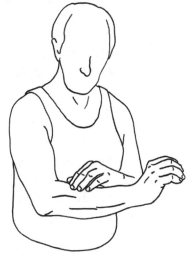

Figure 6.12 Locating extensor carpi radialis brevis by isolated contraction

Any work or sports activity that requires grasping strongly with the hands and fingers will tire the extensor carpi radialis brevis muscles. At the computer keyboard, the short extensors are among the muscles that have to stay contracted to hold your hands up in position for typing. The wrist rest on your computer keyboard is supposed to take the strain off the extensor muscles, but it doesn't always accomplish what's needed: the wrist rest supports the weight of the forearms but often does little to support the weight of the hands.

Try using the wrist rest in a new way. Between spurts of typing, turn your hands to face one another and rest the *sides* of your hands on the wrist rest. This little trick gives all the extensors a break and can make a difference in how much pain you have at the end of the day. Make it your automatic rest position, returning to it as often as you can.

Trigger points are found three or four inches down from the elbow, right against the shaft of the radius. To confirm the location of the short extensor, place your fingers on your forearm as shown in Figure 6.12 and feel the muscle contract when you bend your hand straight back at the wrist. Massage can be done with the supported thumb or even with the opposite elbow, but a tennis ball or hard rubber ball against the wall does the best job. The forearm should be at a right angle to the upper arm, with the palm up and the thumb toward the wall (Figure 6.13). Lean against your arm and roll the ball slowly and repeatedly over the trigger points with as much pressure as you can stand. This deep stroking

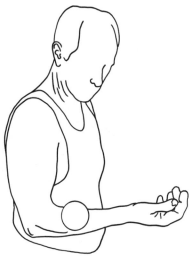

Figure 6.13 Extensor carpi radialis brevis massage with ball against the wall. Use body weight against the arm to apply pressure.

massage should move along the forearm toward the elbow. You need to roll the ball over the trigger points six to twelve times to do an adequate treatment, but come back to it several times a day if these muscles are in a lot of trouble.

The wrist braces that so many people are wearing now effectively take the strain off extensor muscles that have been disabled by trigger points, but the inactivity they impose tends to let the muscles stiffen. In the end, they can make the problem worse. If you pay proper attention to ergonomics, modify some of your work practices, and learn to self-treat extensor trigger points, wrist braces won't be needed (1999, 709–710).

Extensor Carpi Ulnaris

The *extensor carpi ulnaris* (ex-TEN-sur CAR-pee uhl-NEH-ris) attaches to the lateral epicondyle and to the base of the metacarpal bone for the little finger (Figure 6.14). Trigger points in the extensor carpi ulnaris muscle are the most common cause of pain in the ulnar side (the pinky side) of the wrist and hand. It will feel like you've sprained your wrist.

Note that your wrists are normally cocked toward the ulnar side when you're typing at a standard keyboard, requiring the ulnar extensors to stay contracted to keep the hands in this position. The new ergonomic keyboards with angled rows of keys allow you to keep your wrists straighter and are much easier on the ulnar extensor muscles.

The use of most hand tools necessitates cocking the wrist in an ulnar direction. As a consequence, the ulnar extensors are normally conditioned for hard work and are usually very strong, but any muscle can be overworked. Let ulnar wrist pain be your signal that you need to change the position of your hands to give the ulnar extensors

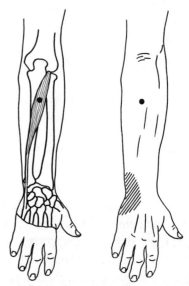

Figure 6.14   Extensor carpi ulnaris trigger point and referred pain pattern

some relief.

Trigger points can be found just below the elbow on the outer side of the forearm, alongside the ulna. To find the belly of the muscle, feel it contract when you bend your wrist in the direction of the little finger (Figure 6.15). Massage the ulnar extensor with a ball against the wall (Figure 6.16). The palm should be facing down, and the thumb side of the hand should be away from the

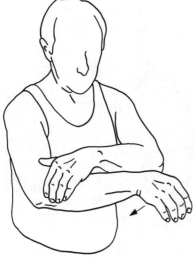

Figure 6.15   Locating extensor carpi ulnaris by isolated contraction

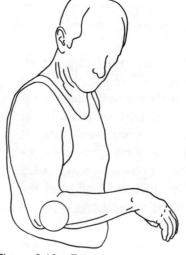

Figure 6.16   Extensor carpi ulnaris massage with ball against the wall

wall. The arm can be either straight down or held horizontally as shown in the illustration. Use your body weight for pressure and stroke repeatedly toward the elbow.

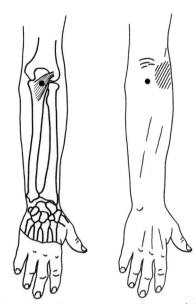

Figure 6.17 Anconeus trigger point and referred pain pattern

Anconeus

The *anconeus* (an-CO-nee-us) is a small muscle found right at the elbow, near the extensor carpi ulnaris (Figure 6.17). It attaches to the ulna and to the lateral epicondyle and works with the triceps to straighten the elbow. Trigger points in the anconeus refer to the lateral epicondyle and can contribute significantly to the pain of tennis elbow (1999, 670).

Find the anconeus in the soft area between the point of the elbow and the lateral epicondyle. To confirm the location of the anconeus, place your finger in this area and feel the muscle contract when you pronate your hand strongly (Figure 6.18).

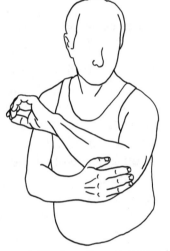

Figure 6.18 Locating anconeus by isolated contraction

(Pronation is when you turn your hand over, palm down.) Use only the fingertips for massage, since a vulnerable ulnar nerve also runs through this space. This nerve is better known as your funny bone.

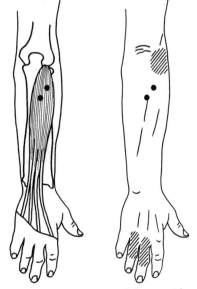

Figure 6.19 Extensor digitorum trigger points and referred pain pattern

Extensor Digitorum

The *extensor digitorum* (ex-TEN-sur dih-jih-TAW-rum) attaches to the lateral epicondyle and to the bones of the fingers (Figure 6.19). Its job is to straighten or extend the third, fourth, and fifth fingers, which it can do selectively because the muscle has a separate tendon for each finger. Although the index finger also attaches to the extensor digitorum, it is primarily controlled by another muscle, the *extensor indicis* (ex-TEN-sur IN-dih-sis) (Figure 6.20).

Trigger points in the extensor digitorum are the prime cause of stiff fingers. They also send pain to the outer elbow and the second knuckle of the third and fourth fingers. The referred pain in your knuckles can be mistaken for the pain of arthritis. You may sometimes have an ache in the back of your forearm and a

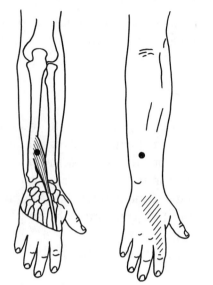

Figure 6.20   Extensor indicis trigger point and referred pain pattern

spot of pain on the inner wrist (not shown). Trigger points in the extensor indicis refer pain to the back of the wrist, hand, and index finger (1999, 718).

When you make a fist or grasp something strongly, the finger extensors are called upon to help keep the wrist from bending when the fingers bend. The harder you grip something, the harder the finger extensors have to work. Activities that call for repetitive gripping or twisting with the hand can overwork the extensor digitorum muscle. Repetitive actions of individual fingers can overtire different parts of the muscle.

At the computer keyboard, the extensor digitorum muscles keep the fingers up when they're not actually making keystrokes. With the hands in typing position, the finger extensors stay tight continuously, with virtually no relief. The operation of the mouse creates the same problem with whatever finger presses the buttons. If you're at the computer a lot, trigger points in your extensor digitorum muscles are probably the cause of that oppressive tightness you feel on the backs of your forearms. Give these muscles a break as often as you can by resting your hands on their sides or by putting them in your lap. This may seem a little compulsive at first, but it won't be the least bit inconvenient once you make a habit of it, and it can be a lifesaver for these extremely vulnerable muscles. Don't expect rest to help much, however, until you get ahead of the trigger points.

Locate the extensor digitorum on the outer or hairy side of the forearm, two or three inches down from the elbow. You can feel the separate parts of the muscle contract independently when you raise the third, fourth, or fifth fingers one at a time (Figure 6.21). You can feel the extensor indicis contract a couple of inches above the bony knob on the outer side of your wrist when you raise your index finger (Figure 6.22).

Massage the extensor digitorum with a ball against the wall, with the back of the hand parallel to the wall and the forearm horizontal (Figure 6.23). Roll the ball slowly along the

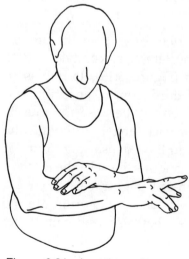

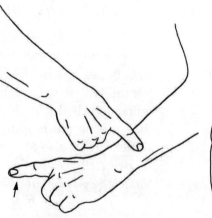

Figure 6.22   Locating extensor indicis by isolated contraction

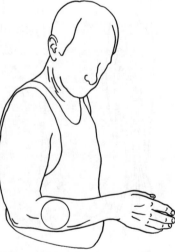

Figure 6.21   Locating extensor digitorum by isolated contraction

Figure 6.23   Extensor digitorum massage with ball against the wall. Roll the ball repeatedly all the way to the elbow.

muscle, from the middle of the forearm to the elbow, leaning hard into it. The trigger points are usually very deep, right at the bone. To access the extensor indicis, pronate the hand (turn it palm down). The extensor indicis will be buried between the radius and ulna bones if you try to massage it with a ball against the wall, so use a supported thumb or a Knobble on it.

Remember that multiple sessions throughout the day work best, each no more than a minute or two in length. Stay ahead of pain by having a session before and after the activity that's causing the trouble.

Hand and Finger Flexors

The hand and finger flexors occupy the inner forearm, most of them attaching to the medial epicondyle, the bony projection at the inner elbow. Their job is to bend the hand inward at the wrist, to cup the hand, and to curl the fingers and thumb in toward the palm.

Pain caused by trigger points in the flexor muscles is sent to various locations on the inner side of the forearm, wrist, hand, and fingers. There are three thick layers of muscle on the inner forearm, making trigger points somewhat harder to isolate and massage than on the back of the forearm.

Massage to the inner forearm can be done broadly but not to any great depth with a tennis ball or lacrosse ball on a desk or dresser top. A ball against the wall is more effective, with your back to the wall and both the ball and your arm behind your back. Deep work can be done on specific trigger points with a Knobble or a supported thumb. Remember to use the Knobble through a cloth.

Flexor Carpi Radialis

The *flexor carpi radialis* (FLEX-ur CAR-pee ray-dee-AH-liss) attaches to the medial epicondyle and the metacarpal bone of the index finger (Figure 6.24). The flexor carpi radialis works with the flexor carpi ulnaris to bend the hand inward.

Pain from trigger points in the flexor carpi radialis is sent to the inner wrist near the base of the thumb. This pain is commonly mistaken for a wrist sprain. The muscles in the ball of the thumb itself also refer pain to this same spot (1999, 753–754, 776).

The hand flexors are abused by excessive use of gripping, twisting, and pulling actions with the hands. Sleeping with the wrists bent severely inward keeps the flexors in an abnormally shortened state and will tend to set up trigger points in them (1999, 762).

The flexor carpi radialis runs right down the center of the inner forearm. Locate the belly of the muscle about three inches below the elbow. Some of the worst

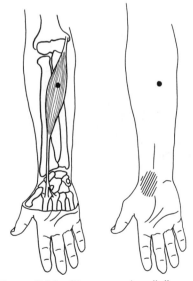

Figure 6.24 Flexor carpi radialis trigger point and referred pain pattern

trigger points are near the elbow. Feel the muscle contract in isolation by bending the hand inward (Figure 6.25). The supported thumb works well for massage of all the flexors (Figure 6.26). The Knobble used through a layer of cloth is also a good tool. A ball and the arm behind the back against the wall is the best way to get the pressure needed to go deep into these thick muscles (Figure 6.27). To be most effective, start the ball two or three inches below the elbow and roll it along the forearm all the way to the elbow.

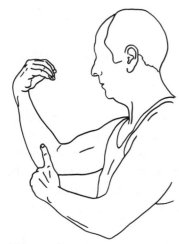

Figure 6.25   Locating flexor carpi radialis by isolated contraction

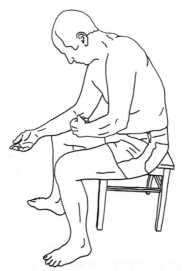

Figure 6.26   Flexor carpi radialis massage with supported thumb

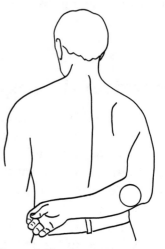

Figure 6.27   Flexor carpi radialis massage with ball against the wall

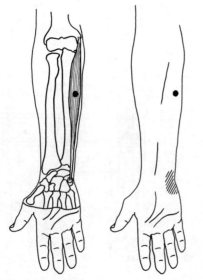

Figure 6.28   Flexor carpi ulnaris trigger point and referred pain pattern

Flexor Carpi Ulnaris

The *flexor carpi ulnaris* (FLEX-ur CAR-pee uhl-NEH-ris) attaches to the medial epicondyle and to a small round bone in the heel of the hand called the pisiform bone. This muscle functions to help bend the wrist inward; it also aids the extensor carpi ulnaris in bending the wrist toward the ulnar side (the pinky side).

Flexor carpi ulnaris trigger points send pain to the ulnar side of the wrist (Figure 6.28). Note that pain in the ulnar side of the wrist can come from either the flexor carpi ulnaris or the extensor carpi ulnaris, or both. Trigger points here can also make the the heel of the hand and inner elbow hurt (not shown). When this muscle is tight, it can compress the ulnar nerve, causing a weakened grip and a sensation of burning or numbness in the fourth and fifth fingers (not shown).

To find the muscle, make it contract in isolation by bending the wrist toward the pinky side of the hand (Figure 6.29). Observe that it runs along the inner edge of the shaft of the ulna. For massage, use a supported thumb or a ball against the wall. There may be more than one trigger point, the worst one being roughly halfway between elbow and wrist.

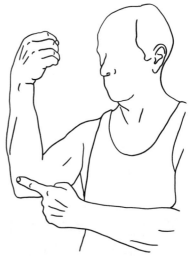

Figure 6.29 Locating flexor carpi ulnaris by isolated contraction

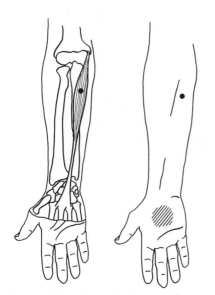

Figure 6.30 Palmaris longus trigger point and referred pain pattern

Palmaris Longus

The *palmaris longus* (pahl-MEH-ris LON-gus) attaches to the medial epicondyle and to most of the tendons in the palm of the hand. The function of the palmaris longus is to cup the hand and assist in flexing the wrist.

Trigger points in the palmaris longus cause a burning or prickling sensation in the palm of the hand (Figure 6.30). Using tools that exert pressure on the palm can be extremely painful when trigger points are present in the palmaris longus. Pain may also be felt in the lower half of the inner forearm (not shown). Trigger points in this muscle don't cause finger pain but are often associated with Dupuytren's contracture, a condition that makes the fourth and fifth fingers stay curled into the palm and resist straightening. (1999: 746)

The palmaris longus is a narrow muscle lying between the flexor carpi radialis and the flexor carpi ulnaris on the inner forearm, a little toward the ulnar side. To locate the belly of the muscle, feel it contract in isolation when you bring the tips of your fingers and thumb tightly together (Figure 6.31). Trigger points in the palmaris can be found from midarm to the bony projection of the inner elbow (the medial epicondyle). Massage them with the same techniques as with the other flexors: supported thumb, Knobble, or ball against the wall.

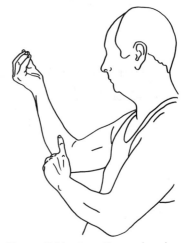

Figure 6.31 Locating palmaris longus by isolated contraction

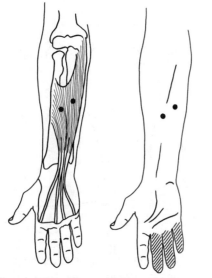

Figure 6.32 Flexor digitorum trigger points and referred pain pattern

Flexor Digitorum

There are two parts to the *flexor digitorum* (FLEX-or dih-jih-TAW-rum): the *profundis* and the *superficialis*. One lies over the other and together they make up the second and third layers of muscle in the inner forearm. The lower attachments of the tendons of the flexor digitorum are to the bones of the fingers (Figure 6.32). At their upper ends, they attach to both bones of the forearm and to the medial epicondyle.

Trigger points in the flexor digitorum send sharp pain to the inner sides of the fingers, which is commonly misinterpreted as arthritis or carpal tunnel syndrome. Uncontrolled twitching of the fingers can be due to trigger points in the flexor digitorum muscles (1999, 765).

Trouble in the flexor digitorum comes from overuse of the grasping function of the hand with tools and sports equipment, such as tennis racquets, golf clubs, and oars. A long car trip with a hard grip on the steering wheel can put them into a bad state. A job employing the constant use of scissors is bad for these muscles. Hard use of the fingers in playing a musical instrument also promotes trigger points in the flexor digitorum muscles.

The bellies of both layers of the flexor digitorum are difficult to distinguish by contracting them. Search for trigger points in the upper half of the inner forearm; expect them to be very deep. Massage this area with a supported thumb or a Knobble. Massage with a lacrosse ball against the wall, with your arm behind your back, gives broad but very deep pressure (see Figure 6.27).

The condition known as "trigger finger," where a finger becomes locked in the flexed position, can sometimes be helped by deep massage to a tender spot on the palm side of the knuckle where the finger joins the hand. Trigger finger can occur in any finger and even in the thumb. It may be due to the flexor tendon becoming stuck within its sheath. According to Travell and Simons, trigger finger can be "promptly and permanently" eliminated by a single procaine injection (1999, 769).

Pronator Teres and Pronator Quadratus

The *pronator teres* (PRO-nay-tur TEHR-eez) attaches to the top of the ulna and the medial epicondyle and then runs diagonally across the inner forearm to attach about halfway down the radius (Figure 6.33). A companion muscle, the *pronator quadratus* (PRO-nay- tur qua-DRAY-tus), connects the radius to the ulna at the wrist. The action of the pronators rotates the radius around the ulna, bringing the hand into a palm-down position, a movement called "pronation." The opposite

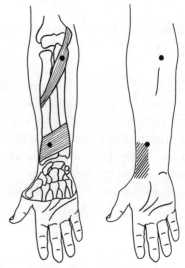

Figure 6.33 Pronator teres and pronator quadratus trigger points and referred pain pattern

action is supination, which turns the palm up. (Supination is accomplished by the supinator and the biceps.) Trigger points in the pronators send pain to a large area on the thumb side of the wrist. Pain may extend into the base of the thumb and up the inner forearm (not shown) (1999, 754, 757). Pronator teres trigger points can cause the muscle to squeeze the median nerve. The resulting numbness in the hand can be falsely attributed to carpal tunnel syndrome.

Any sport or job that requires strong repetitive pronation will overtire the pronator muscles and set up trigger points. In tennis, for example, the hand must pronate strongly when the wrist is used to put topspin on the ball with

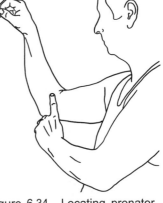

Figure 6.34 Locating pronator teres by isolated contraction

the forehand stroke. Loosening screws with a screwdriver in the right hand requires strong action by the pronators. With the screwdriver in the left hand, the pronators are active in tightening screws.

To find the pronator teres muscle, pronate the hand: turn it over hard, palm down, as far as it will go. Locate the muscle by feeling it bulge up as it contracts, just down from the inner elbow (Figure 6.34). To find the belly of the pronator quadratus, pronate hard while feeling the place on your wrist where you take your pulse (Figure 6.35). The supported thumb works for massaging both muscles. Pronator teres also can be massaged with a ball against the wall with your arm behind you (see Figure 6.27).

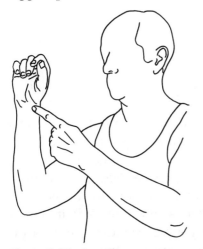

Figure 6.35 Locating pronator quadratus by isolated contraction

Flexor Pollicis Longus

The word *pollicis* (PAH-lih-sis) comes from the Latin for "thumb." The *flexor pollicis longus* attaches to the last segment of the thumb on the surface opposite the nail (under the thumb pad). The other end of this surprisingly large, strong muscle attaches to most of the length of the radius (Figure 6.36). Its action is to bend the thumb toward the palm, an important part of a power grip.

Trigger points in the flexor pollicis longus cause pain and tenderness in the last segment of the thumb. They can make your writing grip feel awkward, weak, or clumsy even in the absence of pain They can cause the last thumb joint to lock or to catch or pop when you bend it (1999, 754, 757).

Locate the belly of the flexor pollicis longus about a third of the way up from the wrist on the radial side

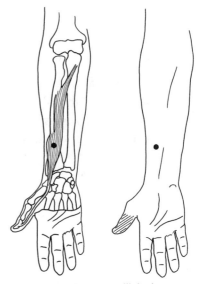

Figure 6.36 Flexor pollicis longus trigger point and referred pain pattern

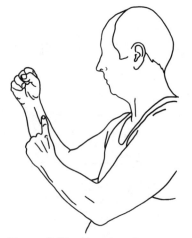

Figure 6.37 Locating flexor pollicis by isolated contraction

(thumb side) of the inner forearm. Feel the muscle contract when you make a hard fist, pressing strongly with your thumb against the middle finger (Figure 6.37). Execute massage against the radius with a supported thumb or with a lacrosse ball against a wall with your arm behind you. Because of the varying length of the fibers in this muscle, there may be several trigger points all along the radius.

Muscles of the Hand

When people have pain, numbness, and other symptoms in their hands, only three possible causes generally come to mind: arthritis, tendinitis, and carpal tunnel syndrome. If any of these are your guess, suspend final judgment until you've checked for trigger points. And look first in distant places. When you're troubleshooting hand symptoms, leave the examination of the hands themselves until last. Deactivation of trigger points in your forearms and at sites further away will very possibly solve the problem. Always use the Trigger Point Guide at the beginning of this chapter to organize your search. After you've excluded referral from other places, symptoms that remain in the hands will be easy to figure out and treatment is straightforward.

There are eighteen muscles in the hand. The four largest operate the thumb. Three modest sized muscles operate the little finger. Four tiny ones in the palm, the lumbricals, help control the tendons. The remaining seven are the interosseous muscles between the bones in the hand. Only tendons are found in the fingers themselves.

Opponens Pollicis

Three of the four short thumb muscles make up the ball of the thumb. The *opponens pollicis* (uh-POH-nenz PAH-lih-sis) will stand for all three to simplify the discussion, since the *flexor pollicis brevis* and *adductor pollicis brevis* overlie the opponens pollicis and the trigger points of all three muscles effectively coincide. Their patterns of referred pain are also similar. All three muscles attach to the thumb bones and to the carpal and metacarpal bones of the hand and wrist (Figure 6.38). The opponens and the flexor move the thumb toward the fingers. The adductor moves the thumb away from the fingers.

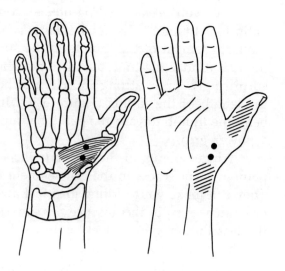

Figure 6.38 Opponens pollicis trigger points and referred pain pattern

Three longer thumb muscles are hidden away in the lower forearm under the mass of extensor tendons. They have the less stressful job of moving the thumb away from the fingers and are rarely afflicted with trigger points.

Trigger points in the opponens pollicis and its companions send pain to the radial side (the thumb side) of the inner wrist, making it feel like you've

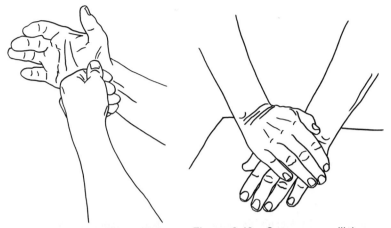

Figure 6.39 Opponens pollicis massage with supported thumb

Figure 6.40 Opponens pollicis massage with 35 mm high bounce ball on tabletop. (The ball is on the table beneath the hands.)

sprained your wrist. They also refer pain to the side of the thumb. They make your pincer grip (the grip between your thumb and fingertips) feel awkward. As a consequence, it may be difficult to write with a pen or pencil or do fine manipulations with your hands (1999, 774–777).

The thumb can be overworked in such mundane activities as weeding the yard, sewing, doing needlepoint, writing with a pen, or playing a musical instrument, and in all craft work and many jobs in industry. Many massage therapists have to quit the profession and seek another way to make a living because of thumbs crippled by overuse.

Search for trigger points all over the fleshy base of the thumb. There are usually more than one. Use a supported thumb for massage, resting the hand on your thigh or your desk for support (Figure 6.39). To give the supported thumb a break, use the Knobble, keeping a layer of cloth between this tool and the flesh. The safest and most efficient way to massage the ball of the thumb may be to roll it back and forth over a small, hard rubber ball on the top of a table or desk (Figure 6.40).

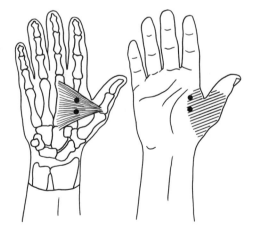

Figure 6.41 Adductor pollicis trigger points and referred pain pattern

Adductor Pollicis

The *adductor pollicis* (uh-DUK-tur PAH-lih-sis) is the fourth short thumb muscle. It makes up part of the web (the fan of flesh between your thumb and the side of your hand) and attaches to the first and third metacarpal bones (Figure 6.41). Its job is to move the thumb across the hand. To verify its location, place a finger of the opposite hand on the adductor pollicis as shown in Figure 6.42. You should feel the muscle contract when you squeeze the thumb against the base of the index finger. This will give you an idea of how it participates in the grasping function of the thumb.

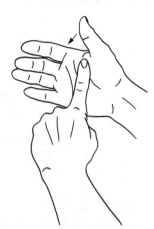 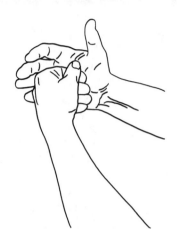

Figure 6.42   Locating adductor pollicis. To feel the muscle contract, press the thumb against the side of the index finger.

Figure 6.43   Adductor pollicis massage with supported thumb

Trigger points in the adductor pollicis refer pain to the base of the thumb; they refer very little pain to the web. Keep in mind that pain can also be referred to both the web and the base of the thumb by the scalenes, brachialis, extensor carpi radialis longus, supinator, and brachioradialis (1999: 774).

Adductor pollicis trigger points can be worked by pinching the web. A less tiring massage technique employs a supported thumb to press the adductor pollicis against the index finger's metacarpal bone in the hand (Figure 6.43). There can be more than one trigger point in this large, thick muscle.

Interosseous Muscles

The *interosseous* (in-tur-AW-see-us) muscles fill the space between the four metacarpal bones in the hand (Figure 6.44). Note that these small muscles occupy only the half of the hand nearest the fingers. The heel of the hand is filled with carpal bones. There are two sets of interosseous muscles. The four *dorsal interosseous* are accessible from the back of the hand. They move the index, fourth, and fifth fingers away from the middle finger and move the middle finger from side to side. The three *palmar interosseous* muscles are accessible through the palm. They bring the fingers together by moving the index, fourth, and fifth fingers toward the middle finger. All seven interosseous muscles have a role in the grasping function and in the many subtle manipulations of the fingers and hand.

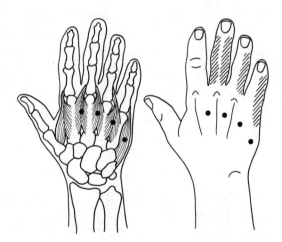

Figure 6.44   Dorsal interosseous trigger points and referred pain pattern

Trigger points in the interosseous muscles refer pain to the sides and undersides of the fingers and the last finger joints. They contribute to finger stiffness, weakness, and awkwardness. Interosseous muscles can cause numbness in the fingers when they compress the digital nerves, which also lie between the metacarpal bones. The digital nerves are sensory nerves for the fingers (1999, 786–788).

The bulky, highly developed *first dorsal interosseous* muscle makes up most of the web between the index finger and thumb (Figure 6.45). Its trigger points have a much wider referral pattern, sending pain to the palm, the little finger, the back of the hand, and all surfaces of the index finger. They frequently refer a deep ache to the entire ulnar (pinky side) side of the hand. To locate the first dorsal interosseous muscle, see and feel it bulge up as you press the index finger against the thumb (Figure 6.46).

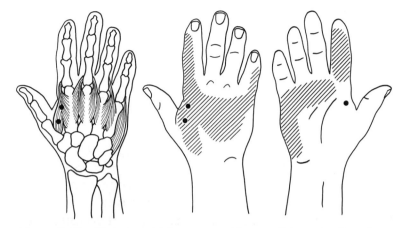

Figure 6.45   First dorsal interosseous trigger points and referred pain pattern

If writing with a pen or pencil gives you pain in the underside of your middle finger and its last knuckle, look for a trigger point in the second dorsal interosseous muscle, between the metacarpals of the index and middle fingers. This muscle helps the middle finger push against the thumb to grip the pen between them. Fixing writer's cramp is often only a matter of finding the hand muscles that have the trigger points. The short thumb muscles and the first dorsal interosseous are the usual source of writer's cramp, but don't overlook the others.

The interosseous muscle of the little finger is located on the outer edge of the hand. Trigger points in this muscle can refer pain to the little finger but aren't usually the source of pain in the edge of the hand. Keep in mind that pain can be sent to the fourth and fifth fingers by many muscles, including the serratus posterior superior, serratus anterior, latissimus dorsi, pectoralis major and minor, extensor carpi ulnaris, flexor carpi ulnaris, and triceps. Numbness in these two fingers and in the ulnar side of the hand comes from the flexor carpi ulnaris, pectoralis minor, triceps, teres minor, and scalenes (1999, 794).

Heberden's nodes, bumps on the sides of the last knuckles, are thought to originate with trigger points in overused interosseous muscles. Bumps on the middle knuckles are called *Bouchard's nodes*. It may be possible to eliminate both kinds of nodes by trigger point therapy to the interosseous muscles, if intervention comes early enough. Even if fully developed, nodes can often be reduced. The same stresses in the interosseous muscles that create nodes on the knuckles may contribute to the development of arthritis (1999, 786-792).

Players of musical instruments like the piano, violin, or guitar, who must often spread their fingers to extreme positions to reach notes, are especially prone to overuse of the interosseous muscles. Repetitive powerful gripping with the fingers on the job or in a sports activity also risks overloading these small muscles.

Your computer mouse puts both the first dorsal and first palmar interosseous muscles at extreme high risk of overuse if you use your index finger to click the buttons. The mouse also predictably overworks the extensor indicis and part of the extensor digitorum, which work together to lift the finger between downstrokes. If you position your mouse to the side of your keyboard, you're likely to create trigger points in your infraspinatus, teres minor, trapezius,

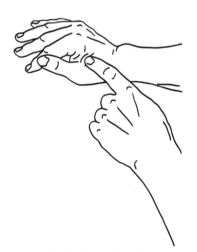

Figure 6.46   Locating first dorsal interosseous by isolated contraction

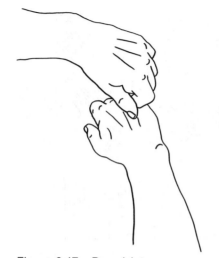

Figure 6.47   Dorsal interosseous massage with supported thumb

rhomboid, and anterior deltoid muscles because of the continuous outward rotation and forward flexion of the arm. A good solution to the mouse problem may be an ergonomic keyboard with a built-in touchpad mouse. Some laptops have a touchpad centered in front of the keys, which is an excellent way to take the strain off many muscles.

The tip of a supported thumb can be used to massage the interosseous muscles (Figure 6.47). Deeper massage can be done with a wedge-shaped rubber eraser, held in a small spring clamp to save your fingers. Figures 6.48 and 6.49 show two different kinds of erasers that can be found everywhere. One is a big pink eraser; the other fits over the end of a shortened pencil, which is then gripped in the clamp. The inexpensive plastic spring clamp shown in the illustrations can be found at many variety, department, and hardware stores.

Massage the thick first dorsal interosseous by pressing it against the metacarpal bone with the supported thumb (Figure 6.50). It works well to massage this muscle by pinching the web, but it can be extremely tiring for the thumb muscles of the hand doing the massage.

Trouble with the interosseous muscles can be difficult to resolve. They're not easy to massage and your activities may be keeping them under continuous stress. Give serious thought to changes you can make in the way you use your hands that will give these special muscles a break. You may even want to think about a job change. In severe cases, the only solution may be to have your trigger points injected by a physician in the approved Travell and Simons manner.

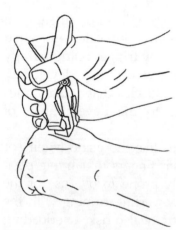

Fig. 6.48   Eraser massage of interosseous

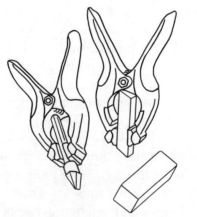

Fig. 6.49   Spring clamps and erasers for massage of interosseous muscles

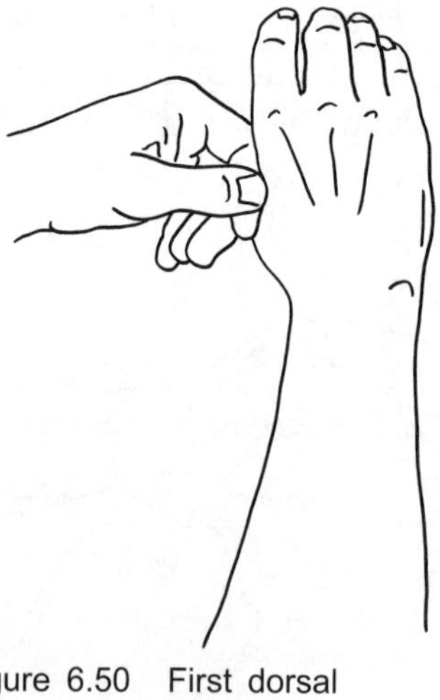

Figure 6.50   First dorsal interosseous massage with supported thumb

CHAPTER 7

Chest, Abdominal, and Genital Pain

Trigger Point Guide:
Chest, Abdominal, and Genital Pain

Chest Pain
    pectoralis major (134)
    pectoralis minor (139)
    scalenes (78)
    sternocleidomastoid (51)
    sternalis (138)
    intercostals (144)
    superficial spinal muscles (165)
    subclavius (137)
    rectus abdominis (146)
    diaphragm (144)

Side Pain
    serratus anterior (141)
    abdominal obliques (146)
    intercostals (144)
    latissimus dorsi (98)
    diaphragm (144)

Abdominal Pain
    rectus abdominis (146)
    abdominal obliques (146)
    superficial spinal muscles (165)
    deep spinal muscles (162)
    quadratus lumborum (169)

Genital Pain (Both Genders)
    rectus abdominis (146)
    abdominal obliques (146)
    intrapelvic muscles (155)
    adductor magnus (207)
    psoas (151)
    piriformis (180)
    bulbospongiosus (156)

Massage Guidelines at a Glance

1. Use a tool if possible and save your hands.

2. Use deep stroking massage, not static pressure.

3. Massage with short, repeated strokes.

4. Do the massage stroke in one direction only.

5. Do the massage stroke slowly.

6. Aim at a pain level of seven on a scale of one to ten.

7. Limit massage to six to twelve strokes per trigger point.

8. Work a trigger point three to six times per day.

9. If you get no relief, you may be working the wrong spot.

Trigger Point Guide
Chest, Abdominal, and Genital Pain

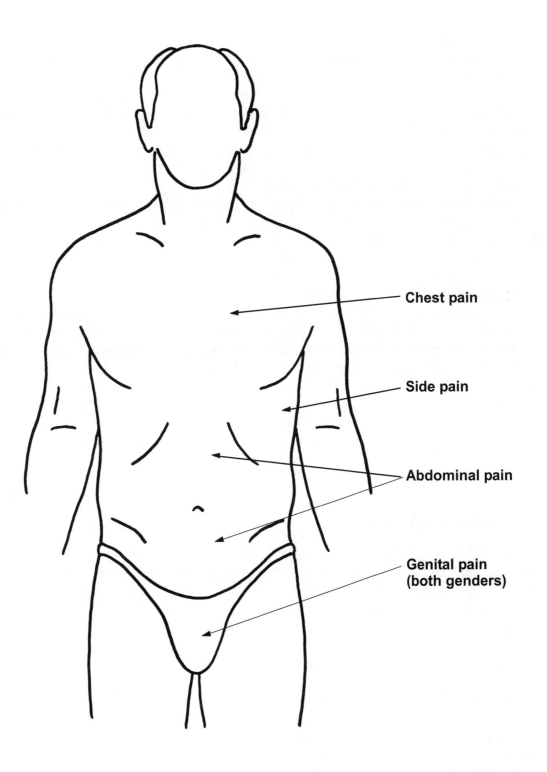

Chest pain

Side pain

Abdominal pain

Genital pain
(both genders)

Chest, Abdominal, and Genital Pain

Symptoms from trigger points in chest and abdominal muscles may be subject to more misdiagnosis and misdirected treatment than those in any other part of the body. This is especially regrettable because the solutions are so simple when trigger points are to blame. Trigger point therapy is the appropriate treatment for many kinds of symptoms in the chest, back, side, stomach, shoulder, arm, and hand that originate in chest and abdominal muscles (Travell and Simons 1999, 830–833, 848–851, 875–879, 894, 905, 951–959).

Trigger points in chest muscles can cause distortions of your posture that promote shallow breathing and shortness of breath. Tenderness, pain, and breathing difficulties caused by these trigger points are often mistaken for symptoms of emphysema, hiatal hernia, or lung disease. Pectoral trigger points can cause back pain, heart arrhythmia, and false heart pain. They may contribute to development of a dowager's hump. Their indirect effects on neck and upper back muscles sponsor headaches, jaw pain, and other symptoms of the head, face, and neck. The numbness they cause in hands and fingers often leads to false diagnoses of carpal tunnel syndrome (1999, 830-833).

Abdominal trigger points cause heartburn, menstrual pain, false appendicitis, diarrhea, nausea, vomiting, food intolerance, bloating, and gas. They commonly produce pain and other false symptoms in the esophagus, kidneys, bladder, colon, and other internal organs, including bogus heart attacks. Colic in babies and stomachaches in both children and adults can be produced by abdominal trigger points. They're even thought to cause bed-wetting in older children (1999, 940–945, 956–959).

Myofascial pain from lower abdominal and intrapelvic trigger points is commonly felt in the groin, rectum, ovaries, uterus, vagina, penis, and testes, resulting in much needless worry and discomfort. Prostate symptoms and impotence in males from the effects of intrapelvic trigger points is not unusual. Painful intercourse for both sexes can have the same source (1992, 118–121).

Mistaken conclusions regarding many of these symptoms can lead to unnecessary surgery and hugely wasteful payments by health-care insurers and by the uninsured. When any of these symptoms are caused by myofascial trigger points, all but those inside the pelvis are easily self-treatable.

Pectoralis Major

The *pectoralis* (pek-tur-AH-liss) *major* muscles are the muscular part of the breasts in both men and women. *Pectoralis* comes from *pectus*, Latin for "breast." *Major* means it's the largest of the four pectoral muscles.

Symptoms

Pain from pectoralis major trigger points may be felt in the chest and the front of the shoulder; down the inner arm, the inner elbow, and the ulnar side of the hand; and into the fourth and fifth fingers. The exact location of the pain depends on the location of the trigger point in several sections of this complex muscle. A trigger point in the lower border of the pectoralis major can cause an irregular heartbeat. You might think a trigger point affecting the heart would be on the left side, nearer to the heart, but this arrhythmia trigger point occurs only on the right. The pattern of pain referred from the pectoralis major and other pectoral muscles can be frighteningly like the pain of a heart attack. Confusion regarding chest pain is compounded by the fact that genuine heart disease can set up trigger points in the pectoral muscles. Long after an afflicted heart has recovered you can still have severe chest pain that in reality is coming not from the heart but from the muscles of the chest (1999, 819–821).

Anna, age seventy-three, an unknowing victim of pectoral trigger points, strapped on a TENS unit every day for her chronic mid back pain. Unable to wear the unit at night, she regularly had to take a pain pill to enable her to sleep. Trigger points had shortened her pectoral muscles to such an extent that she couldn't pull her shoulders back to stand up straight. After her first massage she was able to go to sleep without taking her pain medication for the first time in years. Though she's never eager to massage her own pectoral muscles, which are still very tender, her back always feels better when she does.

Tightness from trigger points in the pectoralis major keeps the shoulder pulled forward, making it difficult to reach back and putting a constant strain on the upper back muscles. This round-shouldered posture also causes the head and neck to be constantly projected forward, which sponsors trigger points in the sternocleidomastoid and scalene muscles. This can make the pectoralis major indirectly the ultimate source of the many symptoms that come from these two troublesome muscles. The overload imposed on shoulder and upper back muscles by a shortened pectoralis major can lead to the development of secondary trigger points throughout the region, progressively limiting movement of the arm and ending in a frozen shoulder (1999, 833).

The round-shouldered posture fostered by pectoral trigger points can have many unanticipated effects, including excessive pressure on spinal disks, compression of nerves, jaw problems, restricted breathing, chronic fatigue, neck pain, and headaches (1999, 809).

Unfortunately, attempts to force a correction of your posture generally fail unless you first find and deactivate the specific trigger points that are keeping the pectoral muscles tight. Efforts to stretch these sensitive muscles without releasing their trigger points can make all your symptoms worse. After the trigger points are gone, stretching and postural retraining are quite appropriate and can be expected to have a beneficial effect.

When your muscles are limber, pain free, and responsive, the best posture is attained simply by raising the crown of your head and standing tall. In the absence of pectoral trigger points, your shoulders will find their own good place. Never aim at keeping your shoulders back in a soldierly stance, which is neither normal nor healthy (1999, 809–810, 833).

Causes

There are three distinct sections of the pectoralis major. The clavicular (upper) section attaches to the collarbone, the sternal (middle) section to the breastbone, and the costal (lower) section to the ribs and stomach muscles. All come together to attach to the front of the humerus. These attachments allow the pectoralis major to rotate the arm inward and to pull it across the chest. The upper section also helps raise the arm; the lower section helps pull the arm and shoulder down. In vigorous sports activities and many kinds of work, the pectoralis major can be overused by any of these movements done with excessive force or repetition.

Carrying a heavy backpack can be a contributing cause, or possibly the sole cause, of trigger points in muscles of the chest, abdomen, upper back, and neck. Tune in to any muscle tension you feel when you have the backpack on. Having to walk with your head and body thrust forward to balance the weight of a backpack should give you a clue to the strain it imposes. Part of your trigger point therapy should be to figure out how to lighten your load or find another way to carry it (1999, 847–953).

Treatment

In men, the pectoralis major is directly accessible through the skin. In women, the upper half is similarly accessible, but the lower half must be approached through breast tissue or by moving the breast aside as much as possible.

Trigger points will be found in four areas of the pectoralis major. You can locate them by distinguishing their different patterns of pain. Trigger points in the clavicular section send pain to the front of the shoulder (Figure 7.1). Trigger points in the sternal section refer pain to the inner arm and the inner elbow (Figure 7.2). They also cause pain in the central part of the pectoralis major muscle itself. Sensitivity in the nipple and pain in the breast comes from trigger points in the thick lateral border of the muscle (Figure 7.3) (1999, 819–821; Long 1956, 102–106).

The trigger point for a fluttery kind of heart arrhythmia is found between the ribs, a couple of inches to the right of the end of the breastbone (Figure 7.4). Pressing on this one is sharply painful, but the heart rhythm straightens out right away if the trigger point is to blame. Massage the arrhythmia trigger point with the fingertips. The trigger point can be difficult to resolve if emphysema engages you in a constant battle to expel your breath (1999, 838).

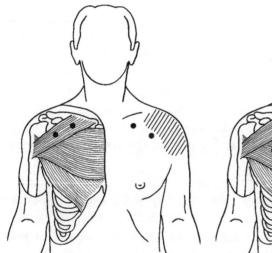

Figure 7.1   Pectoralis major, clavicular section: trigger points and referred pain pattern

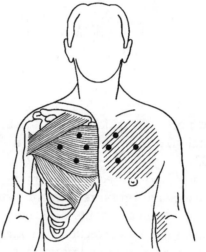

Figure 7.2   Pectoralis major, sternal section: trigger points and referred pain pattern

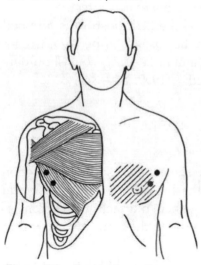

Figure 7.3   Pectoralis major, costal section: trigger points and referred pain pattern

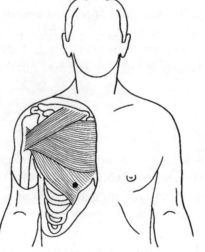

Figure 7.4   Pectoralis major, arrhythmia trigger point

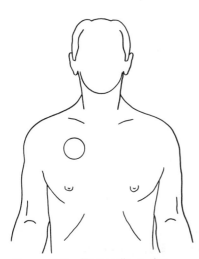
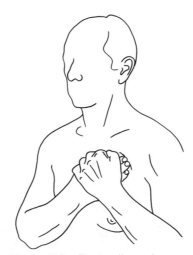

Figure 7.5   Pectoralis major massage with ball against the wall

Figure 7.6   Pectoralis major massage with supported fingers

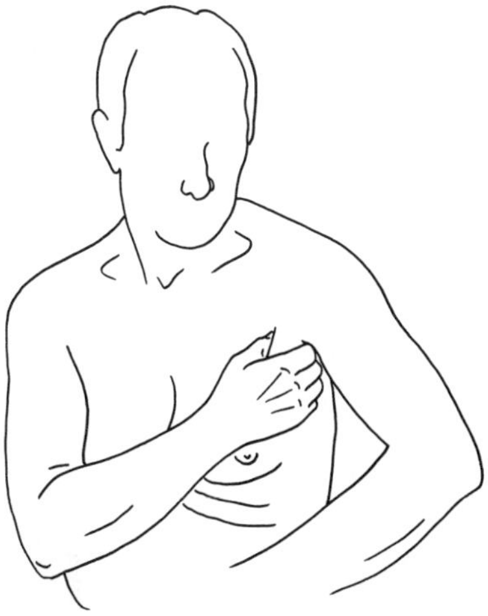

Figure 7.7   Pectoralis major massage of lateral border

Massage with a tennis ball against a wall is very effective for the entire pectoral region (Figure 7.5). Some like the Thera Cane for this and supported fingers also work very well (Figure 7.6). Save your fingers by exerting most of the pressure with the supporting hand. Use short, slow, repeated strokes. For very specific massage of trigger points in the lateral border of the pectoralis major, you'll have to use your fingers and thumb (Figure 7.7).

Don't let large breasts be an impediment to massage: lying on your back will let gravity move both breasts aside, allowing you access to broad areas of the pectoralis muscles that they normally cover. Gravity will also aid you if you lie on one side and then the other to massage the lateral (outer) borders. Large-breasted women are usually well aware of the connection between the weight of their breasts and the aching in their upper back, but they are often unaware of the strain heavy breasts can place on their pectoral muscles.

Pain in or around the breasts can be a serious cause of concern for women, because it naturally arouses fears of breast cancer. Great efforts are being made by health-care agencies to get women to do regular self-examinations in order to familiarize themselves with the natural state of breast tissue and to learn to recognize changes that may represent potential tumor growth. However, physicians, and others who monitor women's health, believe that most women don't do self-examinations, either because they're terrified at the thought of what they might find or because they don't clearly understand what they're looking for (Hackett 2000).

This is very unfortunate, because the breast self-exam is an ideal time to learn to distinguish among normal and abnormal lumps in breast tissue and the sometimes lumplike trigger points in the underlying muscles. Very often, pain in the breast area is nothing more serious than pain from trigger points in the chest muscles. A breast self-exam, if done thoroughly and with attention to possible trigger points, should allay fear, not increase it. Working with a doctor or nurse who understands both myofascial pain and the anatomy of the breast itself can be enormously helpful (Hackett 2000).

Subclavius

The *subclavius* (sub-CLAY-vee-us) muscles lie just under the clavicles, or collarbones. They attach to the middle of the collarbones and to the ends of the first ribs near where they

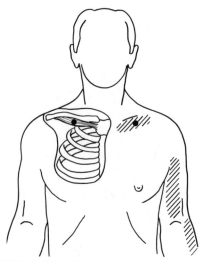

Figure 7.8   Subclavius trigger points and referred pain pattern

join the sternum, or breastbone. The specific function of the subclavius muscles has not been established, but they're most likely to be overworked by the same actions that overwork the pectoral muscles.

Considering their small size, the subclavius muscles have a disproportionately widespread referred pain pattern (Figure 7.8). Subclavius trigger points cause pain just below the collarbone. They also send pain to the biceps and the radial side (thumb side) of the forearm. Sometimes they cause pain in the thumb side of the hand, the thumb, and the index and middle fingers (not shown). When trigger points shorten a subclavius muscle, it can keep tension on the collarbone, squeezing the subclavian vein and artery against the first rib and restricting circulation in the arm and hand (1999, 821, 830).

You won't be able to feel the subclavius directly, hidden as it is behind the clavicular section of the pectoralis major. Search for the exquisite tenderness of its trigger point just below the middle of the collarbone. Supported fingers make an ideal massage tool here.

Sternalis

Sternalis (stern-AH-liss) muscles are present in only about 5 percent of the population and have no obvious function. When present, their configuration is quite variable. You may have a sternalis on only one side. If you have both, they may overlap or cover the breastbone. Sternalis muscles can be thin or thick. Their name derives from the muscles' location, right alongside the sternum (1999, 857-860).

Pain caused by sternalis trigger points is felt strongly in the center of the chest (Figure 7.9). Lesser pain may radiate across the chest, the front of the shoulder and down the inner side of the upper arm (not shown). Trigger points high up in the sternalis near the lower end of the sternocleidomastoid muscles may promote a dry, hacking cough. These symptoms are easily misinterpreted and can result in unneeded treatment for heart disease, lung disease, bronchitis, or sinus infection. It's so easy to check for sternalis trigger points that it's a shame they'd ever be missed. Awareness of them would have saved one woman a great amount of worry.

Angela, age fifty, a registered nurse, weighed 240 pounds, almost twice her ideal weight at her height of five feet, four inches. Although she had chronic pain in several places, her recent unexplained "heart scare" concerned her the most. "I went to the emergency room in the middle of the night with horrible pain in the center of my chest. It had all the signs of a typical heart attack, but none of the tests showed anything. I'm supposedly all right, although anybody

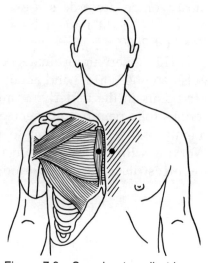

Figure 7.9   Sample sternalis trigger points and referred pain pattern

can see I'm at risk of heart disease with this weight problem. I was really pretty scared."

Trigger points in all Angela's pectoral muscles, including both sternalis muscles, were so bad that she winced and held her breath with the lightest touch. She was surprised. "I've had a lot of bodywork," she said, "but nobody's ever checked my front." Her trigger points were bad enough to have caused her terrifying chest pain, although she still had reason enough to be concerned about her heart. Lying on her back, she found self-applied trigger point massage easy to do, despite her heavy breasts, and felt better equipped to cope with such an event the next time.

Trigger points in the sternalis, when the muscle exists, may come about in association with trigger points in the pectoralis major or sternocleidomastoid muscles. Unsuspected trigger points in the sternalis can be to blame for pain that persists after a heart attack. To find sternalis trigger points, search along the full length of the breastbone on both sides, using supported fingers (1999, 859–860; Epstein, Gerber, and Borer 1979, 2793–2797).

Pectoralis Minor

The *pectoralis minor* (pek-tur-AH-liss) muscle lies completely hidden under the pectoralis major and has a different orientation and very different attachments. Though generally a smaller muscle, it can still be very strong and thick. The pectoralis minor attaches at its upper end to the coracoid process, an odd little piece of the shoulder blade that sticks through to the front of the shoulder (see Figure 5.8). With your arm at rest in your lap, you can feel the coracoid process as a hard roundness, something like a marble under the skin, just below your collarbone right next to the ball of your shoulder (the head of the humerus).

The other end of the muscle divides into three or more sections, which attach to individual ribs in the center of the breast area. The action of the pectoralis minor is to pull down on the coracoid process to fix the shoulder blade in place for various operations of the arm. A secondary function is to pull up on the ribs to assist expansion of the chest during forced breathing, such as in vigorous sports activity.

Trigger points in the pectoralis minor cause symptoms similar to those of pectoralis major trigger points, but a troubled pectoralis minor can have peculiar effects all its own, as illustrated by Aaron's case.

Aaron, age fifty-two, an executive with an automobile company, had had recurrent pain in the front of his left shoulder ever since he'd "messed it up" in a volleyball game ten years earlier. He also had numb fingers most of the time. "Man, I've tried everything, including a lot of physical therapy, but it just doesn't go away." In an effort to strengthen his shoulder, Aaron had been doing hydroaerobics in the pool at the YMCA. So far, it had only made the pain worse.

Active trigger points were found in Aaron's scalene and pectoralis minor muscles. All were far more tender on the left side than on the right. Pressure on his left pectoralis minor accentuated the pain in the front of his shoulder and the numbness in his hand. He could hardly believe that the problem and its solution were so simple. After a single professional massage and instruction in self-applied massage, Aaron got rid of his chronic, long-term pain and numbness in less than three weeks.

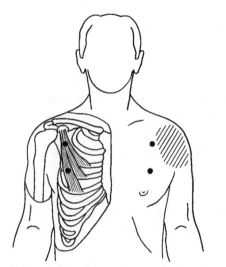

Figure 7.10   Pectoralis minor trigger points and referred pain pattern

Symptoms

The referred pain pattern for the pectoralis minor is nearly the same as for the clavicular section of the pectoralis major, being felt primarily in the front of the shoulder (Figure 7.10). Pain sometimes spills over to the entire breast area and the inner arm, inner elbow, ulnar (pinky) side of the hand, and third, fourth, and fifth fingers (not shown). As with trigger point symptoms in other pectoral muscles, this distribution of pain can be mistaken for signs of heart disease (1999, 844–852).

Tightness from trigger points often causes the pectoralis minor muscle to compress the axillary artery and the brachial nerves, which go to the arm and which are major neurovascular pathways. Blood flow to the arm and hand can be restricted in this manner by the pectoralis minor, even to the point of making the pulse at the wrist hard to detect. Swelling in the hand and fingers, however, is not a symptom of pectoralis minor trigger points, but is caused rather by tight scalenes compressing the axillary vein, which runs under the scalenes but not under the pectoralis minor (1999, 847–851; Rubin 1981, 107–110).

Numbness in the forearm, hand, or fingers caused by a taut pectoralis minor squeezing the brachial nerves may be misdiagnosed as carpal tunnel syndrome or peripheral neuropathy. Recall that the scalenes provoke similar numbness and a similar misinterpretation. Pain from the scalenes is often sent to the chest, to the exact location of the pectoralis minor, and can be one reason for development of its trigger points (1999, 848–851).

The round-shouldered posture imposed by shortened pectoralis minor muscles can cause an ache in the mid back due to strain on the lower trapezius muscles. Excess tension in the pectoralis minor pulls the shoulder blade forward and causes it to stick out in back. This "winging" of the shoulder blade is made worse when the lower trapezius is weakened by trigger points and can't resist the pull of the pectoralis minor. This tightness in the pectoralis minor also restricts movement of the shoulder blade on the chest wall. As a consequence, it may be difficult to raise your arm above your head or reach for something behind you. Attempts at therapeutic stretching of the pectoralis minor are not advisable because of the stress placed on its vulnerable attachments (1999, 852; Lewit 1991, 198–199).

Causes

Hyperventilation or a tendency to do chest breathing can seriously overtax the pectoralis minor, as can a chronic cough. Whiplash injuries can overstretch the pectoralis minor muscles and set up trigger points. Pressure from the straps of a backpack or a heavy purse can cause them by cutting off circulation. Repetitive, forceful, downward motions of the arms in sports or in the workplace can wear these muscles out and promote trigger points. As with the pectoralis major, an habitually slumped, round-shouldered, head-forward posture can also set up trigger points in the pectoralis minor and make them very persistent.

If you have recurrent trouble with your pectoralis minor muscles, start watching for circumstances that tend to cause or perpetuate their trigger points. Under stress, you may be unconsciously holding your breath, hyperventilating, or breathing very shallowly with your chest and not your abdomen. A hunched posture could be keeping the chest muscles shortened and tight.

Heavy lifting will get you in trouble with the pectoralis minor, just as with the scalenes. Working for long periods with your arms out in front of you or up overhead will do the same. Together, trigger points in the scalenes and pectoralis minor cause much of the pain, numbness, tingling, and so on that occur in the arms and hands. Check regularly for trigger points in both the pectoralis minor muscles and the scalenes. It takes only a second or two. These muscles shouldn't hurt when you touch them; tenderness indicates latent trigger points that can be activated by the least abuse.

Treatment

You can locate the pectoralis minor by feeling it bulge up when it contracts. To make the pectoralis minor contract without contracting the pectoralis major, put your hand behind your back, then push back with your hand against a wall or the back of your chair. While doing this, put your other hand on your chest as you would for the pledge of allegiance; your fingertips will then be in the right position to feel the pectoralis minor contract (Figure 7.11).

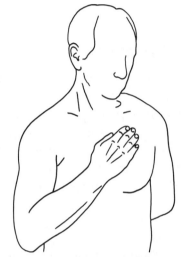

Figure 7.11 Locating pectoralis minor. The hand behind the back is pushing against the wall.

There may be more than one trigger point in pectoralis minor muscles because of the varying length of muscle fibers in the different heads. Execute massage with supported fingers, beginning at the coracoid process and pulling downward on a diagonal line across the chest with very slow, deep, short strokes (see Figure 7.6). The fingertips of the hand opposite to the side you're massaging will be on the trigger points. The supporting hand helps exert pressure. Pectoralis minor muscles are normally high enough on the chest to not be hidden by heavy breasts. If breast tissue is in the way, just lie down to do the massage, as described for the pectoralis major muscles.

Better for the fingers is a tennis ball against the wall. If your nose bumps into the wall, try the technique next to a doorway, letting your head hang through the opening. A Knobble will also save your fingers, as will supported knuckles. Be sure to go clear to the edges of your chest: the area covered by the pectoral muscles is quite large, even on a small person.

Serratus Anterior

Although the *serratus* (seh-RAY-tus) *anterior* is located under the arm, it's actually a shoulder muscle. The muscle's attachments to your ribs and to the inner border of the shoulder blade give it leverage for rotating the shoulder blade so that the socket of the shoulder joint faces more in an upward direction, allowing you to raise your arm. Without this ability to reposition the shoulder blade, you wouldn't be able to raise your arm above your head. The serratus anterior muscles also aid inhalation by assisting expansion of the ribs when you need more air than usual. They cause trouble for chest breathers like Judy, who habitually overwork them.

Judy, age twenty-seven, a social worker, got such a sharp pain in her sides when she was under stress that it was almost impossible to breathe. In her job, she was under stress every day. "When I've got that pain, I feel like I can only use about 10 percent of my lung capacity and I have to breathe quicker. I can't climb stairs, I can't move, I can't do anything. It's like I've got a metal band strapped around me. I can't take a deep breath at all, and if I laugh or cough or sneeze, it's just awful. I feel like I can't get enough air. I start getting dizzy. When it gets really bad, I get back spasms, too."

Extremely tender latent trigger points were found in Judy's serratus anterior muscles. She was shown how to do serratus anterior massage with her fingertips when she feels an episode coming on. Even when the attack is severe, she's usually able to get rid of the pain in her sides within a couple of hours. As a preventative measure, she's trying to learn to relax and breathe with her abdomen.

Symptoms

Pain from trigger points in the serratus anterior muscles is usually felt in the side and often in the mid back at the lower end of the shoulder blade (Figures 7.12, 7.13, and 7.14). Sometimes pain spills over to the inner side of the arm and forearm and to the pinky side of the hand (not shown). This pain pattern can suggest lung disease or a heart attack, and its true source can remain a mystery unless you're wise to myofascial pain (1999, 887–892).

With serratus anterior trigger points, you can't take a deep breath without pain, nor can you exhale completely. Diaphragmatic breathing hurts, so you're limited to shallow chest breathing. A troubled serratus anterior can be a cause of the painful "stitch in the side" so familiar to runners. Side stitch can also come from diaphragm or intercostal trigger points. Tightness in the serratus anterior muscles makes it hard to reach back behind yourself or pull your shoulders back. The pull on your ribs can make your breasts feel abnormally sensitive. Serratus anterior trigger points can add to pain associated with a heart attack (1999, 887–892).

Emphysema isn't thought to promote trigger points in the serratus anterior, but when trigger points are present for other reasons, they can add significantly to the pain felt by emphysema sufferers and to their difficulty in expelling air. When the serratus anterior is in trouble, additional stress is put on the scalene, sternocleidomastoid, and serratus posterior muscles, all of which aid in forced breathing. This can result in a growing cascade of symptoms, from headaches and jaw pain to dizziness and numb hands, making a whole list of mistaken diagnoses possible (1999, 894).

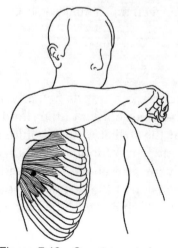

Figure 7.12   Serratus anterior primary trigger point on sixth rib. Trigger points may be in any of the muscle's branches.

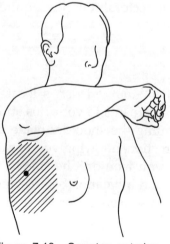

Figure 7.13   Serratus anterior referred pain pattern (side stitch)

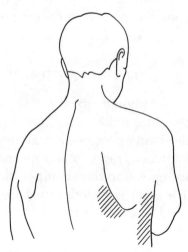

Figure 7.14   Serratus anterior referred pain pattern in the back

Causes

When you need extra breath quickly, as in vigorous sports activity, the serratus anterior muscles assist respiration by pulling on the ribs to expand the chest. For this reason, athletic exertion, especially when you're out of shape, can quickly overtax these muscles. It's usually the amateur or weekend athlete who gets the stitch in the side, not the well-tuned, resilient professional. Since the serratus anterior is so active in movements of the arm and shoulder, it's particularly vulnerable to unaccustomed participation in tennis, swimming, running, chin-ups, push-ups, weight lifting, and workouts on the pommel horse or the rings.

Respiratory illness that involves strenuous coughing can activate trigger points in the serratus anterior muscles. The pain in your sides and back can make you think you're progressing to pleurisy or pneumonia.

Habitual tension and hyperventilation when under emotional duress can activate latent trigger points in serratus anterior muscles. The pain they cause can make you fear the problem is worse than it really is, but if you have the right information, the problem can be remarkably easy to fix. The serratus anterior responds exceptionally well to self-treatment.

Treatment

You can find the primary serratus anterior trigger point on the most prominent rib on your side, three or four inches straight down from your armpit. Generally, this will be the site of greatest tenderness. When this trigger point is very active, you won't like touching it: this one can really hurt. Luckily, it doesn't take much pressure to have an effect. Be aware, however, that trigger points can exist on any of the nine ribs this muscle attaches to. If you have trouble getting rid of the pain in your side, search the whole rib area under the arm, clear up into the armpit. Trigger points in the abdominal obliques that attach to your lowest ribs also cause pain in the side.

Part of the extreme discomfort experienced when you reach into your armpit to massage a subscapularis muscle may come from inadvertently applying pressure to trigger points in nearby parts of the serratus anterior. The back half of the serratus lies between the subscapularis and the ribs. To get the picture, imagine that your shoulder blade and your back ribs are the two slices of bread in a ham and cheese sandwich. Then visualize the subscapularis as the ham and the serratus anterior as the cheese. When your fingers are in the slot in back of your armpit searching for the subscapularis, they are between the ham and the cheese. In this position, your nails contact the subscapularis and the flats of your fingers are on the serratus anterior (see Figure 5.26).

The fingertips can be used for deep stroking massage of serratus anterior muscles (Figure 7.15). To save your fingers, try using a tennis ball against the wall (Figure 7.16). Or just hold the ball in your hand and pull it slowly across the trigger point. Additional pressure can be applied by clamping the ball and the hand against your side with your arm.

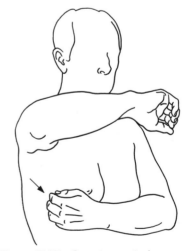

Figure 7.15 Serratus anterior massage using fingertips or tennis ball. The arm is up for clarity. Keep it down for massage.

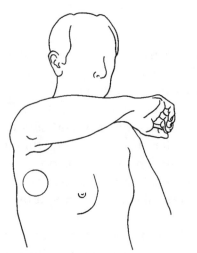

Figure 7.16   Serratus anterior
massage with ball against the wall

Simply being informed about the serratus anterior can keep you out of trouble. Stay alert for early symptoms like the classic sharp stitch in your side when you take a deep breath, or the sense that you can't get enough air. Early intervention with the serratus can stop trouble in its tracks. If you want to avoid trouble in the first place, be mindful of the fact that emotional stress promotes habitual muscle tension, which predisposes serratus anterior muscles to trigger points. Learn to be aware of when you're holding your breath or breathing with your chest. It's also wise to avoid overdoing vigorous athletic activities, especially running, before you're in proper condition. To learn practical ways to reduce habitual muscle tension, read chapter 12.

Diaphragm and Intercostal Muscles

There are a number of muscles that are not treatable with massage, because they are simply too deep inside to be accessible. Muscles inside the chest fall into this class. Luckily, the real troublemakers are on the outside. The *diaphragm* and the *intercostal muscles* are on the borderline. The intercostal muscles are between the ribs and can be massaged with your fingertips. The edge of the diaphragm can be reached under the ribs in front. There's precious little access to these important muscles, but it's enough to do a significant amount of good.

Symptoms

Pain from an intercostal trigger point is usually felt right around the trigger point, although it can refer a short distance toward the front of the body. The pain can be bad enough that you may not be able to turn your body or raise your arm. Trigger points in the diaphragm cause pain under your ribs in front near the diaphragm's attachments behind the bottom ribs (Figure 7.17). Pain typically occurs on exhalation. With trigger points in either the diaphragm or the intercostals, you may experience the same "stitch in the side" and shortness of breath as with the serratus anterior.

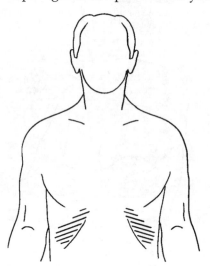

Figure 7.17   Diaphragm referred
pain pattern. Trigger points are
hidden behind the lowest ribs.

Myofascial pain associated with the ribs may be mislabeled "costochondritis," or inflammation of the ribs. You may be told you have a separated rib, ulcers, or gallbladder trouble. Treatment for these conditions is not likely to solve the problem when trigger points are the cause (1999, 862–879).

Causes

The diaphragm is a thin muscle inside the body that separates the organs of the chest from those of the abdomen. It attaches to the inside of the lowest ribs all the way around your body. At rest, the diaphragm has a dome shape, bowing up into the lower chest. When you inhale, the diaphragm contracts and pulls down, flattening out and creating a vacuum in the chest that causes the lungs to inflate. To exhale, ordinarily all you do is relax the diaphragm. When you're breathing heavily, your intercostal muscles are called on to help force the air out. To inhale properly, you have to allow the abdominal organs to move out of the way to make room for the diaphragm to come down. If you strive to keep your stomach flat at all times for the sake of appearances, you unnecessarily hamper the mechanics of natural breathing.

Anxiety, chest breathing, and overexertion in athletics cause trigger points in the diaphragm and the intercostal muscles. Direct trauma or chest surgery can leave the intercostals with trigger points, as can a chronic cough. Any condition that makes you struggle to get your breath can cause trigger points to develop in the diaphragm (1999, 863–864, 875–876; Bonica and Sola 1990, 1114–1133).

Intercostal trigger points can also come from excessive twisting of the body. They may come on after a case of shingles. A slumped posture can foster and perpetuate trigger points in both the diaphragm and the intercostals (1999: 876).

Treatment

As with the serratus anterior, intercostal trigger points derive benefit from only light-pressure massage. That's good, because you won't be able to stand very much pressure when they're at their worst. Use the tips of your fingers and search between the ribs in the area where you have the pain. You may have to work on intercostal trigger points in a number of short sessions over several days to get them under control.

For diaphragm trigger points that are accessible, dig under your bottom ribs in front with your fingers and do as much deep stroking massage as you can manage (Figure 7.18). Your hands and fingers will tire quickly with this, so do short sessions and keep coming back to it. Easier access is gained by pulling the stomach in and exhaling completely. This also stretches the diaphragm, which can be beneficial when done along with the massage. For deepest penetration, sit and lean forward, or lie on your back with your knees up. Any work you do on the diaphragm's peripheral trigger points will benefit any you may have in its unreachable central dome by releasing the general tension on the muscle. Note that taking a deep breath can overcontract your diaphragm, so it's wise to avoid athletics until some progress is made.

A slumped, head-forward posture contributes to problems with the diaphragm and intercostal muscles. Remember, however, that slumped posture may be difficult to correct until trigger points are deactivated in the abdominal and chest muscles. To help all your breathing muscles, learn to breathe with the abdomen instead of the chest. Stop smoking, and take any other action necessary to inhibit chronic coughing.

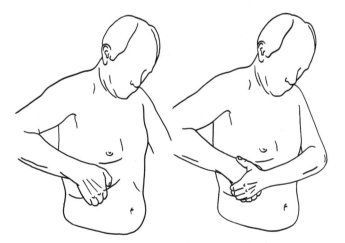

Figure 7.18 Diaphragm massage with supported fingers digging up behind the lowest ribs in front. For deepest penetration, sit and lean forward.

Abdominal Muscles

The abdominal muscles cover the front and sides of the abdomen. The *rectus abdominis*, the vertical central slab of abdominal muscle, attaches to the lower ribs and to the pubic bone. The *abdominal obliques*, the muscles on the sides of the abdomen, attach to the ribs, the rectus abdominis, and the crest of the pelvis. The abdominal obliques are composed of three layers of muscle, each with fibers running at a different angle, like the plies of a tire.

The abdominal muscles function as a unit to arch the body forward, to twist it, or to bend it to the side. They serve as a checkrein when you lean over backward. They help stabilize the spine and support the body during every kind of activity. In both normal and forced breathing, they help expel air from the lungs. Interestingly, their respiratory actions also alternately squeeze and release the large veins in the abdomen, assisting the heart in pumping blood up from the legs. Abdominal muscles also provide the pressure for childbirth, vomiting, urination, and defecation. The extreme exertion of natural childbirth can leave a woman with a belly full of trigger points (1999, 940–959).

Trigger points in the abdominal muscles not only cause pain in the stomach, sides, and back, but also send pain to the organs inside the abdominal cavity and to the sexual organs of both men and women. Travell and Simons call the diverse and often very indirect effects of abdominal trigger points "diagnostically very misleading" (1999, 940). The ways in which abdominal trigger points can mimic other conditions is well illustrated by the following two case histories.

Bruce, age sixty-nine, still active in his hardware business, had severe pain on the left side of his abdomen that felt like it was in his bottom ribs. The pain had started six weeks earlier, just after he began a new set of stomach-strengthening exercises that he'd hoped would help his chronic back pain. He wore a broad elastic back brace and his posture was very stooped and hunched, with rounded shoulders and an upward-tilted pelvis that gave him the shape of a large letter C.

The pain in his ribs increased when he was getting dressed, especially when he lifted his legs to put on his pants. The doctor's opinion was that Bruce had costochondritis, or inflammation of the ribs. "We don't really know what causes it," the doctor said. "All we can do is let the body heal itself. In the meantime, we'll give you a good analgesic to help with the pain." But the pain pills didn't take away very much of Bruce's pain, in either his ribs or his back, and they didn't improve his stooped posture. Disgusted with his doctor and desperate for help, he tried a massage therapist.

Exceptionally painful trigger points were found at several places in Bruce's abdominal muscles, especially where they attached to the ribs. Massage to his abdominals not only eased his rib pain but also diminished the pain in his back. Four weeks later, after daily self-applied massage, he reported that he was able to stand straighter and that the rib pain was completely gone. His back had improved so much from the abdominal massage that he was able to go without the elastic back brace he'd worn for so long.

Gary, age forty-one, an insurance agent, swam and biked regularly to keep himself in shape and to help with his chronic back pain. In the locker room at the Y he confided to a friend that he did stretches constantly, though they didn't really seem to help very much. "What really worries me is this ache I get all the time in one testicle. I seem to get it when my back is acting up. They tell me it's nothing to worry about, but you have to wonder. What if down the road they find out it's cancer?" The friend gave him the name of a massage therapist who had done his own back some good.

Fortunately for Gary, the therapist had recently taken a seminar on myofascial pain where testicular pain, what men call "stone ache," had been discussed. She found an exquisitely tender trigger point on one side of his lower abdominal muscles just above his pubic bone that she felt certain was causing his testicular pain. She found trigger points a little higher in his stomach muscles that her charts indicated could be causing his back pain. She suggested he do self-applied trigger point massage to his stomach muscles before and after his athletic activities, with special attention to the spot just above his groin that she suspected was referring pain to the testicle. Following the therapist's advice, Gary has been able to keep his back pain in check and his "stone ache" has not come back.

Symptoms

Abdominal trigger points cause both external and internal abdominal pain. Pain and other abdominal symptoms are usually assumed to have internal causes, however, and mistaken diagnoses are common. A broad range of medication is prescribed on this basis, with frequently disappointing results. People have been subjected to unnecessary abdominal surgery when myofascial pain has gone unrecognized (1999, 957).

Pain in the upper abdomen from trigger points (Figure 7.19) can be mistaken for heartburn, acid reflux, esophagitis, hiatal hernia, gallstones, stomach cancer, peptic ulcers, heart disease, or simple indigestion. These upper trigger points also cause nausea and projectile vomiting, loss of appetite, and anorexia. There's no way to know whether these symptoms originate in myofascial trigger points or something more serious until any active trigger points have been deactivated. Diagnosis becomes more accurate and treatment of abdominal symptoms becomes more effective when the physician knows about trigger points and can treat them and take them out of the equation (1999, 951–952, 956–957).

Trigger points in the midabdomen (Figure 7.20) can be to blame for colic, stomach cramps, and chronic diarrhea. Excessive gas and a sense of bloating, fullness, swelling, or burning in the abdomen can be due solely to trigger points in the mid and upper abdominal muscles. When a trigger point occurs on the right side of the abdomen in the area of the

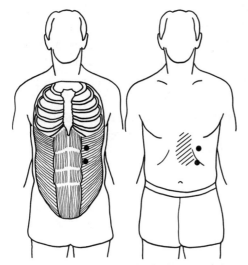

Figure 7.19 Upper abdominal trigger points and referred visceral pain pattern

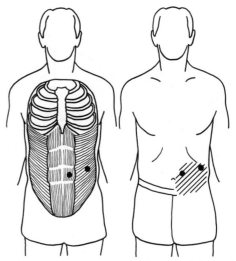

Figure 7.20 Mid abdominal trigger points and referred visceral pain pattern

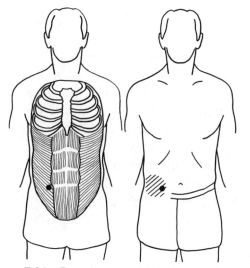

Figure 7.21   Pseudoappendicitis trigger point and referred pain pattern

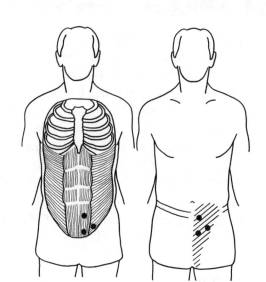

Figure 7.22   Lower abdominal trigger points and referred groin and genital pain (both genders)

appendix, it can do a convincing job of mimicking appendicitis (Figure 7.21). The lack of an elevated temperature and blood tests that come up negative for appendicitis are good reasons to look for trigger points in the nearby abdominal wall. When your doctor doesn't recognize that your symptoms may be from mid and lower abdominal trigger points, you may be told you have irritable bowel syndrome, colitis, or endometriosis (1999, 956; Good 1950, 348–353).

Lower abdominal trigger points can make you think you have an inguinal hernia (Figure 7.22). They also cause painful spasms in the urinary bladder and may affect urine retention, making urination difficult in some cases and hard to control in others. The exasperating and frustrating bed-wetting in older children can be due to trigger points in the lower abdominal muscles. The stress imposed by scolding a child about "accidents" can only make abdominal trigger points worse. Adults who unexpectedly wet themselves may have trigger points that are contributing to the problem (1999, 956–957).

Lower abdominal trigger points also cause a great deal of unnecessary distress when they refer pain to the sexual organs. Much of the menstrual pain felt in the lower abdomen, and in the ovaries, uterus, and vagina, may come from trigger points in the lower abdominals. Pain in the penis and testicles may be nothing more serious than these same lower abdominal trigger points (1999, 956–957).

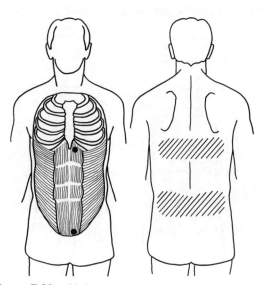

Figure 7.23   Abdominal trigger points and referred pain patterns in the back

Pain in the abdominal muscles themselves usually comes from trigger points. The referral isn't always easy to trace, however, because a trigger point on one side of the abdomen can cause symptoms on both sides or even in another part of the abdomen (1999, 943–945; Melnick 1954, 1324–1330).

Referral of pain to the back from abdominal muscles is quite common and is felt in broad horizontal bands (Figure 7.23).

When your mind is entirely focused on the ache in your back, it may never occur to you that it might be coming from your stomach muscles. Back pain that gets worse when you take a deep breath can be a sign of trigger points in the abdominals (1999, 944; Gutstein 1944, 114–124).

Twisting or bending or turning the body makes abdominally generated myofascial symptoms worse. For this reason, discomfort from trigger points in the abdominals encourages chest breathing and a hunched posture, which then keep the stomach muscles shortened. Shortened muscles, of course, perpetuate trigger points.

Causes

Overexertion on the job or in athletic activity can promote trigger points in the abdominal muscles. Overexercising a soft stomach with sit-ups and leg-ups is famous for making trouble. Sitting in a twisted position, sitting too much, a chronic cough, and emotional stress can all provoke trigger points in the abdominals. The abdominals are among the muscles that are overworked carrying a heavy backpack.

Too much worry and too much sitting do more to predispose you to developing abdominal trigger points than almost anything else. Overexertion in athletic activity comes a close second. Overexercise of the stomach muscles in a frantic effort to get trim is practically guaranteed to set up trigger points. Strong, limber stomach muscles help the lower back and improve your sense of well-being, but it's a mistake to exercise them at all until you've successfully dealt with their trigger points.

Trigger points can be initiated in the abdominal muscles by internal disease and can be the reason for continuance of pain after the disease is cured. As an example, gallbladder trouble can create and perpetuate trigger points in abdominal and superficial spinal muscles. A distressed gallbladder itself can refer pain to the abdomen and to the shoulder blade area. Conversely, pain from abdominal trigger points can feel like gallbladder pain. Pain that persists long after abdominal surgery can often be traced to trigger points that the surgery itself created. Trigger point therapy should always be part of follow-up care (1999, 953).

Most people have latent trigger points in their abdominal muscles and never suspect it until they look for them. The first step in preventing future problems is to get rid of the hidden problems that already exist. Take the time to search out and deactivate latent trigger points in this troublesome area. Get acquainted with your tummy.

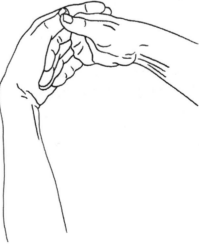

Treatment

Three regions of the abdomen will need attention: the upper, lower, and middle. Trigger points in the upper abdominals should be treated with deep stroking massage with your fingers supported in a way different from the usual position (Figure 7.24). Search all along the ribs, from the center clear out to the sides. Trigger points may be found on the ribs or just under them. You may work this area while sitting, standing, or lying down.

The lower abdominal trigger points will all be found below belt level. Massage them with supported fingers

Figure 7.24 Supported fingers for upper abdominal massage

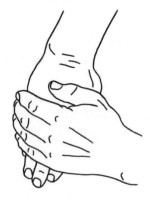

Figure 7.25 Supported fingers for lower abdominal massage

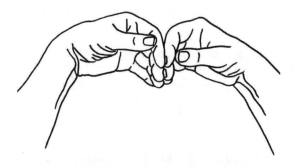

Figure 7.26 Supported fingers back-to-back for mid abdominal massage. The third and fourth fingers of both hands are the primary tools and are placed as much as possible on the same spot.

with your hands in the usual position (Figure 7.25). Push the muscles down against the top of the pubic bone and the hip-bones. Search all along the bones, from the middle on out to the sides. Massage to the lower abdominal region is best done while you're lying down.

In doing abdominal massage, remember how important it is to support your fingers to avoid straining them. For the safest and most effective massage, cut and file your nails to the quick and use the very tips of your fingers, not the flats, on the trigger points. Do the massage through a layer or two of your clothing to protect the skin from abrasion. Use slow, deep strokes in one direction only, moving the skin with the fingers.

According to Janet Travell, women can minimize their menstrual discomforts by massaging the lower abdominal area regularly between periods, daily if necessary (1999, 967). If abdominal massage is made a habit, there's really nothing to it. It only requires a minute at bedtime and another minute first thing in the morning. Any tenderness in these muscles is good evidence of latent trigger points lying in readiness to activate during the stress of the monthly event.

Mid abdominal trigger points should be addressed with the fingers back-to-back (Figure 7.26). This tool works exceedingly well in all areas of the abdomen but works best when you're lying on your back. Make note that the third and fourth fingers of both hands are the primary tools and are placed as much as possible on the same spot. This lets them work like a gang of fingers, and it makes their job much easier.

Trigger points in the midsection and sides of your stomach can also be kneaded with opposing thumbs (Figure 7.27). This can be done standing or lying. Move your hands up and down in opposite directions, squeezing the knots in between (Figure 7.28). Move your hands into different positions, vertically and horizontally, to trap different trigger points. This is a surprisingly effective technique and can cause pain to subside significantly in less than a minute when it's due to trigger points in the muscle. Common

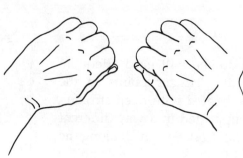

Figure 7.27 Supported thumbs in opposition for mid abdominal massage

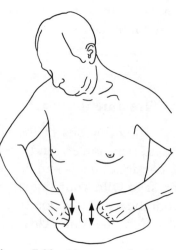

Figure 7.28 Massage of mid abdomen with tummy squeeze. Move hands up and down in opposite directions.

stomachaches often respond very well to this "tummy squeeze." It can be used on a colicky baby if done gently. Older children can be shown how to do it for themselves.

It's important to point out that the presence of abdominal trigger points doesn't exclude genuine internal trouble. However, even when an internal condition can be confirmed, symptoms from abdominal trigger points are likely to be part of the problem. Internal distress does foster myofascial distress. It would be good to check for abdominal trigger points as a part of treatment for internal problems, certainly in any case where the diagnosis is unsure (1999, 956–959; Good 1950, 285–292).

Psoas

The *psoas* (SO-az) muscles are properly called the *iliopsoas* (ILL-ee-oh-SO-az), because they include, as a branch, the *iliacus* (ill-ee-AH-cus) muscles that line the front of the hip bones. Your psoas muscles themselves lie buried behind your abdominal muscles and your intestines.

The psoas muscles attach to the sides of the vertebrae, beginning at the level of your last rib and continuing down to the pelvis. The psoas combines with the iliacus in the groin, and then descends to attach to a bump on the inside of the top of the femur (the thighbone). This bump is called the *lesser trochanter* (tro-CAN-tur). The upper attachment of the iliacus is to the inner rim of the hip bone.

The primary action of the psoas is to flex the hip; that is, to raise your thigh toward your stomach or to bring it forward, as when you walk or run. The psoas muscles also play a large role in raising your body to a sitting position when you're lying down.

Trigger points in the psoas muscles are a common cause of pain in both the low back and the groin. They can also contribute to gynecological symptoms (1992, 95–97, 101; Dobrick 1989, 130–133). Despite their seeming inaccessibility, psoas muscles are actually very easy to massage. If self-treatment of the psoas muscles had been taught in massage school, one woman could have saved herself and her clients much unnecessary misery.

Dawn, age thirty-nine, was a massage therapist and the owner of her own massage clinic, employing several other therapists. She also taught a daily aerobics class that included vigorous stair-climbing routines. To her great annoyance, the exercise that she depended on to maintain her health usually left her with low back pain. She also had pain and stiffness in her groin when she walked. She told a friend, a fellow therapist, about her concern. "I know it's classic repetitive strain, but no way am I going to give up aerobics. If I don't keep myself in shape, I balloon up like you wouldn't believe. I do lots of stretching, but it doesn't seem to be doing what it should."

During a massage, her friend discovered that Dawn's psoas muscles, which did so much of the work in the stair-climbing routines, were as hard as rocks and extremely hypersensitive to touch. Pressure on the trigger points actually reproduced her groin pain. The friend showed her a technique for massaging her own psoas. Within days, the pain in her low back and groin was gone. She was able to help a client with a related problem right away.

Sue, thirty-three, a computer programmer, had just started coming to Dawn for massage. She had been miserable and nearly nonfunctional for several days each month because of severe low abdominal and low back pain. She had told Dawn, "I'd almost undergo a hysterectomy just to get rid of this. I'm serious!"

Massage to Sue's psoas muscles reproduced her low back pain exactly. It also referred pain to her ovaries, making them ache just like they did during her period. Sue massages her own abdominal and psoas muscles now every day between periods. Her back pain is gone and the menstrual distress is much diminished.

Symptoms

Psoas trigger points refer pain to the low back on the corresponding side of the body. (Figure 7.29). The pain pattern is distinguished by being oriented vertically, unless both psoas muscles are referring, in which case the verticality may not be so apparent. When the trigger points are really bad, back pain can extend from the lower shoulder blade area to the upper gluteal region (the upper part of the buttocks). Pain is worse when you're standing. Sit-ups are impossible and you may have difficulty getting up out of a chair. Severely troubled psoas muscles may prevent you from standing or walking at all, leaving you able to get around, literally, only on your hands and knees (1992, 95).

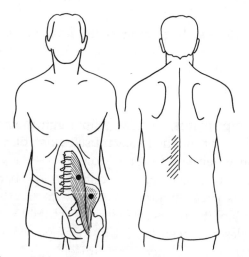

Figure 7.29   Psoas and iliacus trigger points and referred pain pattern in the back

A trigger point in the iliacus branch of the psoas also refers pain to the back in the same pattern as shown in Figure 7.29. A trigger point near the lower attachment refers pain to the groin and upper thigh (Figure 7.30). A fourth trigger point is possible in the psoas minor, a muscle that is present in only about half the population. This small muscle is in front of the psoas major at the level of the belly button. You won't be able to distinguish one from the other by touch. Any of the trigger points in these areas can refer pain to the abdomen and genitals in both men and women (1992, 90–91, 95–97; Dobrick 1989, 130–133).

Tight psoas minor muscles can tilt the pelvis backward, taking the curve out of the lower back. Psoas major muscles, when disabled with trigger points, tilt the pelvis forward, giving an exaggerated curve to the lower back. Both muscles tend to pull the midspine to one side when only the muscles on that side are affected, and may be a significant cause of lateral scoliosis. The effects of psoas trigger points on the spine can be very serious. Shortened psoas muscles keep continuous pressure on the intervertebral disks in the lumbar region and may be at the heart of many otherwise unexplained disk problems (1992, 89–101).

A stooped posture or habitual leaning to one side may be an indication of psoas trigger

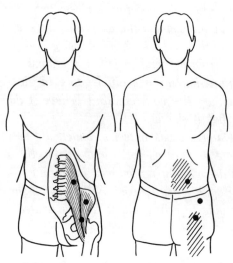

Figure 7.30   Psoas and iliacus trigger points and referred pain pattern in the abdomen, groin, and thigh

points. They can cause you to limp or walk splayfooted. If you have low back pain along with stiffness in your hips or groin in the morning and have trouble standing up straight, you are likely to find trigger points in your psoas muscles. When one of your hips seems to be positioned forward of the other, check for trigger points in the iliacus muscle on the inner surface of that hip (1992, 97–99; Porterfield 1985, 553).

Extending your leg behind you requires the psoas to lengthen. This is what makes walking so difficult when trigger points afflict your psoas muscles. Contraction of the psoas muscles also rotates the legs outward, which will make you walk with your feet turned outward when psoas muscles are tight. Some of the gluteal muscles (in the buttocks) have the same effect.

Causes

The psoas muscles can be overloaded in a fall, by strenuous running or climbing, or by any exercise that overworks the midsection. Sit-ups, leg-ups, or other abdominal exercise can be disastrous for psoas muscles already handicapped by trigger points. On the other hand, abdominal exercise can be greatly beneficial to both the psoas and abdominal muscles if you're scrupulous about keeping them free of trigger points.

Sitting all the time, especially sitting with the knees up, is bad for the psoas muscles because it keeps them shortened. Bucket seats in automobiles make a lot of trouble for these muscles. A strained posture is another source of trouble with psoas muscles. An erect and balanced posture doesn't require any particular muscle or muscle group to work hard maintaining it. However, if you habitually stoop, lean, or slouch, there will be muscles—including the psoas—that have to stay contracted continuously just to keep you from falling over.

Postural distortions caused by tight psoas muscles also tend to overload the muscles of the neck and back, which have to stay tight to keep your head up and your eyes level. Any muscle that's overworked in this way is bound to develop trigger points. The cascade effect of one muscle promoting trigger points in another can eventually leave you with trigger points everywhere in your body.

Treatment

Primary psoas trigger points will be found deep in your abdomen about two inches to each side of your belly button. Search an area halfway between your belly button and your hipbone. The fingers will work back-to-back as shown in Figure 7.26.

Get into position for psoas massage by lying on your back with your knees drawn up. Then let your knees fall over to the side away from the psoas muscle you want to work on. This will bring your hip up and allow your intestines to move to the other side out of the way. The path will then be clear, straight down to the psoas (Figure 7.31). This position with the knees to one side is an excellent way to make all of the muscles on one side of the abdomen easier to massage. Use the fingers back-to-back for the entire area.

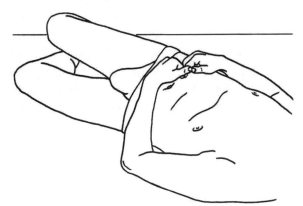

Figure 7.31 Psoas massage with supported fingers back-to-back (see also Figure 7.26)

To confirm the placement of your fingers for psoas massage, raise your head for a moment to contract the rectus abdominis, the central slab of stomach muscle. Your fingers should be just off the outer edge of the rectus abdominis to be properly positioned on the psoas. Press deeply in and feel for a rounded firmness running parallel to the rectus abdominis. A tense psoas will feel like a long pepperoni or kielbasa sausage. If the muscle doesn't have trigger points, it will be soft and you may not be able to find it.

You will recognize the exquisite tenderness of trigger points in the psoas when you touch it. When they're bad, even light massage can be nearly unbearable, but don't let the discomfort make you quit. Trigger points in psoas muscles must be dealt with and direct massage is the most effective way to handle them. You're the best one to do the work, because you have absolute control over the level of pain. Do what you're able to do and come back to it repeatedly.

You will have a better sense of the shape and location of the psoas if you stroke laterally across it (that is, from side to side). Once you're sure of where it is, you can massage the muscle lengthwise. Use a short, one-inch stroke, moving very slowly and moving the skin with your fingers. Check for trigger points from just below your lowest ribs all the way down to your groin.

If you encounter the heavy pulse of the descending aorta when working on your left psoas, just move a fraction of an inch away from the body's midline. The aorta is the body's largest artery and comes directly out of the heart. It's usually closer to the midline than either psoas muscle. If you're lying in the right position to get your intestines out of the way, you shouldn't run into anything else down in there and the psoas should feel like it's right under the skin.

Unless you have chronic pain in your groin or upper thigh, you probably won't have the trigger point in the iliacus. If you think you may, search the front side of each hipbone with either paired thumbs or supported fingers. Massage any trigger points that you find with short, slow strokes.

Tenderness near the muscle attachment at the top of the thigh ordinarily doesn't need attention, because it can be expected to go away when you release the primary trigger points up near the belly button. If it doesn't, lie flat with your legs out straight and look for this attachment trigger point one inch below your groin, slightly to the inside of your thigh. You can feel the psoas contract at this point by rotating your leg outward and raising it just a bit. The trigger point will be clear down at the bone so press your fingers in deeply.

Muscles in the lower torso always tense up to help one another when afflicted by trigger points. If you feel an increase in pain in another area after the psoas muscles are released, look for trigger points in the quadratus lumborum, rectus femoris, tensor fasciae latae, the gluteal muscles, and the hamstrings.

To prevent problems with your psoas muscles, be aware of your posture. Avoid sitting for long periods with your knees up. Long-distance drivers or people who must sit all day at their jobs should take frequent breaks to stand up and walk around, giving their psoas muscles and other hip flexors a chance to lengthen. For sedentary people, this can't be done too often. Sleeping with your knees up in a fetal position keeps the psoas muscles in a shortened state all night long. Train yourself to sleep with your legs down.

Don't try to strengthen your midsection without first attending to all trigger points in the abdominal region. Overworking and overcontracting the psoas muscles, in particular, when they're already in trouble can only make them worse. Also, remember that you can't rely on conventional stretching techniques to get rid of trigger points. Stretching therapy is safe only when done in the Travell manner: conscientiously desensitizing the skin first with refrigerant spray and following up with hot packs. Exercise and conventional stretching are both good ideas only when used at the appropriate time, after the trigger points are gone.

Intrapelvic Muscles

The intrapelvic muscles are hidden away inside the pelvis and are not accessible for self-treatment by massage, except for the muscles immediately inside the anus and one or two that are reachable in women near the opening of the vagina.

Massage of muscles deeper inside the pelvis is described by Travell and Simons in volume 2 of the *Trigger Point Manual* (1992, 127). It requires a rubber glove and a long finger, since massage can be done only through the anus or the vagina. You may find a massage therapist or other professional here and there who is experienced with intrapelvic massage. When it's needed, nothing else will do.

Symptoms

Pain from the intrapelvic muscles is referred to the genitals, perineum, bladder, urethra, very low back, rectum, tailbone, and high on the backs of the thighs. The vagina is commonly affected. A fullness or heavy feeling in the rectal area or prostate is a typical symptom of intrapelvic trigger points. In women, they can contribute to menstrual pain. In men, they can contribute to prostate problems and impotence. They may cause urinary difficulty in both men and women (1992, 110–129).

Intrapelvic trigger points can cause painful bowel movements. They can make you uncomfortable sitting upright and you may favor them by sitting on one cheek on the edge of the chair. You're apt to sit restlessly and pain may increase as you get up from the chair (1992, 118–119; Pace 1975, 107–113).

Since the intrapelvic muscles constitute the floor of the pelvis, their function is to support the contents of the abdomen. As a consequence, they are under terrific strain in late pregnancy and early labor. Much of the low back pain experienced by women at these times may be due to intrapelvic trigger points (1992, 119; Malbohan, Mojisova, and Tichy 1989, 140–141).

Tight intrapelvic muscles are capable of pulling the bones of the sacroiliac joints out of position, resulting in pain in the low back and groin. (The sacroiliac joints are where the wings of the pelvis—the hip bones—attach to the sacrum, the large bone at the base of the spine.) Osteopaths, chiropractors, and some massage therapists are trained to reset these joints. A stable adjustment is assured, however, only by getting rid of the trigger points in the muscles themselves (1999, 121; Kidd 1988, 103–105).

It's important not to make a premature assumption that intrapelvic trigger points are the cause of your problem. Get rid of accessible trigger points first. If you do have intrapelvic trigger points there's always the chance that they are simply satellites of trigger points in external muscles, in which case the internal ones may go away when the external ones do.

Causes

Bad falls, auto accidents, pelvic surgery, hysterectomies, pregnancy, and childbirth can create trigger points in the intrapelvic muscles. Strenuous or intense sexual activity can set up trigger points in muscles inside the pelvis that are specifically associated with the action and function of the genitals (1992, 118–122).

Habitually slouching down in chairs to sit on the end of your spine promotes trouble in the intrapelvic muscles. Pressure imposed on that area strains the many muscles that attach to the underside of the tailbone. Children as well as adults can have pain in the pelvic area caused solely by habitually sitting back on the tailbone.

In middle-aged men, sitting on the tailbone in a recliner for hours watching television can affect the prostate enough to make it hard to urinate. Trigger points in nearby muscles tend to aggravate prostate trouble. Heavy lifting also affects the prostate by adversely affecting muscles in the area. Conversely, an enlarged prostate can promote trigger points. Prostate massage done by proctologists would be more effective if it included specific trigger point massage of the intrapelvic muscles.

Other conditions that promote intrapelvic trigger points are chronic pelvic infections, endometritis, intrapelvic cysts, fibroids, surgical scarring, and hemorrhoids (1992, 121–122; Lilius and Valtonen 1973, 93–97).

Treatment

A pair of muscles in the vaginal wall at the entrance to the vagina can be self-treated with massage. Voluntary tightening of the vagina will contract these muscles and give a clue to where to search for trigger points. By now, after working on other parts of the body, you should be able to recognize the characteristic exquisite tenderness of a myofascial trigger point. The strategy is always to "search and destroy." Any muscle that can be reached can be massaged and will benefit from massage.

Muscles that encircle the inside of the anal opening can also be self-treated with massage. Trigger points in these readily accessible muscles cause difficult bowel movements and may be involved in the creation of internal hemorrhoids. Bearing down will relax the muscles enough for easier insertion of a lubricated, gloved finger (1992, 122–123).

To locate trigger points, press against the sides of the anal opening all the way around. Massage with slow strokes just as you would with any other muscles. Hemorrhoids or trigger points themselves can make this extremely painful, but any little bit you can do will be of benefit. Be patient and persistent. As the trigger points get better, the massage will get easier.

The *perineum* (peh-rih-NEE-um) is also an area where you can get to intrapelvic muscles that are near the surface. In women, the perineum is between the anus and the vagina. In men, it's between the anus and the base of the penis. The perineum feels muscular because it's made of muscle. Search the whole area for trigger points just as you would any other place.

The muscle that surrounds the base of the penis is comparable to the pair of muscles just inside the vaginal opening. If you'd like to learn another word, the muscle is called the *bulbospongiosus* (bul-boh-spun-gee-OH-sis). Trigger points in this muscle cause painful intercourse for women. In men, they can cause impotence. In both sexes, they can cause pain in the perineum after intercourse. Fortunately, for both genders, the bulbospongiosus is the most easily self-treated muscle of the whole intrapelvic group (1992, 125–126).

For muscles deeper inside the pelvis, you will need help and you may want to seek out an experienced professional. Otherwise, an adventurous, intelligent, gentle partner may be able to do you some good, particularly if this person has taken the trouble to develop some sensitivity through self-treatment of his or her own myofascial problems.

To head off problems in the intrapelvic muscles, give some attention to the way you sit. A habit of slouching down and sitting on your tailbone could very well be responsible for most of the pain you're having in the pelvic area.

Heavy lifting is also a danger to these muscles. It's well-known that lifting is one of the things that cause hemorrhoids. The same forces strain the muscles of the pelvic floor and can be the primary cause of trigger points in them. Women who have pain in the low back or pelvic area that may be coming from intrapelvic or abdominal muscles should be very cautious about what they attempt to carry. Picking up babies and light grocery bags is probably unavoidable, but carrying anything as heavy as a one-year-old child may be too much.

Men or women who do very heavy work or engage in vigorous athletics should gauge the effect these activities may be having on the intrapelvic muscles. Remember that the pelvic floor muscles have to support the weight of everything that's in the abdominal and pelvic cavities. Activity that results in additional downward force from the strenuous contraction of the diaphragm and abdominal muscles can seriously overload the intrapelvic muscles.

CHAPTER 8

Mid Back, Low Back, and Buttock Pain

Trigger Point Guide:
Mid Back, Low Back, and Buttock Pain

Mid Back Pain

superficial spinal muscles (165)
deep spinal muscles (162)
serratus anterior (141)
serratus posterior inferior (168)
rectus abdominis (146)
intercostals (144)
latissimus dorsi (98)
infraspinatus (90)

Low Back Pain

gluteus medius (174)
psoas (151)
deep spinal muscles (162)
superficial spinal muscles (165)
quadratus lumborum (169)
gluteus maximus (172)
rectus abdominis (146)
soleus (237)

Buttock Pain

gluteus minimus (178)
gluteus medius (174)
gluteus maximus (172)
quadratus lumborum (169)
superficial spinal muscles (165)
semitendinosus (212)
semimembranosus (212)
piriformis (180)
soleus (237)

Hip Pain

vastus lateralis (199)
gluteus minimus (178)
piriformis (180)
quadratus lumborum (169)
tensor fasciae latae (188)
gluteus maximus (172)

Massage Guidelines at a Glance

1. Use a tool if possible and save your hands.

2. Use deep stroking massage, not static pressure.

3. Massage with short, repeated strokes.

4. Do the massage stroke in one direction only.

5. Do the massage stroke slowly.

6. Aim at a pain level of seven on a scale of one to ten.

7. Limit massage to six to twelve strokes per trigger point.

8. Work a trigger point six to twelve times per day.

9. If you get no relief, you may be working the wrong spot.

Trigger Point Guide:
Mid Back, Low Back, and Buttock Pain

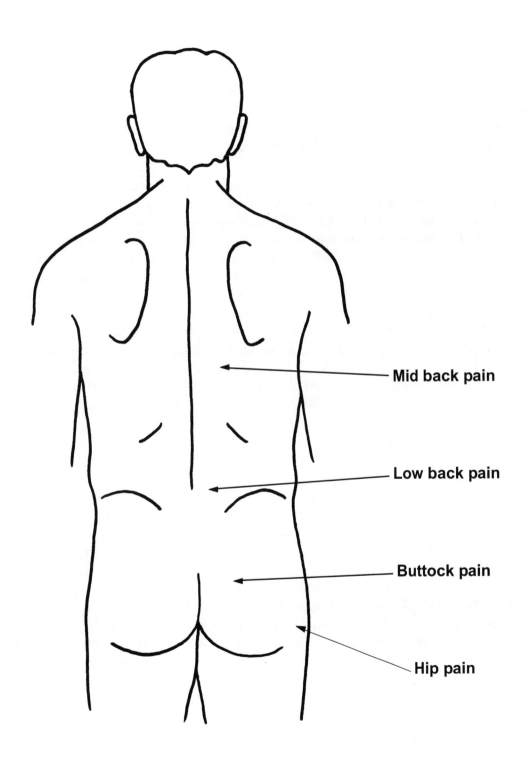

Mid back pain

Low back pain

Buttock pain

Hip pain

Mid Back, Low Back, and Buttock Pain

The solution for your back pain may be simpler than you've been led to believe. Many people are haunted by the fear that pinched nerves, ruptured disks, or arthritis are causing their back pain, when there's a good chance that their pain may be coming solely, or at least in part, from myofascial trigger points in muscles. Even when back pain is due to genuine problems in the vertebral column, myofascial trigger points always contribute a major part of the pain. In fact, there's reason to believe that trigger points are the *root* cause of many spinal problems because of the muscle tension they maintain. Muscle tension displaces vertebrae and causes compression of nerves and disks. When investigating back pain, trigger points should be at the top of the list, because pain that comes from trigger points is usually self-treatable (Travell and Simons 1999, 804–809).

Michael, age fifty-three, a high school band director, was an example of how bad a back problem can get, and yet how simple the solution can be. He suffered from constant pain in his low back and left hip, along with numbness in his left leg and foot. He'd been told he had sciatica and was sure the disks in his back were going bad. Periodic flare-ups were so intense he could hardly get out of bed. During those times, it was impossible to go in to school, or even to stand upright or walk. It hurt almost as much just to sit. Surgery had been recommended, but he wanted to avoid it if he could.

Extremely tender trigger points were found in all the muscles in Michael's buttocks and thighs and in the spinal muscles of his back, especially on his left side. Pressure on a gluteus minimus trigger point in his buttocks accentuated the numbness all the way down his left leg. Most of Michael's back pain and leg numbness disappeared with trigger point therapy. He has maintained and extended the improvement with self-treatment and hasn't had a flare-up—or had to miss work—in nearly a year.

The reason there are so many differing opinions about the cause of back pain is that it's mostly referred pain. This is especially true of low back pain. You may never find the real cause of low back pain if you look for it only in the low back. Surprisingly, trigger points in the buttocks muscles are a frequent cause of low back pain. The reverse is also true: trigger points in the low back often refer pain down to the buttocks and hips. In addition, trigger points in the abdominal and psoas muscles can send pain to the back, though they're easily overlooked, even by people who know trigger points well. For pain in the back and buttocks, the old rule applies more than ever: *Never assume the problem is at the place that hurts!*

Confusing the issue further, back pain is usually a composite, with components sent from trigger points both above and below where you feel the pain. The key to success in self-treating back and buttocks pain lies in your troubleshooting skills. The Trigger Point Guide for this chapter is vital for tracking the various components of your pain to the trigger points that are causing it.

Deep Spinal Muscles

The many kinds of muscles associated with the spine make a confusing array, but it helps to think of them as belonging to two groups: the outer layers and the inner layers. The outer layers are the *superficial spinal muscles*, which are long muscles running parallel to the spine. The inner layers are the *deep spinal muscles,* which are very short muscles oriented diagonally to the spine to gain leverage on individual vertebrae (Figure 8.1).

The names of the various deep spinal muscles are the *semispinalis, multifidi, rotatores,* and *levator costae.* The last group, the levator costae, attaches the vertebrae to the ribs. The others all attach the vertebrae to one another at successively deeper levels (Figure 8.2). Their angular arrangement gives them good leverage for twisting and side bending the spine. When the deep spinal muscles all work together, they help extend the spine, like when you straighten back up after bending over.

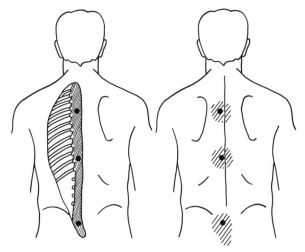

Figure 8.1   Deep spinal muscles; examples of trigger points and pain patterns. (Trigger points can occur anywhere along the spine.)

Symptoms

Pain from trigger points in the deep spinal muscles may feel like it's in the spine itself, as shown in Figure 8.1. Trigger points in the thin multifidi muscles that cover the sacrum at the base of the spine cause sharp pain in the low back. This is one of the few examples of trigger points that cause pain right at the site rather than referring it away. This is because the tension in these small diagonal muscles tends to pull one or more vertebrae out of line to one side. When vertebrae are not perfectly seated together, they send out pain signals of their own, adding to the pain from the muscles. The illustration shows only representative trigger points. They can occur adjacent to any vertebra. Trouble with the deep spinal muscles and their associated vertebrae can be extremely disabling, restricting all motion—front, back, or sideways. Your back typically feels as stiff as a board. Turning your body is next to impossible (1999, 916, 921, 924).

Trigger points in the deep spinal muscles of your lower back can send pain forward to the abdomen and downward into the buttocks. Your tailbone can be quite tender because of

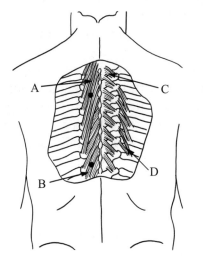

Figure 8.2   (A) semispinalis; (B) multifidi; (C) rotatores; (D) levator costae

referred pain. Your sacroiliac can be put "out of joint" by trigger points at the base of your spine. This is because tension in the deep spinal muscles twists the *sacrum,* the broad bone that joins the spine to the pelvis, causing a slight disarticulation. It's likely that when chiropractic or osteopathic adjustments to the spine succeed, it's because trigger points in the deep spinal muscles are incidentally deactivated. When an adjustment fails to affect the trigger points, the vertebrae are pulled right back out of place again. When trigger points are deactivated directly with deep massage, clients often feel vertebrae popping back into place on their own (1999, 924–925, 929–930).

Extreme tension in the deep spinal muscles can result in damage to the intervertebral disks.

Nerves can also be squeezed by the compressed vertebrae, causing pain, numbness, and other symptoms in the parts of the body served by the nerves. Chronic, long-term tension in the deep spinal muscles can be a cause of scoliosis curves in both children and adults. A proper understanding by physicians of the myofascial source of back pain could make many back operations unnecessary (1999, 924–925).

Osteoarthritis is given the credit for much back pain, especially when it shows up on X-ray. The problem with a medical diagnosis of arthritis is that it shuts off all further inquiry and leaves you with painkillers as your only solution—and they are a poor solution to pain when trigger points are the cause. Back pain is banished by trigger point therapy a very high percentage of the time, even in the presence of "provable" arthritis. It's a fact that osteoarthritis doesn't always cause pain. Active trigger points always do (1999, 925; Crow and Brodgon 1959, 97).

Causes

Valerie, age twenty-six, was addicted to her new computer and it had given her a terrible pain in the middle of her back, just to the left of her spine. The pain was constant but became worse when she moved. Sleep made it go away but only temporarily.

In reality, it wasn't the computer that hurt Val's back. She revealed that she had been sitting sideways at the computer with her body twisted so she could reach the keys. She did this so the cat could be on her lap and not pester her for attention while Val was occupied by what was on the screen. Staying in this twisted posture for hours at a time kept her deep spinal muscles continuously contracted, a sure road to muscle exhaustion and trigger points. Val got rid of the trigger points with her Thera Cane. She also stopped sitting sideways at the computer. She said the cat was annoyed, but not enough to make her leave home.

Maintaining any twisted or unbalanced position like Valerie did at her new computer can leave you open to trouble, but there are many less obvious causes. Weak abdominal muscles can cause an unnecessary load on the back muscles, which may have to work beyond their endurance to compensate. This is why unaccustomed yard work or horsing around with the kids can throw your back out. The deep spinal muscles, being individually quite small, are particularly vulnerable to sudden overload, repetitive motion, or poorly coordinated movement. It's even worse for them when you're cold, tired, or not in good condition in the first place.

It's interesting that the only time the deep spinal muscles are relaxed, except when you're lying down, is when you're standing perfectly upright with your weight evenly distributed on all sides of your spinal column. This fact has profound implications for people who are careless about their posture. The deep spinal muscles are severely overtaxed by slouching. These small muscles must work continuously when you habitually stand or sit with your shoulders hunched, your back rounded, and your head hanging forward.

Treatment

Trigger points in the deep spinal muscles lie very close to the spine (see Figures 8.1 and 8.2). They're found in the shallow trough between the spine and the long vertical mound of muscle on either side. These long mounds are the superficial spinal muscles, which will be discussed in detail in the next section. Skip ahead to Figures 8.4 and 8.5 and take a glance at them. You'll see that each mound is made up of three parallel flat strips of muscle. The innermost, thinnest strip covers the deep spinal muscles. The second strip covers them too, where it begins to broaden in the lower half of the spine.

A tennis ball or lacrosse ball against a wall is generally a good tool for massage of the back, but it may be too large to penetrate to the deep spinal muscles unless you lie on it. If you do the massage in bed, put a book under the ball to keep it from burying in the mattress, or simply do the massage on the floor. Using a ball against the wall gives you more freedom to maneuver, but the ball may need to be smaller and harder than a tennis ball to penetrate deep enough. Deep massage right beside the spine with a 35 mm high-bounce rubber ball is very effective. The 35 mm ball is slightly smaller than a golf ball and is the preferred tool for the bottom of the feet. It can be found

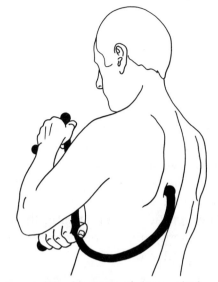

Figure 8.3 Massage of deep spinal muscles with Thera Cane (or use a ball against a wall)

wherever toys are sold. Some people find the Thera Cane or Backnobber effective (Figure 8.3). When using the Thera Cane or any other tool, do not press directly on the vertebrae. You may have to lie down with it, however, and lever it against the bed to get the penetration you need. Whatever tool you use, remember that short, slow strokes have a more beneficial effect than static pressure. Make the stroke in any direction that seems easiest and most ergonomically efficient, but choose a single direction; don't rub back and forth.

Do the massage in short sessions several times a day. Remember that you're working for increased circulation and a direct, focused microstretch of the trigger point tissue. Provided that you succeed in locating all the trigger points that are involved, you can ordinarily expect to significantly diminish, and often eliminate, your pain in two to three days.

To prevent back problems, do something to strengthen your abdominal muscles so that your back muscles don't have to do all the work when you bend and twist and move about. Just remember to be sure your abdominal trigger points are under control before exercising your midsection, or you'll make more trouble for yourself than you already have.

A good way to relieve the strain on your neck and back when you're reading is to sit at a desk and prop the book up. Reading with a book in your lap or flat on a desk requires you to keep your neck and back bent for long periods. It's far better to keep your head up and centered over your body so your neck and back muscles can stay relaxed. College bookstores usually sell a variety of cleverly designed, inexpensive book stands. Put the book stands on a pile of three or four books so that the book you're reading is nearer eye level.

Check to see if your computer screen is too low. You might benefit by raising the monitor with books or magazines or small blocks of wood. You should be able to keep your head level and erect when looking at the screen. Don't spend a minute with your neck bent and your head hanging forward if you can avoid it.

Superficial Spinal Muscles

There are three long, superficial muscles on each side of the spine; the *longissimus* (long-GHIH-sih-mus), the *iliocostalis* (ILL-ee-oh-kuh-STAHL-iss), and the *spinalis* (spin-AH-liss).

See Figures 8.4 and 8.5. They make up the long vertical mounds of muscle that run down between the shoulder blades and the spine. They're thicker in the low back and get progressively thinner as they move up past the shoulder blades. The word "superficial" tells you that they are closer to the surface, covering the deep spinal muscles.

At their upper ends, the longissimus muscles attach to the ribs and the transverse processes (small lateral projections) of the vertebrae. The upper ends of the iliocostalis muscles attach only to the ribs. The lower ends of both muscles attach to the sacrum, the large broad bone at the base of the spine. The spinalis muscles, running right along the spine, attach only to the vertebrae. They're present only in the upper half of the back.

The superficial spinal muscles help with exhalation, bowel movements, coughing, and sneezing. They also function to checkrein the body when you bend forward or to the side. They participate in keeping the body upright and balanced. Like the deep spinal muscles, these long muscles of the spine can be quite relaxed when you're standing still if the body is well centered.

Symptoms

In addition to pain, trigger points cause tightening of the superficial spinal muscles over their entire length. They can bulge out in a hard contraction, giving the impression that one whole side of the back is in trouble, when a single trigger point somewhere is actually the prime instigator. Although this is commonly called a "back spasm," it's not a true spasm that will respond to treatment with heat and stretching. A contraction that's being maintained by trigger points won't give up until you locate the trigger points and deactivate them (1999, 921, 926). Rick's story is an illustration of how misleading a back problem can be.

Rick, age thirty-four, was a muscular power-company lineman who suffered pain and tightness over the entire length of his back, from his tailbone to the base of his skull. He was conscious of his aching back even when asleep. His insurance had paid for CAT scans, MRIs, X-rays, and many visits to two different chiropractors, but there had been no improvement and no definitive diagnosis. Exploratory surgery was being held open as an option. In the meantime, he'd been instructed to exercise and stretch. "I keep doing the stretching," he said, "but it never does any good. My back's so stiff I feel like an old man. It makes me afraid to move."

Rick's superficial spinal muscles were like wooden posts, and trigger points were found in several places along them on both sides. His stiffness resulted from constantly guarding against pain. Trigger point therapy gave him great relief. A month of working on himself with a tennis ball against a wall erased most of Rick's pain. This in turn enabled the muscles to stop guarding. He soon felt loose enough to profit from the stretching exercises that had been prescribed.

Trigger points in the superficial spinal muscles cause a more diffuse kind of pain than trigger points in the deep spinal muscles. The deep spinals cause pain right around the trigger point. Trigger points in the longissimus and the spinalis are found within a couple inches of the spine and send their pain generally downward to the low back and buttocks (Figure 8.4). Iliocostalis trigger points are found three to four inches from the spine and send their pain both upward and downward and a little more to the side (Figure 8.5). Trigger points in the region of the lowest ribs send pain down to the buttocks, no matter what muscle they're in. A trigger point in the longissimus right on the lowest rib is a frequent cause of

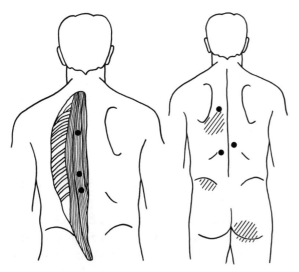

Figure 8.4   Longissimus sample trigger points and referred pain pattern

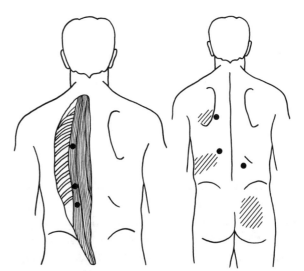

Figure 8.5   Iliocostalis sample trigger points and referred pain pattern

deep pain along the top of the *iliac crest* (hip bone). This is experienced as low back pain and is one of its major causes. This trigger point can occur on either side but is shown low on the left in Figure 8.4 (1999, 914–915).

Pain from iliocostalis muscles may also be projected to the front of the body or to the internal organs, and can be mistaken for the pain of angina, pleurisy, appendicitis, or other visceral disease. Pain from trigger points in any of the superficial spinal muscles can be misinterpreted as a symptom of kidney stones, tumors, rib inflammations, ligament tears, or disk problems. When you do have one of these more serious conditions, remember that myofascial pain from the back muscles is likely to be contributing to your discomfort. Often, trigger points are the only real problem that exists (1999, 924–925).

Part of your low back pain can be coming from trigger points in the soleus muscles in your calves. The soleus muscles actually can maintain a hard, spasmlike contraction in the low back muscles. You may also know that trouble with your feet can make your back hurt (1992, 428–429). See chapter 10 for a discussion of the lower legs and feet.

Stiffness or tightness in the back is a sign of latent trigger points in the back muscles, even when you're not presently having pain. Latent trigger points should be taken seriously because they're an indication that you're verging on trouble. Any little additional stress can quickly turn a latent trigger point into an active one. Trigger points that keep the muscles in one side of the back contracted can cause scoliosis curves. Muscle tension maintained by trigger points can also pull the sacroiliac joint out of place, keeping the pelvis twisted or cocked. When tight superficial spinal muscles squeeze the sensory nerves, the skin on your back may be hypersensitive or have patches of numbness (1999, 923–924).

Causes

Picking up something that is too heavy for you is a major cause of trigger points in your superficial spinal muscles, especially if you lift suddenly or when your body is not straight and centered. The superficial spinal muscles are particularly vulnerable when you do anything strenuous while bending to one side. Lifting something this way puts the full load on just one half of the back, in effect doubling the strain. In all aspects of your work and play, stay balanced on both feet and squarely face the object you're dealing with. Think in terms of distributing the load evenly and you won't go wrong.

Whiplash is another common cause of strain to the superficial spinal muscles. Prolonged immobility or staying in a strained position too long can also create trigger points in these muscles. Repetitive motion on the job is sure to make trouble. Repetitive tasks never give your muscles a chance to rest and catch up.

Treatment

The best approach to massaging the superficial spinal muscles is simply to back up to a wall with a tennis ball. Use a lacrosse ball or hard rubber high bounce ball if you need to penetrate deeper. You can put the ball in a long sock so you'll have a handle for better control of positioning (Figure 8.6). Several other back muscles can be worked on at the same time this way, including the lower trapezius muscles, latissimus dorsi, levator scapulae, rhomboids, and serratus posterior superior.

The Trigger Point Guide at the beginning of this chapter will help you trace referred pain to its source. On the list for your particular problem, check out the muscles one at a time. Simply seek out the exquisitely tender spots and roll the ball repeatedly over them. Use short, slow strokes up and down the back, parallel with the muscle fibers. Rock your pelvis forward and back to roll the ball rather than bending your knees to do it; otherwise, you'll tire rapidly.

Massaging your back with a ball on the floor or on your bed makes good use of the weight of your body. You may have to do it this way to penetrate deeply enough. The disadvantage is the loss of some measure of maneuverability. The Thera Cane is a good tool for the back; many people prefer it for the convenience. The Backnobber may be even more convenient, because it can be taken apart and packed in a suitcase.

If massage of a particular spot seems especially painful, remind yourself that it hurts less when you consciously relax the muscles while you work on them. And don't forget to breathe. When you hold your breath, you also tend to hold muscles tight.

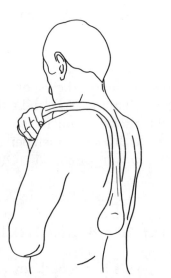

Figure 8.6 Massaging superficial spinal muscles with ball in sock against the wall

Serratus Posterior Inferior

The *serratus* (seh-RAY-tus) *posterior inferior* muscles attach to four vertebrae in the low back and to the four lowest ribs. This gives them the ability to help support the weight of the body during movement and to assist forced exhalation (1999, 908–911).

Pain from trigger points in the serratus posterior inferior usually has the character of a localized ache, which can be mistaken for a sign of kidney distress (Figure 8.7). Trigger points can cause tightness in the muscle that will tend to restrict movement, especially bending or twisting (1999, 911).

In caring for all your serratus posterior inferior muscles, overreaching yourself is bad, both literally and figuratively. Stretching to reach overhead can strain the serratus posterior inferior muscles, particularly if they're cold or are harboring latent trigger points.

Overstretching a muscle is just begging for trouble. Too much twisting of the body or bending to the side is also bad for them. Arrange your work so that you don't have to make strained movements, especially in a repetitive manner.

Give some attention to your bed. A mattress should give a little in the right places to accommodate the curves of the body, but a sagging mattress is bad for the serratus posterior inferior muscles, as well as for the other muscles of the back.

The Thera Cane, Backnobber, or a ball against a wall work well for massage of the serratus posterior inferior muscles. Be aware that in the area around the lower ribs there may be trigger points in several different muscles. Don't be misled by an especially hot one, believing you've found them all:

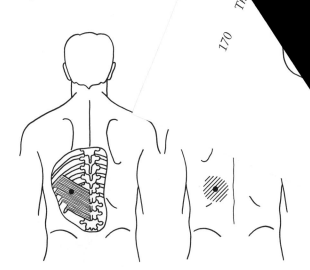

Figure 8.7   Sample serratus posterior inferior trigger point and referred pain pattern

there may be others close by in any direction. It's difficult to differentiate the muscles in the lower back, but it doesn't really matter. Just be meticulous in your search for spots of exquisite tenderness. Troubleshooting for trigger points is a matter of simply getting in the ballpark, then checking the area by feel, inch by inch.

Quadratus Lumborum

The *quadratus lumborum* (kwa-DRAY-tus lum-BOR-um) is a four-sided muscle that connects to the bottom rib and the top of the pelvis on each side. The top rim of the pelvis, which you recognize as your hip bone, is called the *iliac crest*. The iliac crest is an important bony landmark for guiding you to several important muscles. Try tracing it with your thumb from the front of your hip all the way around to the base of your spine. You may enjoy saying "quadratus lumborum"; if not, just call it the "QL."

The quadratus lumborum muscles also attach to the sides of the lumbar vertebrae. All these attachments, right where you do so much bending, give the quadratus the leverage to support the entire upper body. Without them, you'd sway around like a flower on a slender stem. Besides controlling movement at the waist, the quadratus lumborum muscles also participate in forced exhalation, such as in coughing or sneezing.

Symptoms

Eileen, age forty-seven, had suffered spells of excruciating low back pain ever since being hit by a car twenty years earlier. The pain extended downward into her left buttock and hip. Her problem was made worse by her job, which entailed standing most of the day on a concrete loading dock. Only an hour of standing made her back hurt so bad she could hardly keep her mind on her work. Sometimes, she couldn't walk, stand, or even sit upright. Her only relief came from lying down.

"I've had lots of chiropractic and physical therapy but, lordy, it just gives me more pain. I take all kinds of pills just to keep going. How else am I going to be able to work?"

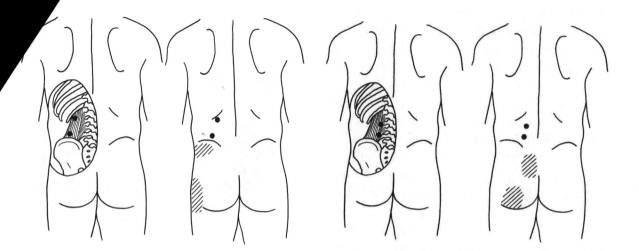

Figure 8.8   Quadratus lumborum superficial trigger points and referred pain pattern

Figure 8.9   Quadratus lumborum deep trigger points and referred pain pattern

Trigger points were found in Eileen's longissimus and quadratus lumborum muscles on her left side, where she felt most of the pain. Three sessions of massage cut her pain by 75 percent. She subdued the rest of the pain herself with a tennis ball and a Thera Cane.

Pain from trigger points in the quadratus lumborum muscles can occur in the hips, buttocks, or around the sacroiliac joint at the base of the spine (Figures 8.8 and 8.9). Coughing or sneezing is likely to bring sharp agonizing stabs of pain. The pain is psychologically paralyzing, making you reluctant to move. You may not be able to turn over in bed or to lie on the afflicted side. Sometimes pain is felt in the groin and down the front of the thigh (not shown). Tight quadratus lumborum muscles restrict pelvic movement, causing trigger points to arise in the gluteus minimus muscle, which in turn can cause symptoms of sciatica. The tension in a quadratus muscle can pull a lumbar vertebra or the sacroiliac joint out of place. It can hold one hip high and put an abnormal curve in your back, making you appear to have scoliosis or a short leg (1992, 28–38, 63).

The pain from quadratus lumborum trigger points is commonly mistaken for arthritis of the spine, disk problems, sciatica, or bursitis in the hip. A physician confronted with these symptoms may feel justified in examining you for kidney stones, urinary tract trouble, and other internal or systemic problems (1992, 28–69).

Causes

A short leg, short arms, or one side of the pelvis being smaller than the other can set up trigger points in a quadratus lumborum muscle. These muscles are often traumatized in falls and auto accidents. They can also be strained if you twist or are otherwise off balance while lifting. Tension from common emotional stress often finds a home in these muscles (1992, 40–41). See chapter 12 for help with habitual muscle tension.

Interestingly, the quadratus muscles are left vulnerable to stress and overuse when the gluteal muscles are stiff and weakened by trigger points. When the gluteals aren't doing their job, the quadratus lumborum muscles must take up the slack. Then they tire out, freeze up, and leave you with twice the trouble you had to begin with. Since the gluteal and quadratus muscles work together, they are usually afflicted with trigger points at the same time.

Treatment

Confirm the location of the quadratus lumborum by feeling it contract when you hike your hip up. The muscle is easier to isolate when you're lying down (Figure 8.10). Pushing your finger or thumb into the side of your back between your hipbone and lowest ribs, you will encounter a solid wall of muscle. This is the edge of both the quadratus lumborum

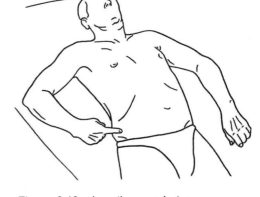

Figure 8.10 Locating quadratus lumborum by isolated contraction with hip hike

and the superficial spinal muscles. The quadratus lumborum is on the front side of this short column of hard muscle. The longissimus and iliocostalis are on the back of it.

If the quadratus lumborum is causing pain, there are likely to be trigger points in several places, especially near the attachments at the hipbone and bottom rib. The supported thumb is a surprisingly good tool for working the quadratus lumborum if you reach across behind you with the opposite hand and grasp the hand that is working. Both hands can then work together to force the thumb into the muscle. Another way to massage between your hipbone and ribs is with a ball against a wall (Figure 8.11). Stand sideways with your arm out of the way in front of your body, and roll the ball from front to back over the short column of muscle.

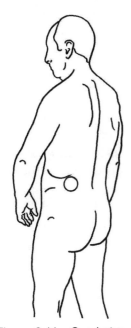

Figure 8.11 Quadratus lumborum massage with ball against the wall

Lying flat on your back in bed with the Thera Cane is an excellent way to massage the quadratus lumborum. To massage the lateral pair of trigger points as shown in Figure 8.12, place the end of the Thera Cane against the front of the muscle, with the cane across your body and the opposite end touching the bed. Pull down with both hands, pressing the muscle against the bed. Execute the stroke downward and toward the outside of the body.

For the medial pair of trigger points, position the knob of the Thera Cane under your back, about halfway across, as shown in Figure 8.13. In the drawing, the left hand stays perfectly still, like a fulcrum or pivot. The right hand executes a rowing motion, pressing toward the ceiling and then stroking toward the face. To massage the quadratus on the right side, simply reverse the tool and the hands.

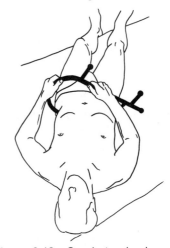

Figure 8.12 Quadratus lumborum lateral trigger points massage with Thera Cane

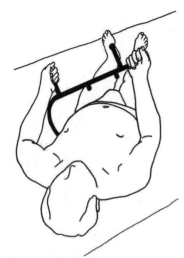

Figure 8.13 Quadratus lumborum medial trigger points massage with Thera Cane

If you have pain from quadratus lumborum trigger points but you're in a situation where you can't stop and work on them, just pinch the skin over the quadratus lumborum hard enough to hurt a little. This distracts the nervous system and quiets the pain signals long enough to get you where you're going. It will at least enable you to walk and get out of the middle of the street.

It pays to stay ahead of the curve with trigger points. Don't wait for them to catch you at a bad time. Troubleshoot your quadratus lumborum muscles from time to time, especially the ones you've had trouble with in the past. Do this even when you don't have pain. Latent trigger points cause muscles to weaken, shorten, and stiffen, but may give no other indication of their presence unless you press on them looking for tenderness. Staying alert for latent trigger points makes it easy to nip trouble in the bud.

Gluteus Maximus

People tend to think of their *gluteus* (GLU-tee-us) *maximus* as simply something to sit on. The truth is that without your gluteal muscles you'd literally fall on your face. You wouldn't be able to walk, run, jump, or even stand up. Of the nine buttock muscles, the gluteus maximus is the largest. Trigger points in the gluteus maximus cause pain in the low back and in the buttocks themselves.

The function of the gluteus maximus is hip extension, which is the action employed in climbing stairs. Jumping, running, and fast walking require the power of these muscles; they're only minimally active during easy walking. The gluteus maximus muscles contract strongly when you lean over with your knees bent or when you squat or do a deep knee bend. They also help you get up from a sitting position.

Symptoms

Gluteus maximus trigger points don't send their pain very far. Depending on the trigger point's location, pain is felt in the low back, outer hip, tailbone, or gluteal fold, or in the sacroiliac joint at the base of the spine (Figures 8.14, 8.15, and 8.16). You may find yourself constantly changing position while sitting due to a general aching and burning in the buttocks. Your hips may feel stiff, you may have difficulty getting up out of a chair, and you may limp. If you can no longer bend over and touch your toes, part of the problem is undoubtedly a shortening of gluteus maximus muscles caused by trigger points (1992, 133–134, 137).

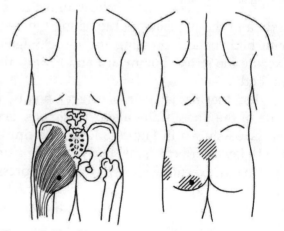

Figure 8.14 Gluteus maximus number 1 trigger point and referred pain pattern

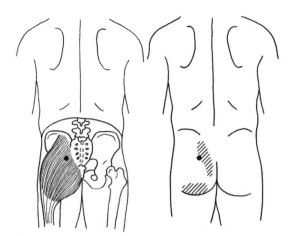

Figure 8.15   Gluteus maximus number 2 trigger point and referred pain pattern

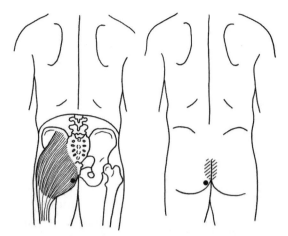

Figure 8.16   Gluteus maximus number 3 trigger point and referred pain pattern in the tail bone

Pain caused by gluteus maximus trigger points is often blamed on bursitis of the hip, a compressed disk, arthritis, sciatica, or a sprung sacroiliac joint. Pain in the tailbone can be mistaken for damage or disease when it's only referred pain from a nearby trigger point (1992, 132–138).

Trigger points in your gluteus maximus can disrupt the comfortable patterns of everyday life, if not make that life completely miserable. A vivid example of this was Kenny, age forty-two, a long-haul truck driver. Kenny wasn't bothered as much by his chronic low back pain as he was by the constant aching and burning in his hips and gluteal area. It was impossible to find a comfortable sitting position. The long hours on the road had become intolerable. "I feel like I ought to look for another line of work. The trouble is, I'd like the job I've got just fine, if it just wasn't for this problem."

Kenny's problem gluteus maximus muscles were adversely affected by sitting day in and day out behind the wheel of his truck. Practical treatment for a traveling man included working on his trigger points with a tennis ball in the sleeper bed in the back of the truck's cab. He also found it helpful to stop more often to get out and walk around.

Causes

Climbing or unaccustomed gym exercise can set up trigger points in gluteus maximus muscles when you're out of shape. Trigger points can also come from a sudden hard contraction experienced in a fall, or even when you catch yourself to keep from falling. Swimmers who use the flutter kick often overtax these muscles (1992, 139).

Sitting on hard surfaces or just sitting too much activates trigger points in gluteus maximus muscles. Office chairs are particularly bad for them, often having only a layer of highly compressible foam rubber over a rock-hard plywood or molded plastic seat. Office workers who must sit all day are guaranteed an eventual chronic backache emanating from gluteal trigger points (1992, 139).

Other hidden factors make trouble. Trigger points can cause enough tension in the gluteus maximus muscles to disturb the sacroiliac joint and add to your low back pain. Stiffness in trigger point–afflicted spinal, abdominal, or thigh muscles can put an extra strain on gluteal

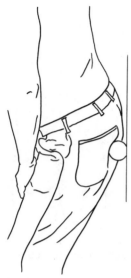

Figure 8.17   Massage of gluteal muscles with ball against the wall

muscles. Unfortunately, the recommended practice of lifting with bent knees to avoid straining your back can overwork gluteus maximus muscles when done repetitively (1992, 141).

To prevent trouble with gluteus maximus muscles, examine your lifestyle. Most people sit virtually all the time. Look for opportunities to be on your feet and active at something. The lack of exercise that comes from too much sitting encourages the development of latent trigger points that make the muscle shorten and stiffen up. Sitting also restricts circulation in the gluteus maximus. Check for latent trigger points before beginning a regime of exercise involving the gluteus maximus, such as stair climbing, deep knee bends, gym workouts, or running. If you know you've had trouble with this muscle in the past, take the time to massage it before and after activities that stress it.

Treatment

There's no mystery about the location of your gluteus maximus. It covers all the other buttocks muscles, except portions of the gluteus medius and minimus near the hip. A tennis ball or lacrosse ball against a wall gives the best maneuverability for gluteus maximus massage (Figure 8.17). For maximum pressure, you may want to lie on the ball in bed or on the floor. When lying on the ball, pull your knee up to facilitate freer movement. The Thera Cane is also good for some quick work, although it can be hard to get enough pressure to go deep (Figure 8.18). Remember that a slow, deep stroke across the trigger point is better therapy than static pressure. A couple of minutes of massage several times a day gets rid of gluteus maximus trigger points within a day or two, and improvement usually begins immediately.

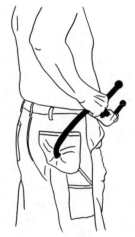

Figure 8.18   Massage of gluteal muscles with Thera Cane

Gluteus Medius

The *gluteus medius* is at the top of the list of the many muscles that cause low back pain. A great deal of low back pain could be ended quickly with proper attention to gluteus medius muscles (1992, 150). The following case history shows how easily back pain can be treated, once you have the appropriate information.

Duane, age thirty-nine, was totally incapacitated with intense low back pain after moving a heavy couch by himself. "It was on the curb. I was afraid somebody else would get it if I took time to go find help." Now he couldn't sleep because of the pain and he hadn't smiled in two days. The curve was gone from his lower back, his pelvis was locked in a forward thrust, and he could hardly walk. He was sure that he'd done horrible damage to his spine. He'd been to the emergency room where he'd been given muscle relaxants and a painkiller; he'd been to the chiropractor twice. Nothing helped.

Three days after deep massage to his buttocks and low back muscles, Duane was walking erect with very little pain. His hips were free and the curve had returned to his back. He was sleeping, too. "If my back starts hurting in the night, I just reach for the tennis ball and work on it right there under the covers," he said. "Why didn't the doctor tell me about that?"

Symptoms

Pain from trigger points in gluteus medius muscles is felt in the low back just above and below the belt line and often extends into the buttocks and hips (Figures 8.19, 8.20, and 8.21). Back pain from this source can be excruciating and disabling, seriously undermining endurance. Pain in the hips can make it hard to find a comfortable sleeping position. Gluteus medius trigger points are a frequent cause of hip and low back pain in the later months of pregnancy. Pain in both the hips and low back can make walking almost impossible (1992, 150–151; Sola 1985, 683).

Afflicted gluteus medius muscles pull the rim of your pelvis down, stiffening and flat-tening your lower back and adding to your disability. Chronic shortening of gluteus medius muscles caused by latent trigger points makes you stand and walk with your pelvis thrust forward (1992, 159).

The common assumption is that pain in the low back is caused by some problem in the lumbar spine, such as arthritis, a her-niated disk, disarticulated vertebrae, a compressed nerve, or a sacroiliac joint dys-function. X-ray evidence of these spinal abnormalities is often used to justify sur-gery for low back pain, although such abnormalities are often found in people who never suffer low back pain. Pain from

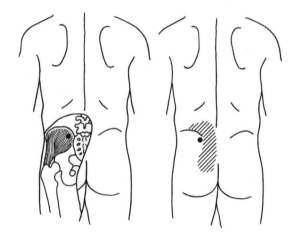

Figure 8.19 Gluteus medius number 1 trigger point and referred pain pattern

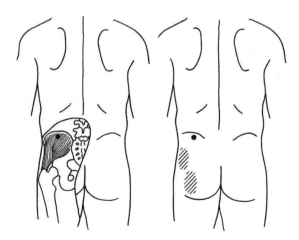

Figure 8.20 Gluteus medius number 2 trigger point and referred pain pattern

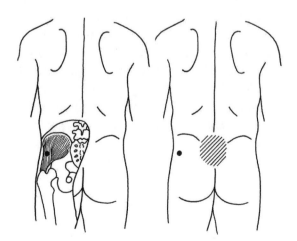

Figure 8.21 Gluteus medius number 3 trigger point and referred pain pattern

myofascial trigger points that remains after surgery can be greatly mystifying and frustrating to both doctor and patient. It's disturbing to think that trigger points may have been the only thing needing correction in the first place (1992, 154–155).

Causes

Although the gluteus medius is no more than half the size of the gluteus maximus, it's still a very thick, strong muscle, whose primary function is allowing you to walk upright. Each time you take a step, the gluteus medius muscle of the opposite hip contracts to keep the pelvis from tilting when you lift your foot. As you walk along, the gluteus medius muscles take turns supporting the entire weight of the upper body. Because of the leverage at the hip, gluteus medius muscles have to alternately generate a force equal to more than *twice* the body weight.

Any additional demand or imbalance is compounded in this same way. For instance, consider that each pound of excess body weight adds two pounds to the workload of the gluteus medius muscles. You may have observed that heavy people often lumber or waddle, throwing their weight from side to side as they walk. This is the body's natural effort to protect itself by moving the weight fully over the leg with each step instead of requiring the gluteus medius muscles to lever it. Waddling may not look great, but don't knock it: it's pretty good body mechanics under the circumstances. Low back pain in pregnancy can be traced to trigger points in gluteal muscles caused by the stress of being temporarily "overweight."

Gluteus medius muscles can be overworked when you carry heavy weight while walking. Lifting while standing in place doesn't overtax the gluteus medius muscles, as long as the weight is distributed evenly between both feet.

Trigger points in the quadratus lumborum can sponsor trigger points in the gluteus medius. This is because the gluteus medius lies in the referral area for the quadratus lumborum. It's wise to search for tender spots in both muscles when you have low back pain.

Other potential causes of overload in these muscles are weight lifting, running, falls, aerobic exercise, and habitual weight bearing on one side of the body, such as carrying a child always on the same hip. Standing or sitting still for long periods of time makes the gluteus medius vulnerable by encouraging stiffness. A common condition called Morton's foot can cause unstable foot placement, which can bring about trigger points in gluteus medius muscles (1999, 155–156). Morton's foot is discussed in detail in chapter 10.

As a safeguard for the gluteus medius muscles, don't stand on one leg to put on your pants. You can easily strain a muscle when you catch a foot in a pants leg and unexpectedly have to catch your balance. Sit down to get both feet through, then stand to finish pulling your pants up. It may seem a little silly at first, but it's a habit that becomes increasingly valuable with the passing years.

You may prefer to take your injections in a hip rather than an arm or shoulder. Just be aware that injections into a gluteus medius muscle can set up trigger points and leave you with an annoying backache. When this happens, it's good to be able to recognize a myofascial problem and know what to do about it.

Sitting a lot with your legs crossed is bad for these muscles, especially if you always cross the same leg. When you exercise, remember that moderate exercise done frequently is much safer and more efficient for strengthening than infrequent hard-driving sessions.

Wearing a wide pelvic belt during strenuous activity and while doing heavy lifting can give the gluteus medius muscles enough extra support to prevent their being overstressed. A six-inch wide elastic band worn over the hips is perfect for this. A man's jockstrap is available in this width. A woman's girdle can also be useful for this purpose. Taking the precaution to wear such things can be the critical factor in warding off an unpleasant backache at the end of the day.

Treatment

The gluteus medius is under the gluteus maximus, attaching along the rim of the ilium, the top of the hip bone. The other end attaches to the *greater trochanter* (tro-CAN-ter), the prominent lump at the top of the thighbone. Many muscles attach to the greater trochanter, because of the great leverage it gives for moving the thigh. This bony landmark sticks out on the side of your hip and you can locate it by feel. The relationship between the hip bone and the greater trochanter is shown in Figure 8.22.

To locate the gluteus medius, shift your weight to one foot while you feel for a contraction just below the top of the hip bone (Figure 8.23). The top of your hip bone may be a little higher in back than you may have thought; it can extend an inch or two above your belt line. You can also feel the gluteus medius contract just above the greater trochanter and

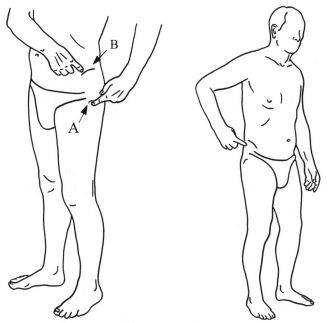

Figure 8.22 Feeling the greater trochanter (A) and the top of the hip bone (B)

Figure 8.23 Locating gluteus medius by isolated contraction with weight shift to right foot

a little to the rear. This is where you can often find an especially bad gluteus medius trigger point overlying a common gluteus minimus trigger point. It's not unusual for all the muscles on one side of your buttocks to have trigger points at the same time.

Trigger points number 1 and number 2 in the gluteus medius may be hard to find, buried as they are under the gluteus maximus and some fat padding. Massage the gluteus medius with the same tools used with the maximus, namely the tennis ball and the Thera Cane. You may have to press fairly hard to get to them. Otherwise, try a lacrosse ball against a wall (Figure 8.24). A short, rolling stroke is most effective; continuous pressure can do more harm than good. Visualize *ironing* trigger points—pressing them flat.

For going really deep into the gluteal muscles, someone else's elbow is hard to beat. For this procedure, you lie on your stomach and the person with the elbow sits beside you. If you let a friend or relative work on you, be sure they either already understand the concepts outlined in this book or are eager (or at least willing) to learn.

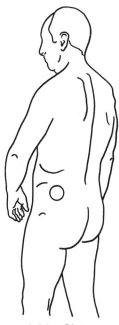

Figure 8.24 Gluteus medius massage with ball against the wall

Gluteus Minimus

The *gluteus minimus* muscle attaches to the lower half of the wing of the hip bone and to the top of the greater trochanter. It functions just like the gluteus medius in supporting the pelvis during walking. The gluteus minimus is the smallest of the gluteal muscles, buried under the maximus and medius, which together are six times as large. Considering its size, you might think the minimus would be of little consequence, but it can create great discomfort over a surprisingly widespread area, leaving you and your doctors full of consternation and puzzlement. This was exactly Karen's experience.

Karen, age sixty-five, was left with severe low back pain in a six-inch band at belt level after a fall on the ice. The pain traveled down the outside of her right leg all the way to her ankle. Her thigh grew numb if she had to stand for any length of time in the grocery line. Shifting her weight to her left leg helped, but then her left hip would begin to hurt. Getting up from a chair caused excruciating pain in her right hip. She had to begin using a cane to help her walk.

Trigger points were found in all of Karen's gluteal muscles, but they were especially bad in the gluteus medius and gluteus minimus muscles of her right hip. Shallow pressure on the trigger points was enough to make her cry out. Despite the frightening severity of her symptoms, two sessions of professional massage and a program of daily self-applied massage with a tennis ball for three more weeks ended most of her pain.

Symptoms

Trigger points in the gluteus minimus muscles cause pain down the back or the side of the thigh and the lower leg as far as the ankle (Figures 8.25 and 8.26). Tracking down the problem can be made difficult by pain from associated trigger points in the quadratus lumborum, gluteus medius, piriformis, tensor fasciae latae, vastus lateralis, peroneus longus, and hamstring muscles. Pain from gluteus minimus trigger points can be excruciating and constant. Numbness can occur anywhere in the referral areas. In addition to leg pain, there is often a diffuse tenderness in the buttocks (1992, 168–169; Zohn 1988, 212).

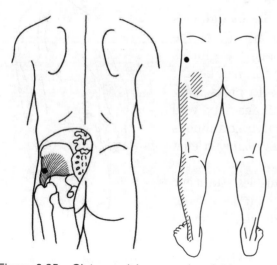

Figure 8.25   Gluteus minimus number 1 trigger point and referred pain pattern

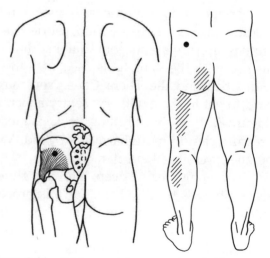

Figure 8.26   Gluteus minimus number 2 trigger point and referred pain pattern

Walking is painful. Getting up from a chair is painful. You may limp to favor the afflicted side or have difficulty crossing your legs. Rolling over on your "bad side" can awaken you at night (1992, 173).

Pain and other symptoms in the buttocks and backs of the legs are collectively called *sciatica*, independent of the cause. Sciatica is a description, not a diagnosis, although it's usually assumed to result from compression of the sciatic nerve or a nerve in the spine. Sciatic symptoms can also be mistaken for evidence of a ruptured disk, arthritis of the spine, bursitis of the hip, or sacroiliac joint dysfunction. Surgery for sciatic symptoms is appallingly common, though it regularly fails to erase the pain when the physician has neglected to consider myofascial trigger points in the diagnosis (1992, 173–175; Sheon, Moskowitz, and Goldberg 1987, 165, 168–169).

Causes

Sitting on a fat wallet is a well-known cause of trigger points in the gluteus minimus, resulting in "back pocket sciatica." Pressure from the wallet inhibits blood flow. Trigger points predictably arise in muscles where circulation is restricted (1992, 182).

Falls, sports activities, prolonged sitting, prolonged standing, and running or walking too much are examples of things that can foster trigger points in gluteus minimus muscles. Low back pain that comes on after standing or walking can usually be blamed on trigger points in these muscles. Limping to favor a bad knee or sore foot places undue stress on this muscle. Carrying your weight on one leg makes the gluteus minimus on that side work double-time (1992, 175).

Chronic sacroiliac joint displacement with its resulting pain is often due to trouble in the gluteus minimus and medius muscles. If frequent sacroiliac adjustments by the chiropractor seem to help but never have a lasting effect, get busy learning about trigger points in your "back pocket" muscles (1992, 175).

Treatment

Shift your weight from side to side to feel the gluteus minimus contract just above and a little behind the greater trochanter (Figure 8.27). Use a tennis ball or lacrosse ball against the wall for massage of the gluteus minimus (Figure 8.28). Penetration must be very deep to reach any of the trigger points in this muscle. Although the Thera Cane or a ball against the wall are effective when skillfully used, you might want to seek the help of a partner's elbow.

If you want to take better care of your gluteus minimus, be careful about overdoing any activity that involves vigorously shifting your weight from side to side or bearing

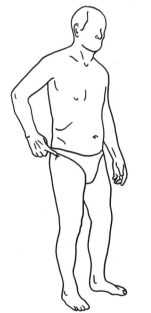

Figure 8.27 Locating gluteus minimus by isolated contraction with weight shift to right foot

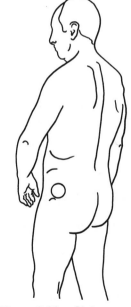

Figure 8.28 Gluteus minimus massage with ball against the wall

your weight primarily on one side. Even jogging and walking can be bad for the gluteus medius and minimus if trigger points are handicapping them. When you must stand for long periods of time, you can keep your gluteus medius and minimus muscles from stiffening up by shifting your weight often. Also, take the time to track down trigger points in the legs, knees, ankles, and feet that may be affecting your posture and gait and thereby contributing to stress on your hips.

Piriformis

The *piriformis* (peer-uh-FOR-miss) is the largest and most important of six short hip rotator muscles that are located between the sacrum and the greater trochanter in the middle of the buttocks. The piriformis muscle attaches just inside the rim of the sacrum and then travels across to attach to the top of the greater trochanter. With the leverage gained by these attachments, the piriformis is able to strongly rotate the leg outward. When the leg is stationary, the piriformis turns the body in the opposite direction. Overdoing either of these rotary movements tends to set up trigger points in piriformis muscles. Piriformis muscles cause an incredible amount of misery, as much from nerve and blood vessel entrapment as from the referral of myofascial pain. When the piriformis is to blame for your trouble, you're lucky if you ever find out, as shown by Steve's story.

Steve, age forty-five, a traveling salesman for a drug company, had suffered for years from a deep ache in his right hip. His discomfort rarely rose to the level of outright pain, but it was unrelenting and oppressive. Sometimes he also had pain, numbness, and tingling in his foot and the back of his leg. "It's pretty obvious it comes from being in the car so much, but I've got to drive to make a living. I like to play handball, which you'd think would help loosen it up, but it actually makes it worse. I've been to physical therapy and do a lot of stretches, but it never gets any better."

Trigger points in Steve's right piriformis muscle were found to be causing his hip pain. An unexpected overload of the muscle during a quick turn while playing handball probably started the problem. Sitting behind the wheel of the car for hours actually wasn't the source of the trouble, but the inactivity did encourage the muscle to stiffen. Self-applied massage to his piriformis muscle stopped the aching in Steve's hip and the occasional pains in his leg. He took steps to keep the muscle flexible by moving his leg into alternate positions while driving. He's also trying to become more aware of body mechanics in his handball games.

Symptoms

Pain and other symptoms in the buttocks are likely to be composite effects from more than one muscle. Nevertheless, in most instances, you can expect the piriformis to be involved. Piriformis muscles make a great deal of trouble, especially for women. For some reason, problems caused by trigger points in piriformis muscles are six times as prevalent in women as in men. Luckily, once you grasp the cause and effect of myofascial pain, these problems aren't difficult to cope with (1992, 193; Pace and Nagle 1976, 435–439).

Referred pain from the piriformis is felt in the sacrum (the base of the spine), the buttocks, and the hip (Figures 8.29 and 8.30). Either trigger point may refer to the entire buttocks area. Occasionally, pain spreads to the upper hamstrings (not shown). Trigger points

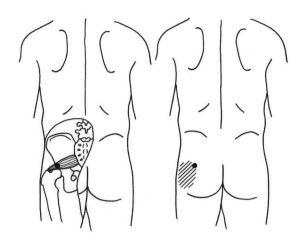

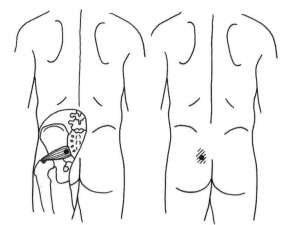

Figure 8.29   Piriformis number 1 trigger point and referred pain pattern

Figure 8.30   Piriformis number 2 trigger point and referred pain pattern

occurring in the other short hip rotator muscles just below the piriformis (Figure 8.31) are believed to have similar referral patterns (1992, 187–188, 192; Retzlaff et al. 1974, 799–807).

Tension in the piriformis can put a twist in the sacroiliac joint, adding to your pain. The resulting tilted sacrum can make you appear to have a short leg. Shortening of the piriformis sponsored by trigger points makes it difficult to cross your legs or rotate your leg inward. Spreading your legs may also be extremely painful. You may limp because of the pain. When trigger points are bad enough, you may not be able to walk. You will be unable to find a comfortable sitting position; you'll tend to squirm and shift

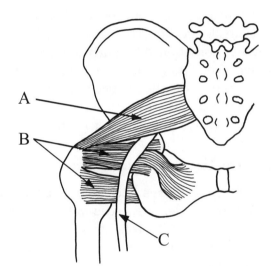

Figure 8.31   (A) piriformis; (B) the other short hip rotators; (C) the sciatic nerve (posterior view)

around constantly. Sitting aggravates afflicted piriformis muscles. Lying down brings little relief (1992, 194).

A shortened piriformis muscle also grows in diameter, causing compression of the sciatic nerve, which results in an entirely separate set of symptoms. Pain from sciatic nerve compression is harsher than pain produced by trigger points and is felt in the back of the thigh, the calf, and the sole of the foot. There may also be other abnormal sensations, such as numbness, tingling, burning, or hypersensitivity, in any of these areas. A familiar example of the effects of pressure on sciatic nerves is the prickly tingling you get in your legs and feet after sitting too long on a toilet seat. The relationship between the sciatic nerve and the piriformis is shown in Figure 8.31 (1992, 194; Hallin 1983, 69–72).

For decades, the medical profession has known this collection of sciatic symptoms as "piriformis syndrome," although the cause of the piriformis enlargement remained speculative. Surgical release of the muscle (cutting it in two) for the treatment of sciatica was once a common treatment. This operation is still performed by surgeons who are unaware of the effects of myofascial trigger points (1992, 193; Shordania 1936, 999–1001).

A piriformis muscle that is shortened and swollen by trigger points can entrap numerous other nerves and blood vessels coming out of the pelvis, making all kinds of trouble. One result can be a sense of swelling in the buttocks, leg, calf, and foot. Even worse, a tight piriformis muscle can impinge upon the pudendal nerve, causing impotence in males and pain in the groin, genitals, or rectal area of either gender. Piriformis muscles compressing gluteal nerves and blood vessels are believed to be responsible for gluteal muscle atrophy, wherein one or both buttocks waste away (1992, 194; Rask 1980, 304–307).

Pain and all other symptoms caused by piriformis trigger points are commonly misinterpreted to be the result of inflammation of the sciatic nerve, intervertebral disk protrusion, arthritic spur formation, or spinal nerve root compression. Wider recognition of the myofascial causes of "piriformis syndrome" could eliminate many unnecessary spinal operations (1992, 194–195).

Causes

Quick changes of direction in sports activities such as tennis, handball, soccer, football, basketball, and volleyball constitute a special risk for the piriformis muscles. When you're not well conditioned for such activities, vulnerable muscles like the piriformis are the first to suffer. Work that requires twisting while lifting also can stress them unduly.

On the other hand, inactivity, especially too much sitting, can promote the development of trigger points in piriformis muscles. In the young, piriformis trouble results from too much activity. In the old, it results from too little.

Treatment

You must have a clear understanding of how to find the bony prominence of the greater trochanter to succeed in finding the piriformis muscle. If you're unsure, take another look at Figure 8.22. Visualize the path of the muscle crossing on a slightly upward slant from just above the greater trochanter to the edge of the sacrum. To locate the piriformis by feeling it contract in isolation, you need to keep the gluteus maximus from contracting at the same time. You can do this by rotating your leg outward while lying down (Figure 8.32). The exquisite tenderness of a trigger point in the piriformis will confirm its location.

There may also be trigger points in the other hip rotators found just below the piriformis. Search the area between the top of the femur and the sit bone. A good way to locate a sit bone is simply to sit on your hand. You will feel it.

As you can see in Figure 8.31, the sciatic nerve, after leaving the pelvis, ordinarily passes beneath the piriformis, then travels straight down the back of the leg. Prolonged or excessive pressure on the sciatic nerve can damage it. With self-treatment, such risks are minimal because of the immediate feedback you get when you're overdoing it. In massaging below the piriformis, you may inadvertently press on the sciatic nerve,

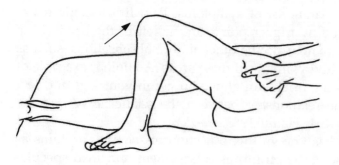

Figure 8.32   Move the knee strongly outward to locate the piriformis by isolated contraction

in which case you will feel very uncomfortable electric sensations in your leg. Simply move the massage a tiny bit to one side.

Self-applied massage of piriformis muscles is done with a tennis ball or lacrosse ball on the floor or against a wall (Figure 8.33). Piriformis trigger points are hidden by the thickness of the gluteus maximus, so penetration must be very focused and very deep. A smaller ball may be needed, but not so small as to get completely lost in the overlying muscle and fat padding. Some people prefer using the Thera Cane or Backnobber in bed. An elbow employed by a family member or sympathetic friend can really get to it.

Since part of the piriformis is inside the pelvis and inaccessible for self-applied massage, a hidden trigger point may persist near the pelvic attachments after all the others have been taken care of. In this situation, your only recourse may be an attempt to gently stretch the muscle (Figure 8.34). Note that the foot is placed on the outside of the opposite leg. The opposite hand pulls on the knee. Don't attempt this stretch if you haven't succeeded in bringing the accessible trigger points below the level of exquisite tenderness. And go easy: don't forget that forced stretching can reactivate the trigger points you've just gotten rid of.

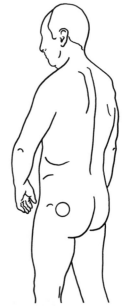

Figure 8.33 Piriformis massage with ball against the wall

Intrapelvic massage with a gloved finger in the rectum can be done as a last resort for this interior piriformis trigger point when it fails to respond to stretching. Persistent symptoms, especially those of sciatic nerve impingement by a swollen piriformis muscle, can be serious enough to justify this unusual mode of treatment. According to Travell and

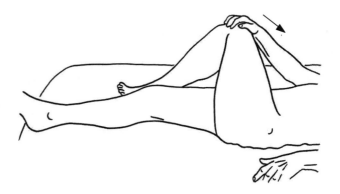

Figure 8.34 Piriformis stretch

Simons, intrapelvic massage can be very effective if done by an experienced and knowledgeable physician, physical therapist, or massage therapist. Note that in some localities the law does not permit massage therapists to do massage inside the pelvis (1992, 206; Thiele 1937, 1271–1275).

A sacroiliac joint that's out of place can cause piriformis trigger points to come right back. In such a case, a manual adjustment of this joint by a chiropractor or osteopath may be required for permanent resolution of the problem. Often, however, a sacroiliac joint will slip back into place with successful inactivation of the trigger points in all the muscles that affect it, which would be most of the muscles discussed in this chapter (1992, 16–18; Lewit 1985, 83–85).

To take better care of your piriformis muscles, be aware that unaccustomed vigorous activity places them in jeopardy. At the other extreme, prolonged immobility can set the piriformis up for trouble. If you find that your job or your lifestyle keeps you sitting all the time, get up on your feet and do something.

Moderate exercise is good for piriformis muscles when myofascial trigger points aren't handicapping them. Remember that trigger points shorten and weaken a muscle. In that condition, overstretching or overworking the muscle can quickly make its problems worse. Get rid of your trigger points before you get too serious about any exercise.

Finally, don't let anyone tell you that rest will solve the problem of myofascial pain. Inactivity is a classic perpetrator of trigger points.

CHAPTER 9

Hip, Thigh, and Knee Pain

Trigger Point Guide:
Hip, Thigh, and Knee Pain

Groin Pain
pectineus (203)
adductor longus (204)
adductor magnus (207)
rectus abdominis (146)
abdominal obliques (146)
psoas (151)
intrapelvic muscles (155)

Outer Thigh and Hip Pain
gluteus minimus (178)
vastus lateralis (199)
piriformis (180)
quadratus lumborum (169)
tensor fasciae latae (188)
gluteus maximus (172)

Inner Thigh Pain
pectineus (203)
vastus medialis (197)
gracilis (209)
adductor magnus (207)

Front of Thigh Pain
adductor longus (204)
psoas (151)
adductor magnus (207)
vastus intermedius (196)
pectineus (203)
sartorius (191)
quadratus lumborum (169)
rectus abdominis (146)

Back of Thigh Pain
gluteus minimus (178)
semitendinosus (212)
semimembranosus (212)
biceps femoris (211)
piriformis (180)
intrapelvic muscles (155)

Inner Knee Pain
vastus medialis (197)
gracilis (209)
rectus femoris (194)
sartorius (191)
adductor longus (204)

Outer Knee Pain
vastus lateralis (199)

Front of Knee Pain
rectus femoris (194)
vastus medialis (197)
adductor longus (204)

Back of Knee Pain
gastrocnemius (235)
biceps femoris (211)
popliteus (214)
semitendinosus (212)
semimembranosus (212)
soleus (237)
plantaris (215)

Numbness of the Thigh
sartorius (191)
psoas (151)
gluteus minimus (178)

Trigger Point Guide:
Hip, Thigh, and Knee Pain

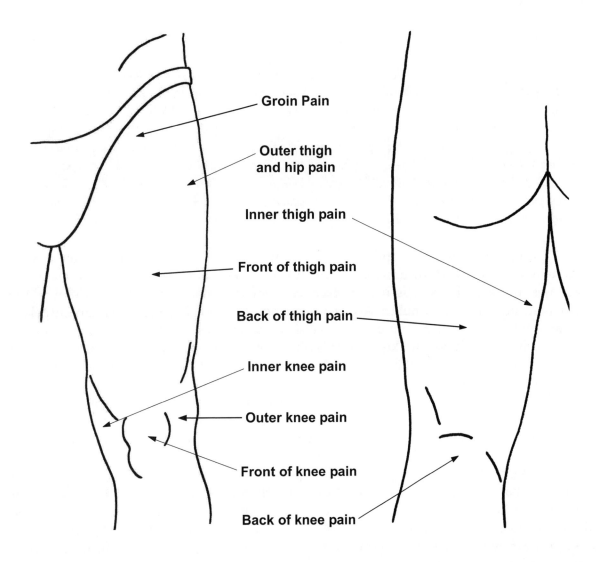

Groin Pain

Outer thigh
and hip pain

Inner thigh pain

Front of thigh pain

Back of thigh pain

Inner knee pain

Outer knee pain

Front of knee pain

Back of knee pain

Hip, Thigh, and Knee Pain

Pain in the hips and knees is a major source of disability, contributing to a diminished quality of life for a great number of people. When your knees and hips hurt, you quit participating in sports, you stop exercising, you begin hiring others to get the yard work done. You stop going for walks on pleasant evenings. You foresee ending up in a wheelchair or having to use a walker or cane because of your bad knee or bad hip. For many, this is a very real but utterly needless outcome, as it was in Deborah's case.

At age forty-four, Deborah was teaching dance in the public schools, traveling from school to school throughout her district. She seemed to spend half the day in her car. When she began the job ten years earlier, she had still been lithe and limber and had been able to demonstrate the dance steps and exercises. Now, because of increasing pain and stiffness in her hips and knees—due to her increasingly sedentary way of life—she was limited to using videos and telling the kids about dance instead of demonstrating the steps herself.

Trigger points were found to be responsible for the trouble in Deborah's hips and knees. Daily self-applied massage of her thigh muscles stopped the pain and she began feeling like exercising and stretching again. Within weeks, in her classes she was able to go back to showing instead of telling. Her students were delighted: Deborah noted a big increase in their interest and enthusiasm when they were able to have a live leader.

Arthritis, ligament injury, and deterioration of joint cartilage are the most usual medical explanations for hip and knee pain. X-rays and other tests often seem to substantiate such diagnoses. But even in the absence of objective evidence, joint pain itself is assumed to be proof that the joint is in trouble. As a consequence, hip and knee replacement surgery is commonplace and heavily promoted (Travell and Simons 1992, 221, 263–264, 300–302).

In reality, pain in hip and knee joints is often nothing more than referred pain from trigger points in the muscles of the thigh; such pain can be every bit as intense and debilitating as pain from a damaged joint. Even when a hip or knee joint has suffered a genuine injury, trigger points in associated muscles nearly always contribute a major part of the pain. Treatment of joint trauma should always include treatment of trigger points in all nearby muscles. Look for trigger points first when you have pain in a hip or knee. You can take care of trigger points yourself.

The Trigger Point Guide at the beginning of this chapter is the key to locating the trigger points that are causing your pain. Begin with the muscle at the top of the list for your pain and explore each one in turn. You may find that more than one muscle is involved, although there's usually one that's causing most of the trouble. Read the chapter and observe your own body to learn how the individual muscles work in the various actions of the hip and knee joints. When you know exactly what action has initiated the problem, you can often go right to the muscle that's causing most of the pain. It would also be a good idea to review the Massage Guidelines on pages 38, 132, or 160 to be sure you're working the trigger points in the safest and most efficient way.

Tensor Fasciae Latae

Ignore the fancy Latin word endings in *tensor fasciae latae* (TEN-sur FAH-shuh LAH-tuh). The name is commonly pronounced as shown. To perform its function, this muscle tightens *(tensor)* the wide sheet of fibrous tissue *(fascia)* that covers the outer side *(lata)* of the thigh. The fascia lata and its thick central tendon, the *iliotibial band*, transmit the power of the tensor fasciae latae and gluteus maximus to the thigh and knee.

The tensor fasciae latae's job is to assist in bending the knee and the hip. It participates in raising the thigh forward or to the side and in rotating the leg inward. The tensor fasciae latae muscles help stabilize both the pelvis and knees during walking and running. In runners and other athletes, the tensor fasciae latae muscles are usually very highly developed. Sit-ups also require the action of these muscles.

Symptoms

Trigger points in the tensor fasciae latae (TFL) muscle cause pain in the hip joint just in front of the greater trochanter (Figure 9.1). There can be two sites for trigger points, one in front immediately below the hip bone, and another an inch or so to the outside. Occasionally, pain may extend down the outer thigh as far as the knee (not shown). You may also have a deep ache behind your hip, between the sit bone on that side and greater trochanter (not shown). The muscle shortening that is sponsored by trigger points makes it difficult to straighten the hip. You may need to walk slowly because of the restriction in the hip. You tend to stand with both your hip and knee partly flexed. Leaning backward is almost impossible when tensor fasciae latae trigger points are at their worst (1992, 218, 221).

The downward pull of a tight tensor fasciae latae on the front of your hip bone can tilt the pelvis forward and give you an excessive curve in your lower back. This same effect may make you appear to have a short leg. It can be difficult to lie on the affected hip because of its tenderness. Pain from trigger points in the tensor fasciae latae may be mistaken for bursitis of the hip. It may also be wrongly blamed on a thinning of the hip joint cartilage (1992, 217–221).

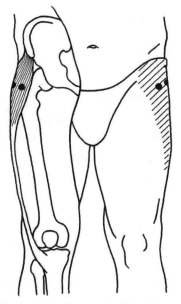

Figure 9.1 Tensor fasciae latae trigger points (in front and on the side) and referred pain pattern

Ryan, age thirty, had such a stiff hip in the morning that he couldn't stand up straight until he'd walked around and stretched for several minutes. He had the same problem at noon after sitting all morning at his desk. His hip was stiff again at the end of the day and after riding any distance in the car. He could do his morning run only if he stretched well beforehand; but if he stretched too much or ran too hard, he got sharp stabs of pain in his groin and thigh.

A trigger point very high on the front of Ryan's hip was discovered to be the source of the stiffness in his hip. Self-applied massage before and after his early morning run soon freed up the restriction. He also found that stretching worked better if he massaged his hip first.

Causes

Too much walking, running, or climbing can overwork tensor fasciae latae muscles. After they've been overstressed, sitting tends to sponsor trigger points by keeping the muscles short. Sleeping with the knees up does the same thing. Tensor fasciae latae muscles are stressed even more by walking or running on uneven ground. They also work harder compensating for worn-out shoes or unstable ankles caused by Morton's foot, which is discussed in detail in chapter 10.

The tensor fasciae latae muscles are always working when you're on your feet. Walking with heavy loads can place needless strain on these muscles. Being overweight makes them work harder. When you have ongoing trouble with them, try to avoid prolonged sitting. If you tend to get stiff in your hips, be careful about sitting with your knees jackknifed up and try not to sleep curled up in a fetal position.

Be mindful that walking, running, jogging, and other exercise and sports activities can be rough on muscles that aren't loose and flexible. Monitor the condition of your hip joints. Stiffness is a clear sign of the presence of latent trigger points. Overworking any muscle that contains latent trigger points can quickly activate them and lead to pain.

Treatment

To locate the belly of the tensor fasciae latae by isolated contraction, first find the greater trochanter, the bony knob on the side of your hip. Figure 8.22 will help with this. Place a finger right in front of the trochanter and shift your weight from leg to leg (Figure 9.2). The muscle will alternately bulge and soften. Simply turning your knee or foot inward also makes the muscle contract, as does raising your leg to the side. The tensor fasciae latae is a very busy muscle.

Supported fingers don't work well for deep massage of the tensor fasciae latae because the leverage is poor. The Thera Cane is excellent however (Figure 9.3), or you can stroke the muscle deeply with a tennis ball or lacrosse ball against the wall (Figure 9.4). Trigger points can be deep in this thick muscle. If your hips are well padded, you might want to use an even smaller, harder ball. Place the ball just in front of the greater trochanter and lean hard against it. Roll the ball across the muscle fibers or along them, whatever works best for you.

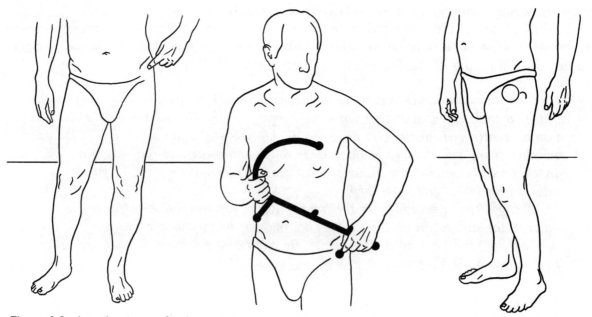

Figure 9.2   Locating tensor fasciae latae by isolated contraction with weight shift

Figure 9.3   Tensor fasciae latae massage with Thera Cane

Figure 9.4   Tensor fasciae latae massage with ball against the wall

Several other muscles are usually in trouble along with the tensor fasciae latae. When there's pain or stiffness in a hip, troubleshoot all the muscles listed in the Trigger Point Guide for "Outer Thigh and Hip Pain."

Be aware that tightness in the iliotibial band on the outside of the thigh is due to tightness in the tensor fasciae latae and gluteus maximus muscles, due of course to trigger points. Apparent tenderness in the iliotibial band is more likely coming from trigger points in the underlying vastus lateralis, which is part of the quadriceps.

Sartorius

The *sartorius* (sar-TOR-ee-us) is the longest muscle in the body. The word comes from the Latin for "tailor." In olden times, tailors often sat in a cross-legged position to do their work. Strong action of the sartorius muscles is needed to get the legs into this posture. The sartorius attaches to the hip bone then descends, crossing the thigh toward the inner side, and attaches again to the tibia on the inner side of the knee. (The tibia is the larger of the two bones in your lower leg.) This arrangement allows the sartorius to participate in raising the leg forward and turning the knee outward. A soccer kick requires strong contraction of the sartorius.

This long muscle is interrupted in several places by strips of connective tissue that break the long muscle fibers into short ones. Each section of muscle has its own belly, creating the possibility of trigger points anywhere along the muscle's entire length.

Symptoms

Trigger points in the sartorius create only localized pain. It can occur anywhere along the muscle on a track that wraps around the thigh from the hip bone to the inner knee (Figures 9.5 and 9.6). The pain doesn't have the deep aching quality that usually typifies myofascial pain. It's felt instead as a burning or tingling sensation just under the skin. A quick movement or excessive extension of the hip (putting the leg too far back) is apt to cause a sharp jab of pain right around the trigger point. Simply sitting down, which slackens the sartorius muscles, can give temporary relief of the symptoms. Standing can make the symptoms worse by keeping the muscles taut (1992, 226–229).

Sartorius trigger points don't send active pain to the knees but they can make the inner knees so hypersensitive to

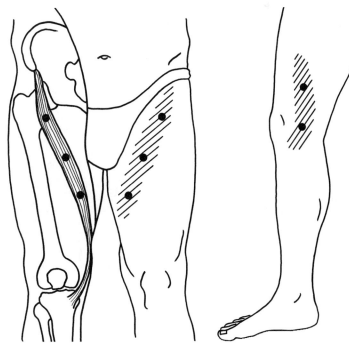

Figure 9.5 Sartorius trigger points and referred pain pattern

Figure 9.6 Sartorius referred pain pattern near the knee

pressure that it's uncomfortable to lie on your side with your knees together. This sensitivity can lead to the mistaken assumption that you have something wrong with your knee joints (1992, 229; Lange 1931, 49).

Compression of sensory nerves by a tight sartorius muscle can also cause superficial burning pain, numbness, itching, and tingling in the skin of the front and outer thigh. This is not referred pain but rather a direct effect on a nerve. These symptoms are often labeled "meralgia paresthetica," which is a fancy way of saying that you have numbness and pain in your leg. This term is merely descriptive and not a true diagnosis, since it leaves the cause unnamed. Look for trigger points in the sartorius if you're experiencing these symptoms (1992, 230–232; Kopell and Thompson 1976, 84–88).

Jonathan, age twenty-four, had typical sartorius symptoms: burning pain and numbness in both thighs. He also got sharp flashes of pain in his inner thighs if he took long strides when he walked. The numbness in his outer thighs seemed related to his yoga exercises, especially when he sat in the lotus position too long.

Trigger points were discovered in both of Jonathan's sartorius muscles on his inner thighs. Self-applied massage before and after his yoga practice greatly diminished his symptoms. After losing ten pounds, he found he was able to maintain the lotus position with less strain, and the pain went away altogether.

Causes

A sudden, vigorous twisting movement with the foot planted can initiate trigger points in the sartorius. They may also be caused by a twisting fall. Maintaining contorted yoga positions and keeping the legs up while sitting or sleeping encourages the development of trigger points in sartorius muscles.

To keep the sartorius out of trouble, avoid extreme extension of the hip when your muscles are tight or cold. Overextension occurs when you take unusually long strides or make an unusual twisting movement. Extreme efforts in athletics can overcontract, overstretch, or overwork any muscle, including the sartorius. Be circumspect about vigorous activity when you're out of shape. Any strains or overuse that cause trigger points in other hip muscles can have a secondary effect on the sartorius. Sartorius muscles are rarely in trouble by themselves. Other muscles usually involved are the rectus femoris, vastus medialis, psoas, tensor fasciae latae, gluteus medius and minimus, piriformis, and the adductors of the inner thigh.

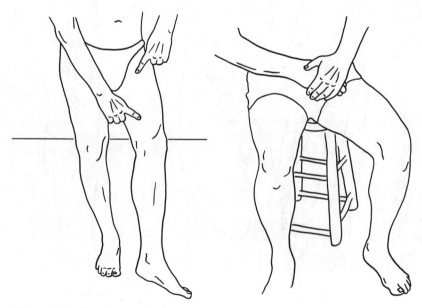

Figure 9.7 Locating sartorius by isolated contraction, by raising the leg forward

Figure 9.8 Sartorius massage with supported fingers

Treatment

Locate the sartorius by feeling it contract when you do the combined movement of hip flexion and lateral rotation (Figure 9.7). This action lifts the leg forward and turns the knee outward. The muscle will contract even harder if you also move the whole leg to the outside.

Search all along the muscle from the front of the hip to the inner knee. Massage trigger points with supported fingers in slow, deep circles (Figure 9.8). Paired thumbs are also effective. Note that the sartorius crosses the vastus medialis. Both muscles are often involved together and can be worked at the same time with the same techniques.

Quadriceps Muscles

Anatomically, the quadriceps is a single muscle with four heads, although only three are visible in Figure 9.9. The quadriceps covers the front and outer thigh and part of the inner side, wrapping almost three-quarters of the way around the upper leg. All four heads of the quadriceps attach to the kneecap by way of a common tendon. The kneecap, or patella, is entirely enclosed within this tendon and moves with it. Free movement of the kneecap is fundamental to free operation of the knee joint. Trigger points in any of the quadriceps heads can inhibit this freedom and make it difficult to bend the knee.

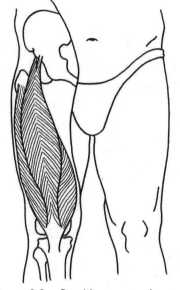

Figure 9.9   Quadriceps muscle

The common tendon attaches to the top of the tibia, allowing the quadriceps muscles to straighten the knee. An additional function of the rectus femoris, the frontmost part of the quadriceps, is to help flex the hip.

The quadriceps muscles are the largest, heaviest, and most powerful muscles in the body. Quadriceps trigger points are *the primary source of knee pain*. A case of jumper's or runner's knee is ordinarily nothing more serious than referred pain from the quadriceps. Growing pains in the legs and knees of children can usually be traced to trigger points in their quadriceps muscles. Quadriceps trigger points may also cause the phantom knee pain felt by amputees who no longer have their knees. Restless leg syndrome, a serious annoyance to its victims and a mystery to their doctors, can be traced to trigger points in quadriceps muscles. Knots in the quadriceps can also cause a locked knee, a trick knee, or a buckling hip (1992, 249–253, 263).

Pain and weakness from quadriceps trigger points are easily mistaken for tendinitis, bursitis, or arthritis of the knee, or for evidence of damaged ligaments or meniscus cartilage. Treatment is unlikely to succeed when the problem is wrongly assumed to be in the joint simply because it's the site of the pain (1992, 248–265).

Knee pain can be extremely debilitating and yet unimaginably easy to get rid of when you understand what's really going on.

At age forty-six, Kurt's latest crisis with his knees made him stop in the middle of mowing his lawn because of the unbearable pain it was causing. He went inside to sit down and rest, but when he stood up again he could barely walk across the room. He'd had recurrent trouble with his knees for twelve years, ever since climbing a mountain in the Adirondacks. His knee pain had begun on the descent and had gotten so bad that he'd been able to continue walking only with the aid of friends. At a medical center, he had been told he'd eventually need both knees replaced, because X-rays showed thinning of the joint cartilage.

Kurt's crisis with lawn mowing motivated him to call a friend who had been studying trigger points. Over the phone, his friend helped him find horribly painful knots in his thigh muscles. Kurt was actually able to knead the knots with one hand while they talked. When he hung up the phone, he found that he could get up and walk across the room with greatly diminished pain. Daily self-applied massage of his quadriceps muscles over the next few weeks ended the twelve-year-long problem with his knees.

The quadriceps muscles are commonly abused by overexercise or overexertion in sports activities, or by carrying heavy loads, walking in high heels, climbing, jumping, kneeling, and squatting. Working all morning in the garden can really get them into trouble. A job that gets you up and down continuously all day will quickly overtax the quadriceps muscles. Keep in mind that favoring other muscles of the hip and thigh due to trigger points can place increased stress on the quadriceps.

For the purpose of tracing specific pain to specific trigger points, the four heads of the quadriceps will be treated as four separate muscles.

Rectus Femoris

The *rectus femoris* (REC-tus FEM-or-iss) muscle is found on the front of the thigh and runs straight from the hipbone to the knee. *Rectus* in Latin means "kept in a straight line."

The rectus femoris muscle attaches, along with the other quadriceps muscles, to the common tendon at the knee, which allows it to participate in extending (straightening) the knee. The other attachment of the rectus femoris is to the pelvis, which makes the muscle a powerful flexor of the hip; it helps you raise your leg or sit up in bed. The dual function of the rectus femoris leaves it vulnerable to types of abuse that have little effect on the other heads of the quadriceps. Symptoms of rectus femoris trigger points are so far removed from the cause that few people would ever make the connection, as illustrated by one young woman's experience with them.

After walking around in platform heels all afternoon at a craft fair, Rene, age twenty-two, felt as though she had bugs under her kneecaps. It was a weird crawly kind of pain. She thought if she could just get under her kneecaps, she could fix it. She always had problems with her knees when she got out and walked around, but she didn't know why. She wasn't athletic and she'd never strained her knees that she knew of.

Rene's "knee bugs" turned out to be from trigger points in her rectus femoris muscles in the fronts of her thighs. Deep massage of these muscles stopped the pain under her kneecaps in less than a minute. A massage therapist told her that her leg muscles were weak and lacked stamina from too much sitting and not enough exercise. Walking in high heels added to the strain on her thigh muscles; this strain quickly tired the muscle and was the immediate cause of the trigger points.

Symptoms

The most common trigger point in the rectus femoris muscle refers pain deep inside the knee; this pain is usually described as feeling like it's under the kneecap (Figure 9.10). A second trigger point is sometimes found just above the knee. This trigger point causes a deep ache above the knee, local to the trigger point (Figure 9.11). Both these trigger points make the knees stiff and weak. They also contribute to restless leg syndrome. Interestingly, tightness in the muscle, in maintaining tension on the patellar ligament, inhibits the knee-jerk response to the doctor's taps with a percussion hammer (1992, 249–250, 267).

Causes

Sitting for long periods of time keeps the rectus femoris shortened, a condition that promotes trigger points. Overdoing any activity that requires strong or repeated hip flexion can put the rectus femoris muscles in jeopardy. For this reason, climbing, cycling, running, and fast walking are rough on them, as are sit-ups and leg lifts. Kicking a football or soccer ball calls for strong action of the rectus femoris. Even the flutter kick in swimming can be an unsuspected cause of knee pain from rectus femoris trigger points. Athletes of all types very frequently have hard knots in this part of the quadriceps.

Walking in high heels or wedge-soled shoes is a frequent, unsuspected cause of trigger points in rectus femoris muscles. You may not want to stop wearing stylish shoes just because someone says they're bad for you, but knowing they may be causing your knee pain at least gives you the option of compensating at the end of the day with some well-placed massage.

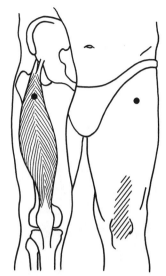

Figure 9.10 Rectus femoris number 1 trigger point and referred pain pattern

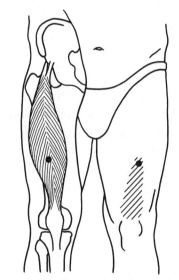

Figure 9.11 Rectus femoris number 2 trigger point and referred pain pattern

If your knee pain comes from athletic activities, you don't have to wimp out and cut back. Just be smart enough to do some preventative maintenance on your quadriceps before and after every session. If you stretch for this purpose, do trigger point massage first; otherwise, the muscles will resist stretching and won't completely release.

Treatment

Locate the rectus femoris by feeling it contract when you raise your leg (Figure 9.12). Notice that it contracts much harder with a straight knee than with it bent; this is because of the muscle's dual function. Massage the rectus femoris with paired thumbs while standing or sitting. Supported fingers are awkward for massaging trigger points near the groin (they offer poor leverage), but they work well on the lower part of the muscle. The Thera Cane is a

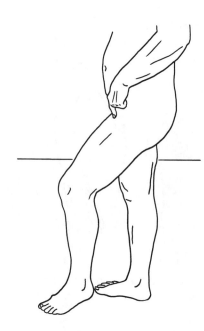

Figure 9.12   Locating rectus femoris by isolated contraction

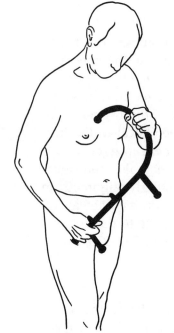

Figure 9.13   Rectus femoris massage with Thera Cane

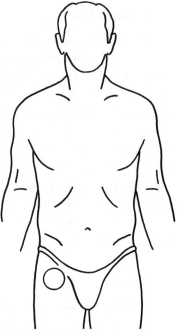

Figure 9.14   Rectus femoris massage with ball against the wall

good tool to use in either place (Figure 9.13). A tennis ball or lacrosse ball against a wall is great since you have the advantage of using your weight for pressure (Figure 9.14).

Be aware that trigger points may be found in other muscles near the groin, including the tensor fasciae latae, sartorius, and pectineus. Any of these can weaken the hip enough to give way when you put your weight on it. It's useful to be able to tell them apart. Learn to find the muscles individually by contracting them in isolation. Your work will be more successful when you know exactly where everything is.

Vastus Intermedius

The *vastus intermedius* (VAST-us in-ter-MEE-dee-us) muscle lies hidden beneath the rectus femoris and is equal to it in size. Overuse of the knee is the primary cause of trigger points in the vastus intermedius. Too much climbing or overexercise of the quads at the gym typically makes trouble for this muscle.

Pain from trigger points in the vastus intermedius is characteristically felt in the midthigh, spreading and radiating down from the trigger point, occasionally as far as the knee (Figure 9.15). Pain increases when you walk, and increases dramatically when you climb stairs. You may have trouble straightening your knee when you stand up after sitting for a long while. Stiffness in the knee may cause you to limp. Vastus intermedius trigger points

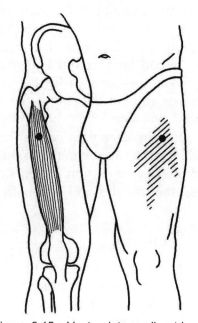

Figure 9.15   Vastus intermedius trigger point and referred pain pattern

combined with those in the upper gastrocnemius of the calf can make your knee weak enough to buckle without warning.

Being completely covered by the rectus femoris, the vastus intermedius is difficult to locate by isolated contraction, particularly since all the quadriceps heads normally contract at the same time. You'll have to massage vastus intermedius trigger points through the rectus femoris. The pain pattern will indicate whether they exist. Paired thumbs or supported fingers are the best tools (Figure 9.16). The Thera Cane also works well. A tennis ball against the wall doesn't really go deep enough but a lacrosse ball will.

Search the front of the thigh a third of the way down from the groin. The knot will be about the size of a quarter and a little lower on the thigh than the rectus femoris number 1 trigger point (see Figure 9.10). It's sometimes possible to push the rectus femoris aside to get to the vastus intermedius if the muscles are relaxed and you are familiar enough with them.

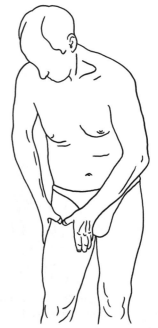

Figure 9.16   Vastus intermedius massage with paired thumbs

Vastus Medialis

The *vastus medialis* (VAST-us mee-dee-AL-iss) is the muscle that forms the oval bulge toward the inner side of the thigh just above the knee. The vastus medialis attaches to the femur and to the kneecap and tibia through the common quadriceps tendon. Contraction of the vastus medialis pulls the kneecap somewhat to the inside, which is important in countering the pull of the vastus lateralis to the outside.

Problems caused by vastus medialis trigger points commonly affect runners.

Linda, age fifty-three, had a right knee that tended to give way unexpectedly. She often fell when walking or running and had once broken her wrist. Pain in her knees and the risk of falling had caused her to give up jogging.

Extremely tender trigger points were found in the quadriceps muscles of both of Linda's legs. Her vastus medialis muscle was especially bad in her right leg, the one that was so prone to collapse. Regular massage to her quadriceps, with special attention to her right vastus medialis, put an end to her buckling knee and enabled her to begin running again.

Symptoms

Trigger points in the vastus medialis send pain to the inner thigh and to the knee (Figures 9.17 and 9.18). The knee pain usually focuses in the lower half of the knee a bit to the inside. Vastus medialis trigger points typically make the knee weak; a buckling knee, in fact, is their signature. People who are elderly or overweight are at great risk for falling when a "trick knee" gives way (1992, 250).

Knee pain and weakness caused by vastus medialis trigger points are frequently mistaken for signs of arthritis, ligament damage, and tendinitis. Ice, rest, and painkillers are typical remedies prescribed for knee pain, although none have any direct effect on trigger

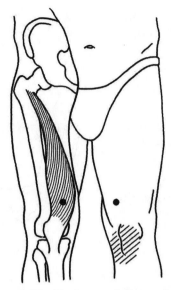

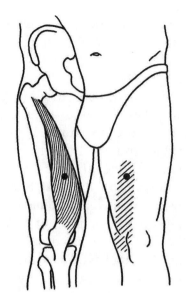

Figure 9.17   Vastus medialis number 1
trigger point and referred pain pattern

Figure 9.18   Vastus medialis number 2
trigger point and referred pain pattern

points. If overdone, physical therapy for knee pain in the form of exercise and stretching can make vastus medialis trigger points worse, resulting in increased pain and weakness (1992, 264–265).

Causes

As with the other quadriceps muscles, overuse and overload cause trouble for the vastus medialis. Deep knee bends and running are two activities that commonly overwork vastus medialis muscles. Unstable ankles due to Morton's foot also adversely affect these muscles. Walking with the ankles turned inward or the feet turned outward are signs of this condition (1992, 266). (See more about Morton's foot in chapter 10.)

Prevent accidental falls caused by a trick knee by keeping up with your vastus medalis trigger points. This sort of preventative maintenance has many benefits. Trigger points keep a constant low-grade tension on muscles which is believed to eventually damage their attachments at the joints. You can help prevent deterioration of your knee joints by keeping your quadriceps muscles free of trigger points.

Treatment

Paired thumbs work well for massage of the vastus medialis (Figure 9.19). Supported fingers are good too (Figure 9.20). You can also do excellent deep massage with an elbow while sitting on the edge of a bed or chair (Figure 9.21). With the vastus medialis, massage done when symptoms first appear can get rid of pain surprisingly fast. Give the trigger points six to twelve deep strokes several times a day.

In an emergency, you can pinch the skin over the vastus medialis to temporarily inhibit pain or weakness in the knee—long enough to get you out of the path of a raging bull. Elastic knee braces use this same effect in squeezing or putting pressure on the muscle. Knee supports, however, have little curative effect. Remember that knee pain is less likely to be

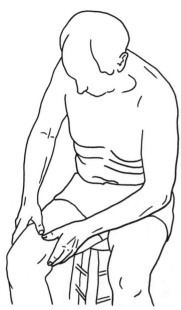

Figure 9.19 Vastus medialis massage with paired thumbs

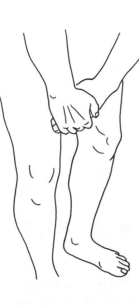

Figure 9.20 Vastus medialis massage with supported fingers

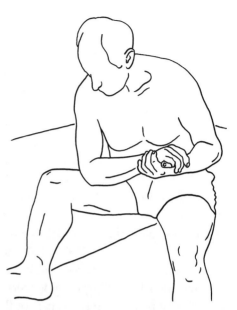

Figure 9.21 Vastus medialis massage with elbow

coming from the knee itself than from the muscles above it. If you're prone to having a buckling knee, check for trigger points every day. Latent trigger points don't cause pain but can still be the cause of dangerous knee weakness.

Vastus Lateralis

The *vastus lateralis* (VAST-us la-ter-AL-iss) covers the entire outer side of the thigh from the greater trochanter to the knee, attaching to the kneecap and tibia through the common quadriceps tendon. It also wraps around the femur to cover part of the front and back of the thigh. It's the largest muscle of the quadriceps group, much larger than you may suspect. It's also the source of a surprising amount of trouble, as exemplified by Chuck's story.

Chuck, thirty-one, had been an athlete all through school, and was an avid skier and rock climber as an adult. Now he had chronic knee pain and both knees had been known to lock (fortunately never at the same time). His knee difficulties were keeping him on the sidelines, annoyed and impatient with his condition. He couldn't even enjoy a little half-court basketball with his friends.

Luckily, the girlfriend of one of Chuck's friends happened to know something about trigger points. She showed him how to look for myofascial knots in his legs that might be causing his knee trouble. Within minutes, he had discovered several very painful spots in his outer thighs that hurt like crazy when he pressed them. To his amazement, the self-applied massage technique she showed him immediately began to relieve his pain. In just a couple of weeks of working every day on his knots, he was able to return to his athletic activities, essentially pain free.

Symptoms

Trigger points in the vastus lateralis can make the hip and outer thigh hurt, and they're an exceptionally common source of knee pain (Figures 9.22, 9.23, 9.24, 9.25, and 9.26). Trigger points in the muscle's back edge can cause pain behind the knees and in the back of the hip (1992, 251–253).

Vastus lateralis trigger points are very common in children, even infants, and probably account for much of their unexplained thigh and hip pain. Healthy children—babies too—are continuously exercising and overexercising their leg muscles. "Growing pains" may be largely undiagnosed myofascial pain that would have a very simple remedy if it were only recognized (1992, 251–252).

Walking can be exceedingly painful with afflicted vastus lateralis muscles. Lying on your side can be very uncomfortable. Tension in the muscle can pull the kneecap to one side, locking it in place and preventing movement in the knee. A locked knee is usually due to a trigger point just above and to the outside of the kneecap. The normal position of the kneecap is maintained by balanced action of the vastus medialis and lateralis muscles. Trigger points in the vastus medialis can weaken its counterbalancing effect on the vastus lateralis and may be of central concern in treating a locked knee (1992, 251–252).

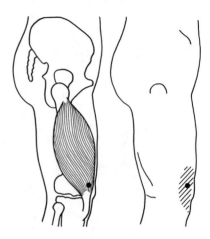

Figure 9.22   Vastus lateralis number 1 trigger point and referred pain pattern

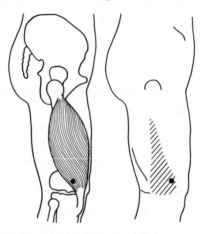

Figure 9.23   Vastus lateralis number 2 trigger point and referred pain pattern

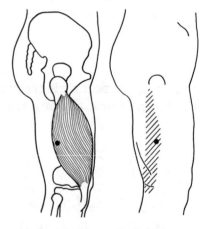

Figure 9.24   Vastus lateralis number 3 trigger point and referred pain pattern

Causes

Overdoing any activity involving the legs will predictably set up trigger points in the vastus lateralis, and the effects are almost always felt in the knees. Because overload of the quadriceps is produced by so many kinds of activity, latent trigger points in the vastus lateralis are present in virtually everyone,

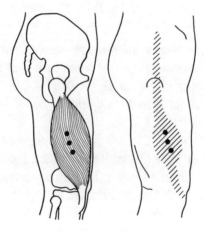

Figure 9.25   Vastus lateralis number 4 trigger points and referred pain pattern

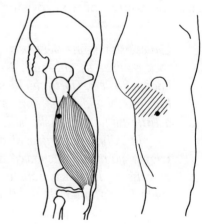

Figure 9.26   Vastus lateralis number 5 trigger point and referred pain pattern

though very rarely recognized. A direct blow to the muscle can set up trigger points. Keeping the leg straight and immobilized can do the same. Ironically, a knee brace or splint meant to be therapeutic by keeping the knee from bending can actually perpetuate trigger points in the vastus lateralis.

Treatment

As seen in Figures 9.22 through 9.26, vastus lateralis referred pain patterns are very diverse. The more aware you are of the exact location of your pain, the more success you'll have in finding the specific trigger points that are causing it. With the vastus lateralis, several may be involved.

Trigger points near the knee are easily massaged with supported fingers. Move the skin with your fingers and pull them toward you over the trigger point. Higher up the leg, adequate leverage is hard to attain with the fingers. An excellent way to massage the central part of this muscle is to lie on your side with a tennis ball under the thigh (Figure 9.27). Move the leg forward and back to execute the stroke. When you are awakened in the night by aching thighs, this gives enough relief to go right back to sleep. The Thera Cane, Backnobber, Knobble, or a ball against a wall are great tools for the vastus lateralis (Figures 9.28 and 9.29). Raking the thigh with the knuckles also can be quite effective when the other hand is put on top to double the pressure.

Be sure not to miss trigger points along the back edge of the muscle, which is on the back of the thigh. Some vastus lateralis trigger points are very deep, seeming to lie right on the bone. Like the vastus medialis, the vastus lateralis responds especially well to massage.

Among athletes, amateur and professional, the ability to find and massage trigger points in their legs should be considered an essential skill. Self-applied massage is a valuable complement to stretching for loosening and warming up the muscles before exercise or an athletic event. Self-applied massage can help prevent athletic injuries because it directly addresses the trigger points that keep muscles shortened and vulnerable.

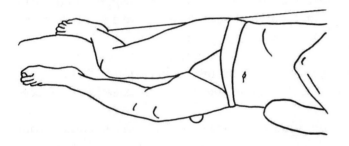

Figure 9.27 Vastus lateralis massage lying on side with ball. Move the leg forward and back over the ball.

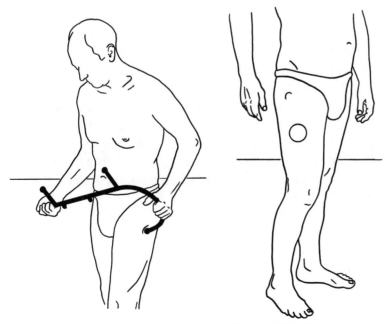

Figure 9.28 Vastus lateralis massage with Thera Cane

Figure 9.29 Vastus lateralis massage with ball against the wall

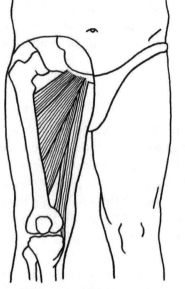

Figure 9.30   Inner thigh muscles

Inner Thigh Muscles

The inner thigh is heavily muscled and highly suscep-tible to the kinds of muscle strain that can establish myofascial trigger points (Figure 9.30). Unfortunately, the inner thigh is unexplored territory for most people and trigger points typically go undetected and untreated. Even professional massage therapists neglect working on the inner thighs, because it seems so invasive. Yet trigger points in the muscles of the inner thigh are extraordinarily common and cause many worrisome problems that are frequently mis-diagnosed. Women have a high risk of straining these muscles during sexual activity, by both overstretching and overcontracting them (1992, 290–291, 300).

Trigger points high in the inner thigh are of spe-cial concern because their pain is felt in the hip joint and deep inside the pelvis. These trigger points can cause painful intercourse for women, leading them to fear they have rectal, bladder, or gynecological problems. When men have these same trigger points, they're likely to believe they have rectal, bladder, or prostate problems or an inguinal hernia. Pain from inner thigh trigger points is often misread as indicating arthritis of the hip or knee joints. When such pain is mistakenly blamed on the loss of joint cartilage, needless hip and knee joint replace-ment can result (1992, 289–306).

The familiar "groin pull" experienced by athletes, dancers, and gymnasts comes from trigger points in muscles of the inner thigh. When your feet move far apart during an acci-dental slip on the ice, the inner thigh muscles are very likely to be strained. Pain from trigger points in these muscles is felt in the inner thigh itself. Sometimes it extends as far as the knee and shin (1992, 302).

The muscles of the inner thighs function primarily to move the legs toward one another or to cross one over the other, an action called "adduction." (Remember the word by think-ing of *adding* one leg to the other.) The inner thigh muscles are important in helping stabilize the hip during walking and running. These muscles are employed vigorously when you go skating, skiing, or horseback riding (1992, 302).

Trigger points in the inner thigh muscles can be initiated by something as seemingly harmless as getting in and out of a car or taking overly long strides. Sitting in deep car seats or sitting with the legs crossed can promote shortening of the inner thigh muscles, which can set up trigger points. Arthritis of the hip often sponsors trigger points in the inner thigh muscles. Persistent pain after hip surgery can be due largely to trigger points in nearby mus-cles of the thigh that have been initiated by the surgery itself (1992, 300–302).

Trigger points are hard to find in the inner thighs, especially deep ones near the groin. Even a normal amount of fat makes the muscles hard to differentiate. It's unlikely that you'll want anyone else taking care of trouble in this area, so it's vital that you learn to do it your-self. Get to know the five muscles of the inner thigh: pectineus, adductor longus, adductor brevis, adductor magnus, and gracilis.

Pectineus

The *pectineus* (pek-tin-EE-us) is the highest muscle of the inner thigh group, lying in a depression just below the groin crease. Interestingly, the name pectineus derives from *pecten*, Latin for "comb." The pectineus has the shape and size of the long-toothed combs that women wore in their hair in olden times. The muscle also has striations or ridges that resemble the teeth of a comb.

The pectineus attaches to the underside of the pubic bone and to the back of the thighbone, near its top. These attachments enable the pectineus to move the thigh inward or forward, or to rotate it outward. This muscle uses these very actions to help you cross your legs.

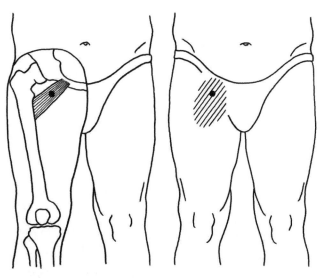

Figure 9.31   Pectineus trigger point and referred pain pattern

Symptoms

Darren, age thirty-six, a massage therapist, had sharp pain in his right groin that typified pectineus trouble. The pain increased when he walked, especially if he took long steps. He knew muscles well, so he recognized the pain as coming from his right pectineus, which he'd strained running after a Frisbee the day before. Deep massage, self-applied, cured the problem in one day.

Pain from a pectineus trigger point occurs deep in the groin just below the crease where the leg joins the body (Figure 9.31). It may be felt as either a sharp pain or a deep ache, often seeming to be coming from the hip joint itself. Extreme extension of the thigh increases pain, but the leg's range of motion is otherwise unrestricted. Note that several other muscles may project pain to the groin, including the psoas, gracilis, and the three adductor muscles (1992, 236–237).

Causes

Unexpected slips and falls can cause the pectineus to be overcontracted or overstretched. Forced stretching or contracting of the pectineus in running games or gymnastics commonly creates trigger points. Doing the splits when you're out of condition is particularly unwise. The crossover soccer kick with the instep can overwork this muscle. Gripping the sides of the horse with your knees while horseback riding is very tiring for the pectineus muscles.

Women who bring their legs forcefully together or apart during sexual activity often develop trigger points in their pectineus muscles and other muscles of their inner thighs. Too much sitting is bad for the pectineus, especially sitting with the legs crossed or held tightly together. Lifting with the legs far apart can strain the pectineus muscles. Hip replacement surgery can leave a pectineus muscle with trigger points and leave the patient with persistent "enigmatic" pain (1992, 236-240).

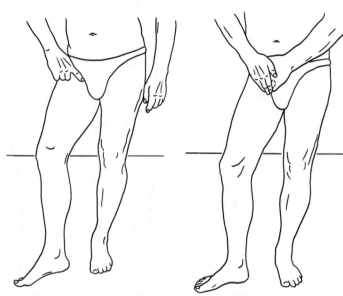

Figure 9.32   Locating pectineus by isolated contraction, raising the inner leg forward

Figure 9.33   Pectineus massage with paired fingers

To safeguard your pectineus muscles, avoid sitting for long periods of time with your legs crossed or held tightly together. If you've pulled a pectineus muscle while running, playing sports, doing gymnastics, or exercising, try to figure out exactly what movement may have over-stretched or overcontracted the inner thigh muscles. Such actions would include vigorously cross-ing one leg over the other or tak-ing overly long strides.

Treatment

Locate the pectineus muscle just below the groin crease. On a heavy leg, this muscle may be too deep to be distinguished by isolated contraction, but it's worth a try. Feel for the muscle in the bottom of the soft triangular depression just to the inside of the sartorius muscle (Figure 9.32). This *femoral triangle* is bounded by the *inguinal ligament* (represented by the groin crease), the sartorius, and the adductor longus (see Figures 9.7 and 9.35 for help in locating the sartorius and adductor longus). When contracted, these two muscles make a muscular V at the top of your thigh, a little to the inside.

Massage the pectineus with the paired fingers of both hands while standing (Figure 9.33). While sitting, you may be able to reach the muscle with the supported thumb of the opposite hand. The femoral nerve, artery, and vein pass through the groin in this area, so don't use a hard massage tool of any sort. Your fingers or thumb should do no harm if you're careful. If you feel the femoral artery pulsing under your fingers, just move a bit to one side. This area will bruise easily, so plan to work conservatively on it over several days.

Adductors Longus and Brevis

Both the *adductor longus* and the *adductor brevis* attach to the pubic bone and to the back of the upper thighbone (femur). The adductor longus and pectineus muscles completely cover the adductor brevis. The adductor longus is a relatively long muscle, extending half-way down the inner thigh. Its lower part is covered by the vastus medialis. The adductor longus is the most prominent and easily located of the inner thigh muscles. Although the adductor longus and adductor brevis are separate muscles, they function essentially as one. For simplicity, we'll refer to them together as the "adductor longus."

Symptoms

Beverly, age fifty-two, had to stop her early morning walks at the mall because of the intense pain she had begun to have deep in her right groin. On an X-ray, the cartilage

in her hip joint appeared to be thin. She was told that without an operation, her hip would only get worse and she'd probably end up in a wheelchair. She was assured that hip replacement was common now and that her insurance would pay for it.

As a last resort before scheduling surgery, and at the urging of a friend, Beverly went to a massage therapist. She was skeptical that anything so trivial as massage could help such a serious condition, but her friend pointed out that she had nothing to lose. Horribly painful places were found in Beverly's inner thighs. Pressure on the trigger points in her right leg sent pain to her hip that was just like the pain she got from walking. The therapist showed her how to massage her own thighs and arranged for two follow-up sessions. In three weeks, the deep pain in her hip was gone and she was able to resume her walking in the mall.

Trigger points in the adductor longus are the most common cause of groin pain. Typically, it's felt deep in the hip joint (Figure 9.34). Occasionally, pain may extend down the inner thigh to the inner side of the knee, as far as the shin (not shown). Pain occurs during vigorous activity and is greater when you're carrying something. Pain also may arise during any hard contraction of the inner thighs, such as might be caused by a sudden twist at the hip. At rest, there may be no pain at all (1992, 290).

Adductor longus trigger points cause stiffness in the hip, tending to limit movement of the thigh in all directions and to restrict lateral rotation (turning your knee to the outside). The inner thigh feels drawn up and tight. Tightness and pain can curb your participation in sports: jumpers are unable to jump; dancers can't

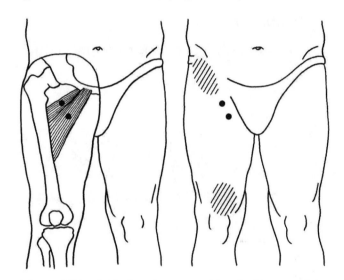

Figure 9.34   Adductors longus and brevis trigger points and referred pain pattern

dance; runners don't run. Professional athletes are apt to be benched for several games when these trigger points flare up (1999, 300).

Groin and inner thigh pain in children is often attributable to trigger points in the adductor muscles. They are among the muscles most likely to be abused in unrestrained play. These "growing pains" are usually left untreated and the child is left to suffer. This is regrettable because trigger points are as easily self-treated by children as they are by adults. Children should be taught about myofascial pain in school. Think how much better the lives of adults would be if they'd learned how to find and fix their trigger points as children (1992, 290).

Osteoarthritis in hip joints is a common problem in older adults and causes pain similar to that caused by trigger points. Arthritis pain is different, however, in that it is felt more in the outer hip than the inner thigh. Nevertheless, pain from adductor longus trigger points is often misinterpreted as arthritis. Massage of the adductor longus quickly differentiates the two conditions. If massage makes the pain go away, it's probably not being caused by arthritis (1992, 302).

Causes

Taking inordinately long steps or moving your legs too far apart can overstretch and strain the adductor longus muscles. Slipping on the ice is a classic way to cause a groin pull. Reaching beyond your limits in sports is particularly risky. Poor conditioning inevitably sets you up for muscle strain and myofascial trigger points. Holding on with your knees and thighs while horseback riding can overwork the adductor muscles.

Remember that extreme movements of the leg at the hip are what cause virtually all the trouble with inner thigh muscles. Don't go near your maximum range of motion until you're certain that you're quite loose and limber, and be mindful of the reasonable limits of your strength. Trigger points can activate very quickly in any muscle when you set out to play or work when you're cold and stiff. Even when you're warmed up and in good condition, be circumspect about quick, impetuous starts before the muscles have done a little easy work. These principles become more important as you grow older.

Treatment

You can easily locate an adductor longus muscle while lying on your side with your leg

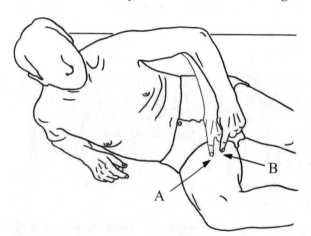

drawn up and lying on its side (Figure 9.35). In the illustration, the ghosted hand is pointing to the adductor longus. The fully rendered hand points to the adductor magnus, which will be discussed in the next section.

Raise your knee slightly off the bed to feel the adductor longus muscle contract. It should stand out clearly as it approaches the groin, and you may be able to grasp it between your fingers and thumb (Figure 9.36). Compare this with how you grasp the adductor magnus, which is immediately behind the adductor longus (Figure 9.37).

Figure 9.35   Locating adductor longus (A) and adductor magnus (B) by isolated contraction, raising right leg from bed

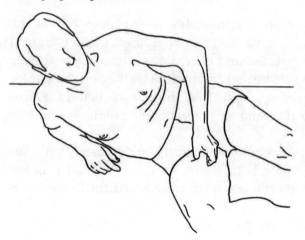

Figure 9.36   Grasping adductor longus between fingers and thumb

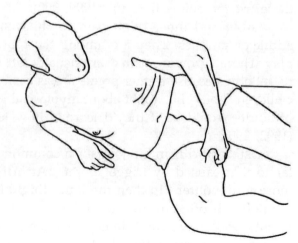

Figure 9.37   Grasping adductor magnus between fingers and thumb

Massage the adductor longus with supported fingers with your leg lying on its side on the bed (Figure 9.38). Supported knuckles or a supported thumb may also work for you. The muscle should be relaxed in this position. If you try to massage the inner thigh muscles while sitting with both feet on the floor, the muscles have to contract to resist the pressure. The Thera Cane can also be used, but with any tool other than the fingers, it's wise to work through a layer of cloth, since the skin of the inner thigh is such a sensitive area.

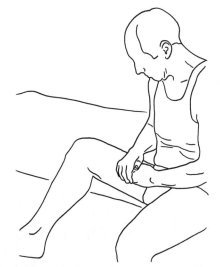

Figure 9.38   Adductor massage with supported fingers or supported knuckles

Adductor Magnus

The *adductor magnus* (uh-DUK-ter MAG-nus) is the third largest muscle in the body. It attaches right in the crotch between the pubic bone and the sit bone and then divides into three parts, which descend to attach all along the back of the femur. The longest segment attaches just above the knee.

The muscle fibers of the different sections of the adductor magnus travel at different angles, giving the muscle the ability to participate in several functions. The main job of the adductor magnus muscles is to strongly adduct the thighs, that is, to bring the legs together. They also help stabilize the pelvis and extend the thighs during walking and running.

The adductor magnus is a complex muscle that's not easy to find, understand, or deal with. This muscle is well worth learning about, however, because its trigger points can be the cause of the kind of worry and grief experienced by Carol.

Carol, age twenty-three, a graduate music student majoring in piano, had gone to a massage therapist for help with pain in her hands. During the third session, she hesitantly asked if massage might help her "sexual pain" too. Encouraged to explain, she said that she had been sexually active for five years and had always experienced extreme pain in her vagina. Having her legs apart made it worse. With further questioning, she remembered that even when she was a child, her inner thighs had always seemed tight and would never stretch well after exercise. She said that she sometimes felt a pulling that verged on pain if she stepped out too far when walking or running.

At the university clinic, they told her she was perfectly fine physically. It was suggested that she get some counseling, and perhaps drink a glass of wine before she got together with her boyfriend. Carol had tried both "prescriptions" but neither had helped.

Massage of Carol's inner thighs revealed excruciating spots of pain very high on both inner thighs, just in front of the gluteal folds. She felt embarrassed to have massage done in that area and asked if it would be possible to do the massage herself. After some experimentation, she was able to massage the tender spots with a tennis ball while sitting on a hard wooden chair.

She later reported a satisfactory outcome.

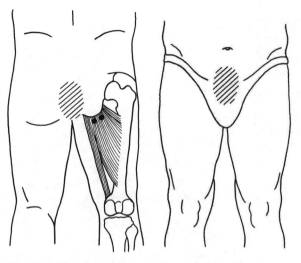

Figure 9.39   Adductor magnus number 1 trigger points and referred pain pattern inside the pelvis

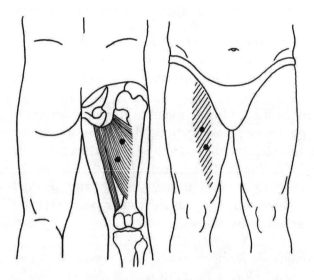

Figure 9.40   Adductor magnus number 2 trigger points and referred pain pattern

Symptoms

Trigger points in the upper part of the adductor magnus cause pain inside the pelvis (Figure 9.39). This deep internal pain may be quite diffuse and unfocused or may be localized as a sharp, sudden explosion of pain at the pubic bone, or in the vagina, rectum, prostate, or bladder. Trigger points in the middle part of the muscle cause pain and stiffness in the inner thigh from the groin almost to the knee (Figure 9.40) (1992, 290–291).

Pain from trigger points in the adductor magnus is increased by extreme abduction of the hip (spreading the thighs). For this reason, internal pelvic pain may occur in women during intercourse, causing great worry about possible visceral or gynecological disease. Unawareness of the myofascial causes of internal pelvic pain can lead to a wide range of mistaken diagnoses and misdirected treatment, including surgery. Examination for myofascial trigger points should always come first when diagnosing pain in the area of the groin. Many concerns can be eliminated if simple massage takes away the pain (1992, 289–301).

Causes

The adductor magnus muscles are employed in such activities as climbing stairs, gripping the sides of the horse while riding, and making quick turns in skiing. Trigger points are likely to arise when these activities are overdone. During exercise, take care not to overstretch muscles that are already inhibited by trigger points.

Other common causes of adductor magnus difficulties are accidental slips of the feet while coming down stairs, or slipping while walking on ice or simply getting in and out of a car. A sudden overload with the legs apart or any movement that suddenly spreads the legs can strain the adductor magnus muscles. A slip of the foot can be the biggest single danger to the muscles of the inner thigh. Be wise about the shoes you wear; high-heeled shoes are not good for these muscles, nor are shoes with the soles and heels worn smooth, because they increase the risk of slipping or falling. At work or play, avoid accidentally overstretching or overloading the adductor magnus muscles by taking care to keep your weight well balanced on both feet.

Treatment

The adductor magnus is behind the adductor longus and brevis muscles. Look again at Figures 9.35, 9.36, and 9.37. Try to differentiate among these muscles by putting your fingers between them on the inner thigh.

The best way to massage the adductor magnus number 1 trigger point is with the Thera Cane (Figure 9.41). As shown in the illustration, this trigger point is most accessible when you place one foot on a chair. First locate the sit bone, then search an inch or so below it on the inner side of the thigh.

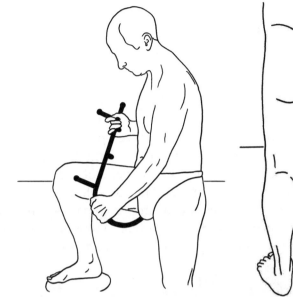

Figure 9.41 Adductor magnus number 1 massage near the sit bone with Thera Cane

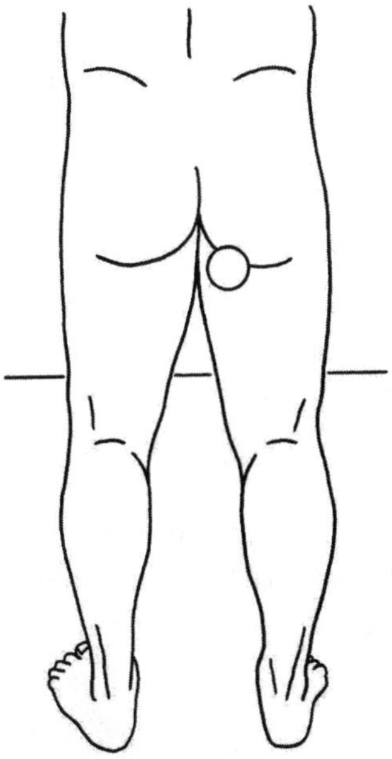

Figure 9.42 Position of ball for adductor magnus number 1 trigger point massage on wooden chair

Alternatively, a tennis ball, lacrosse ball, or a hard high bounce rubber ball can be used to massage this trigger point if you sit on it on the edge of a hard chair or bench. This is difficult to illustrate clearly, so the approximate position of the ball is shown on the vertical body (Figure 9.42). It's also possible to work this place with the fingers, although it can be awkward and the leverage isn't great. The pain from massaging this trigger point can be quite surprising and intense, but persevere: it's a very important trigger point to master.

Massage the adductor magnus number 2 trigger point with supported fingers. Prop the leg up on the bed as shown in Figure 9.38 in the section on the adductor longus.

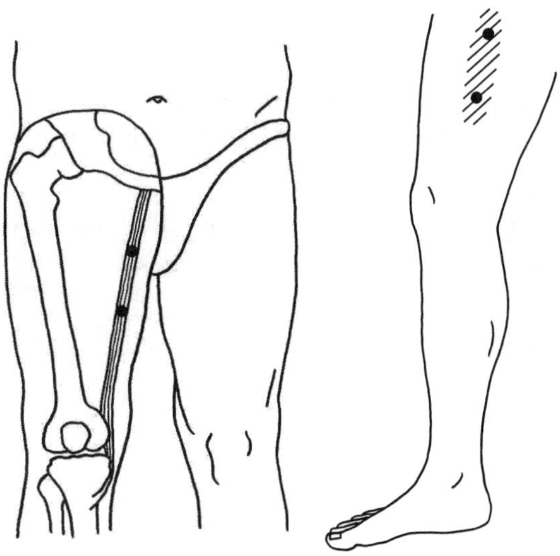

Figure 9.43 Gracilis trigger points and referred pain pattern

Gracilis

The thin, flat *gracilis* (GRAS-il-iss) muscle is the second longest muscle in the body; only the sartorius is longer. *Gracilis* is a Latin word meaning "slender." The gracilis muscle attaches to the pubic bone then descends the full length of the inner thigh to attach again below the knee. These attachments give the gracilis an action at the hip and at the knee, helping flex both joints. Because the muscle is normally slack, it's not easily overloaded. Trigger points in the gracilis are usually induced by referred pain from trigger points in the other inner thigh muscles.

Pain from gracilis trigger points is local to the muscle and is not referred to any other site (Figure 9.43). Although only two trigger points are shown in the drawing, they may be found anywhere along the length of the muscle. The pain is usually a hot, stinging sensation, felt right under the skin along the inside of the thigh. There may also be a sense of diffuse achiness in the same area. Pain is constant at rest and is not relieved by any change of position; however, walking sometimes gives relief (1992, 291, 300).

The gracilis and sartorius muscles produce pain in similar locations on the inner thigh, though the pain from sartorius trigger points is somewhat sharper. Stretching isn't effective for either the sartorius or the gracilis, since both muscles are somewhat slack to begin with and therefore not amenable to therapeutic lengthening.

The gracilis muscle is the most superficial of the inner thigh muscles, lying immediately under the skin. Nevertheless, you may not be able to distinguish the gracilis from the general mass of adductor muscles unless you happen to be very thin. Its trigger points can be located, however, by simply searching for relatively superficial tender spots along the inner thigh. Massage the gracilis with supported fingers or paired thumbs.

Hamstring Muscles

You may not have a clear idea of just what your hamstrings are, or exactly where they are. They're not "strings" at all, but rather three exceptionally strong, slender muscles that cover the backs of the thighs (Figure 9.44). Latent trigger points in the hamstrings, with consequent tightening of these muscles, are extremely common. Pain and stiffness from hamstring trigger points occur as often in children as they do in adults (1992, 316).

You've heard of athletes having "pulled a hamstring," or worse, having torn a hamstring. Such injuries often originate with trigger points that prevent normal lengthening of the hamstrings. Muscles in this state don't respond completely to warm-ups or stretching routines and are very susceptible to strain and physical damage. If athletes were more aware of trigger points and knew how to deactivate them, there would undoubtedly be fewer hamstring injuries. The

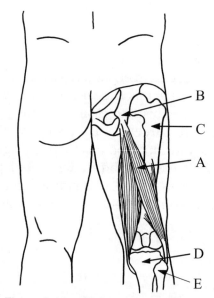

Figure 9.44   (A) hamstrings; (B) sit bone; (C) femur; (D) tibia; (E) fibula

following case history illustrates the long-term effects a hamstring injury can have when treatment doesn't include care for incidental trigger points (1992, 324–326; Brody 1980, 24–26).

Nathan, age twenty-one, experienced a serious low back strain on his job with a package delivery company. The pain sent him to the emergency room, where he was given painkillers and muscle relaxants. The pain persisted, however, and he was unable to resume work.

Several sessions of massage to his back and buttocks muscles got rid of Nathan's back pain, but he still had difficulty bending over to pick anything up because of stiffness in the backs of his legs. He revealed that he'd had that stiffness ever since tearing a hamstring running the hurdles in high school. The injury had ended all participation in athletics. He often had pain in the back of the leg that had been injured and hadn't been able to touch his toes in five years. Stiff hamstring muscles, in making it hard for him to bend over, had made back strain inevitable.

Self-applied massage with a tennis ball on a wooden chair allowed the muscles to begin to lengthen. Nathan was able to return to work with renewed confidence. Despite the scarring that remained in the one hamstring muscle from the old injury, he was eventually able to touch his toes again.

Biceps Femoris

The *biceps femoris* (FEM-or-iss) has two parts and is comparable to the biceps muscle of the upper arm. It is also known as the "lateral hamstring," or the one closer to the outer side of the thigh.

The main part of the biceps femoris attaches to the sit bone and to the back of the thighbone. It then descends to attach to the top of the fibula, the slender outer bone of the lower leg. The biceps femoris has great power to bend the knee, and it also participates in extending the hip. These actions are necessary for walking, running, and jumping. The braking action of all the hamstrings keeps the body from falling forward whether you are moving or standing still. The hamstrings also control the rate of descent when you bend forward at the hip.

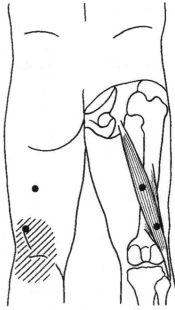

Figure 9.45 Biceps femoris trigger points and referred pain pattern

Symptoms

Pain from trigger points in the biceps femoris muscle is felt as a dull aching behind the knee (Figure 9.45). The pain tends to be toward the outer side of the back of the thigh rather than centered, and sometimes concentrated around the head of the fibula. Discomfort from biceps femoris trigger points sometimes extends up the back of the thigh and down into the upper calf (not shown) (1992, 316).

Causes

Trouble with the hamstrings comes about when the legs are kept bent at the hip and knee joints for long periods. A sedentary lifestyle is bad for the hamstrings, tending to shorten and stiffen them. Chairs that put pressure on the backs of the thighs promote the development of hamstring trigger points. Playing football, basketball, and soccer frequently results in hamstring injuries, particularly when the players are poorly conditioned amateurs. Other sports activities like swimming and cycling can be hard on the hamstrings when latent trigger points are keeping them shortened and weak (1992, 324–326).

The actions of all the thigh and hip muscles are interrelated. Trouble in one muscle spreads quickly to the others. Tightness in the quadriceps muscles, for example, makes the hamstrings work harder by restricting range of motion at the knee. Trigger points in the hamstrings cause the gluteal muscles to be under strain, since both these muscle groups must lengthen to allow you to bend at the hip. The weakening effect of hamstring trigger points also places a greater burden on the sartorius, gracilis, gastrocnemius, and plantaris muscles during knee flexion. You should always expect to find multiple trigger points in the hips and thighs.

Treatment

Differentiate the biceps femoris from the other hamstring muscles by feeling for the groove between them halfway up the back of the thigh. You can do this while sitting. Keep your foot on the floor and contract the back of the thigh as if you were trying to pull your foot back. This will make the muscles stand out. Also, feel at the outer side of the back of the knee for the heavy biceps femoris tendon. This tendon ends at the head of the fibula, the knob at the top of the outer side of the lower leg. Note in Figure 9.45 that the muscle travels diagonally up the back of the leg from the head of the fibula to the sit bone. The lower black dot in each leg represents possible multiple trigger points in the short head of the biceps femoris, which is hidden by the long head.

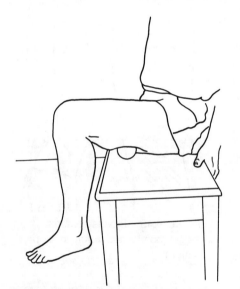

Figure 9.46   Hamstring massage with ball on wooden bench or chair

The hands and fingers tire quickly when used to massage hamstring trigger points, but the Thera Cane works well when you're either standing or sitting. Try levering the Thera Cane against the hamstrings while sitting in a soft chair. Better yet, work them with a tennis ball while sitting on a hard surface, such as a wooden chair or bench (Figure 9.46). You won't be able to massage the hamstrings with a ball against the wall.

To take better care of your hamstrings, note the types of chairs, couches, and car seats that put pressure on the backs of your thighs and make adjustments wherever possible. If your feet don't rest squarely on the floor, use anything you can find as a footrest. The hamstrings of people with short legs are put at risk everywhere they go; car seats and deep couches cause problems even for tall people.

Latent trigger points in hamstring muscles are unusually sneaky: you may never suspect you have them even when they are causing serious trouble. Be alert for stiffness in the backs of the legs, which is a sure sign of hamstring trouble. It pays to check often on the condition of the hamstrings and take the time to work on the trigger points you find. It's the best preventative measure possible for warding off serious hamstring injuries and the effects that shortened hamstrings can have on other muscles.

Semitendinosus and Semimembranosus

The "semi" muscles, *semitendinosus* (seh-me-ten-din-OH-sis) and *semimembranosus* (seh-me-mem-bran-OH-sis), are the other half of the hamstrings, complementing and counterbalancing the force of the biceps femoris. Their names reflect the fact that half the length of both muscles is made up of very strong tendonlike tissue. These muscles act as a unit and will be discussed as though they were one muscle; we'll call them the "semi muscles" for short.

Symptoms

Pain from trigger points in the semi muscles is felt primarily high on the back of the thigh at the gluteal fold (Figure 9.47). The pain pattern sometimes extends down the inner side of the back of the thigh and into the calf (not shown). In this case, the entire back of the thigh from the gluteal fold to the calf may be tender to the touch. When pain from the semi muscles does occur at the knee, it is a sharper sensation than pain from the biceps femoris and is felt more toward the inner side of the knee (1992, 316).

Pain and stiffness caused by trigger points in the semi muscles is frequently mislabeled "hamstring tendinitis." The wide distribution of pain from hamstring trigger points may also lead to a mistaken diagnosis of sciatica. Surgery on the spine exploring for the cause of presumed sciatic nerve impingement is not uncommon. Exploration for trigger points should always be done first (1992, 324–325).

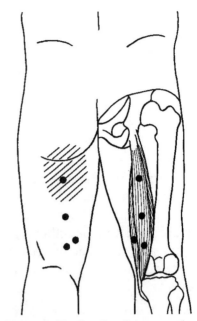

Figure 9.47 Semitendinosus and semimembranosus trigger points and referred pain pattern

In cases of genuine physical injury to the hamstrings, trigger points are always involved in producing part of the pain. They actually may be the root cause of the injury, in having made the hamstrings less resilient and therefore more vulnerable (1992, 325).

Causes

The semi muscles attach to the sit bone and to the inner side of the top of the tibia. Their action is to help extend the hip and flex the knee. Injuries to the semi muscles occur at maximum flexion of the hip and extension of the knee, the position at which the two muscles are at their maximum length. This is the position the leg is in just after kicking a soccer ball or football. When you're running the hurdles or doing the splits in gymnastics, it's the forward leg that is at risk for hamstring injury.

Overstretching causes trigger points in the semi muscles, as does too little stretching resulting from too little activity. Sitting all day and all evening—on the job, in the car, and at home—contributes to shortening of the semi muscles. Constant pressure on the backs of the thighs by the edge of a chair seat cuts off circulation and promotes trigger points in all the hamstring muscles (1992, 326).

Tightness in any of the hamstring muscles is frequently the root of chronic low back pain. Tight hamstrings cause a posterior tilt of the pelvis, flattening the curve of the lower back and distorting the mechanics of back and buttocks muscles. The resulting abnormal posture also encourages the head to be projected forward, resulting in added strain on the upper back and neck. In these ways, the domino effect of tight hamstrings can be the indirect cause of pain in quite distant parts of the body, including the jaws, face, and head. In short, your hamstrings can be involved even if your only complaint is chronic headaches (1992, 328).

Treatment

Locate the semi muscles on the inner side of the back of the thigh. Search the entire area with the tennis ball against the seat of a wooden chair, as with the biceps femoris (see Figure 9.46). Move your leg from side to side over the ball, exploring the full width of the back of the thigh. Most trigger points in the semi muscles will be found in the mid- and lower thigh, although it's not unusual for them to occur right below the sit bone. In Figure 9.47, each black dot in the lower half of the two muscles represents possible multiple trigger points in the semimembranosus, which is hidden by the semitendinosus. You may not suspect you have trigger points in your hamstrings until you take the trouble to look for them.

The most important thing to remember about all the hamstring muscles is that they can't be adequately stretched unless their trigger points are deactivated first: trigger points actively inhibit the lengthening of muscle fibers. The stretching that is routinely done before exercise and sports activities may give you the feeling that you're taking proper care of your hamstring muscles, but if their trigger points are left untreated, they can still be at risk for injury.

Popliteus

The *popliteus* (pop-lih-TEE-us) is a small muscle found at the back of the knee. The word popliteus derives from *poples*, Latin for "ham." The popliteus, being small and hidden, is often overlooked in troubleshooting for trigger points.

The popliteus muscle's upper attachment is to the outer side of the lower end of the thighbone. Its lower attachment is to the top of the back of the tibia. Its function is to unlock the knee so that it can bend. The popliteus also assists the posterior cruciate ligament (inside the knee joint) in preventing the femur from moving forward on the tibia. Damage to this ligament may overload the popliteus, causing pain from trigger points to persist after surgical repairs to the ligament have been made.

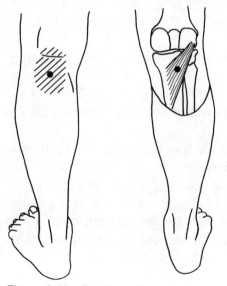

Figure 9.48   Popliteus trigger point and referred pain pattern

Symptoms

Trigger points in the popliteus muscle cause pain behind the knee when you straighten your leg (Figure 9.48). A shortened popliteus will prevent normal locking of the knee. The popliteus may not be suspected until trigger points in the biceps femoris have been deactivated.

Pain is also felt when crouching, running, or walking, and is worse when walking downhill or downstairs. Trigger points in popliteus muscles are often responsible for the acute pain experienced in the backs of the knees by hikers and backpackers on their way back down from a climb.

Knee pain caused by popliteus trigger points can be mistaken for tendinitis, torn ligaments, and damage to the meniscus or other knee joint tissues. While real physical damage to the knee is always a possibility, especially from accidents and in violent team sports, you shouldn't assume that knee pain automatically means knee surgery. The first step should always be to look for trigger points in the muscles that control the knee (1992, 343–345).

Causes

Popliteus muscles are overworked by running, twisting, sliding, and quickly changing direction in running games such as soccer, baseball, and football. Tennis, volleyball, and track competition are other events where popliteus stress may occur. Downhill skiing and downhill hiking are hard on popliteus muscles. Wearing a knee brace for pain relief can be an unsuspected cause of popliteus trouble by immobilizing the muscle and preventing its normal action (1992, 343–345).

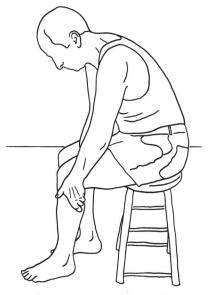

Figure 9.49 Popliteus massage with fingers of both hands

Treatment

Popliteus trigger points are found just below the knee crease between the two heads of the gastrocnemius muscle (this muscle can be seen in Figure 10.23). They're very deep, right on the tibia. Massage the popliteus with the fingers of both hands or with paired thumbs; illustrations 9.49 and 9.50 show the hand positions. It's best not to use a hard massage tool in this sensitive area.

Avoid stretching the popliteus and other muscles of the back of the leg without first massaging trigger points that may inhibit lengthening. Avoid wearing high heels of any kind; they tend to keep the knees flexed and the popliteus muscles shortened.

Remember that a sedentary lifestyle is perfect preparation for myofascial disasters. Be cautious about suddenly going hog-wild about getting into shape, but do find ways to be active in a regular and reasonable fashion.

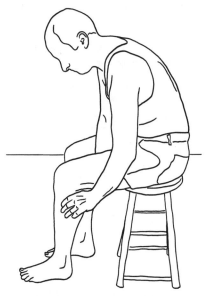

Figure 9.50 Popliteus massage with thumbs

Plantaris

The *plantaris* (plan-TEHR-iss) is also a small muscle found behind the knee. Its name reflects a very different function from that of the popliteus. *Plantaris* comes from the Latin *planta*, meaning "sole of the foot." (You may be familiar with plantar warts, which occur on the bottom of the foot.) With the aid of its incredibly long tendon, the plantaris helps the calf muscles *plantar flex* the ankle. Plantar flexion is when you point the foot down.

The plantaris attaches to the bottom end of the thighbone near the attachment for the popliteus. Its long tendon descends to attach to the calcaneus, or heel bone, joining the

Achilles tendon. A very small muscle, the plantaris is easily overstretched when extreme extension occurs in the knee and ankle at the same time. The knee is straight in extreme extension; the foot is bent upward from the ankle as far as it will go.

Pain from plantaris trigger points is centered behind the knee but may extend down into the upper calf (Figure 9.51). Search for trigger points at the outer side of the back of the knee, right in the crease. Use the same massage techniques as for the popliteus (see Figures 9.49 and 9.50).

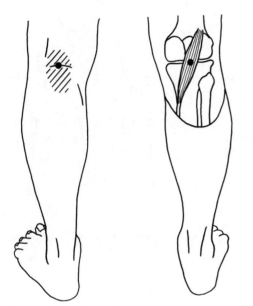

Figure 9.51   Plantaris trigger point and referred pain pattern

CHAPTER 10

Lower Leg, Ankle, and Foot Pain

Trigger Point Guide:
Lower Leg, Ankle, and Foot Pain

Front of Leg Pain
tibialis anterior (223)
adductor longus (204)

Back of Leg Pain
soleus (237)
gluteus minimus (178)
gastrocnemius (235)
semitendinosus (212)
semimembranosus (212)
flexor digitorum longus (241)
tibialis posterior (240)
plantaris (215)

Side of Leg Pain
gastrocnemius (235)
gluteus minimus (178)
peroneus longus (230)
peroneus brevis (232)
vastus lateralis (199)

Front of Ankle Pain
tibialis anterior (223)
peroneus tertius (233)
extensor digitorum longus (226)

Back of Ankle Pain
soleus (237)
tibialis posterior (240)

Outer Ankle Pain
peroneus longus (230)
peroneus brevis (232)
peroneus tertius (233)
abductor digiti minimi (250)

Inner Ankle Pain
abductor hallucis (249)
soleus (237)
gastrocnemius (235)
flexor digitorum longus (241)

Leg and Foot Numbness
gluteus minimus (178)
piriformis (180)
interosseous (245)
soleus (237)
peroneus longus (230)
extensor digitorum longus (226)
abductor hallucis (249)
adductor hallucis (253)
flexor hallucis longus (241)

Trigger Point Guide:
Lower Leg and Ankle Pain

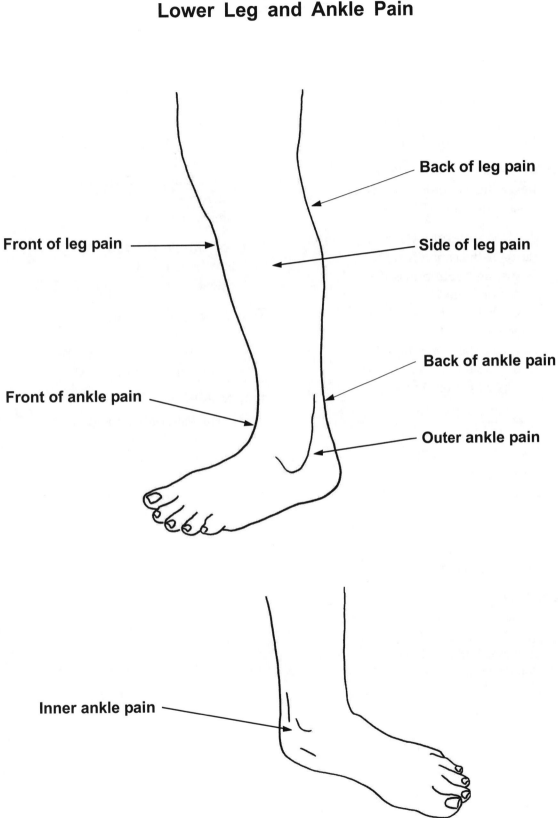

Back of leg pain

Front of leg pain

Side of leg pain

Back of ankle pain

Front of ankle pain

Outer ankle pain

Inner ankle pain

Trigger Point Guide:
Foot Pain

Under Big Toe Pain

flexor hallucis longus (241)
flexor hallucis brevis (253)
tibialis posterior (240)

Under Smaller Toes Pain

flexor digitorum longus (241)
tibialis posterior (240)

Head of Metatarsal Pain

flexor hallucis brevis (253)
flexor digitorum brevis (251)
adductor hallucis (253)
flexor hallucis longus (241)
interosseous (245)
abductor digiti minimi (250)
flexor digitorum longus (241)
tibialis posterior (240)
flexor digiti minimi brevis (254)

Arch and Midfoot Pain

gastrocnemius (235)
flexor digitorum longus (241)
adductor hallucis (253)
soleus (237)
abductor hallucis (249)
interosseous (245)
tibialis posterior (240)

Heel Pain

soleus (237)
quadratus plantae (252)
abductor hallucis (249)
tibialis posterior (240)
abductor digiti minimi (250)
gastrocnemius (235)

Top of Foot Pain

extensor digitorum brevis (245)
extensor hallucis brevis (245)
extensor digitorum longus (226)
extensor hallucis longus (226)
flexor hallucis brevis (253)
interosseous (245)
tibialis anterior (223)

Top of Smaller Toes Pain

interosseous (245)
extensor digitorum longus (226)

Top of Big Toe Pain

tibialis anterior (223)
extensor hallucis longus (226)
flexor hallucis brevis (253)

Toe Numbness

flexor hallucis longus (241)
interosseous (245)
peroneus longus (230)
abductor hallucis (249)
adductor hallucis (253)
extensor digitorum longus (226)

Trigger Point Guide:
Foot Pain

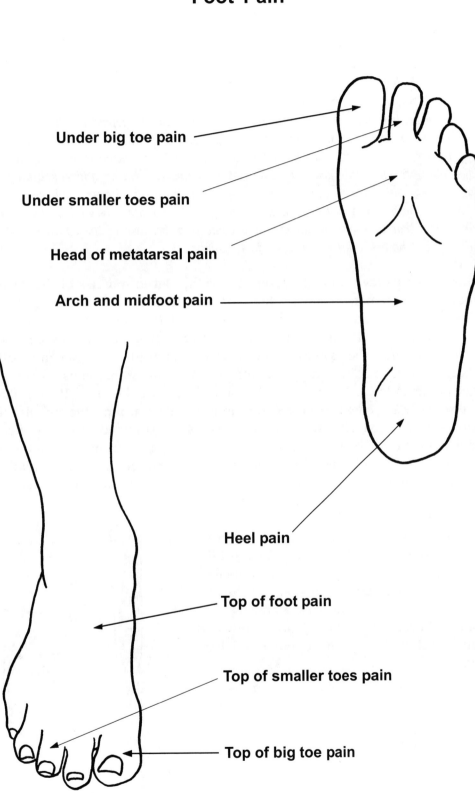

Under big toe pain

Under smaller toes pain

Head of metatarsal pain

Arch and midfoot pain

Heel pain

Top of foot pain

Top of smaller toes pain

Top of big toe pain

Lower Leg, Ankle, and Foot Pain

Laura, age twenty-five, in New York City on vacation, developed incapacitating foot pain after walking all day on the concrete sidewalks, seeing the sights. She had to take a cab to an emergency treatment center, where she was advised to just take some Aleve and get off her feet. Even after resting and taking the pills, Laura's feet still hurt and she could barely hobble around her hotel room. She was very annoyed that each day "off her feet" was a day lost from her vacation.

A massage therapist who had an office in Laura's hotel showed her how to massage her lower legs to get rid of her foot pain. She'd already spent a great deal of time massaging her feet, but it hadn't helped very much. After massage to her calf and shin muscles, however, she could walk with almost no pain. By resting and continuing the massage throughout the evening and again the next morning, she was able to go out again on a somewhat reduced schedule, planning to take more cabs and do less "hoofing it." She knew that the pain would probably come back because of the continued strain of walking, but now she knew what to do to combat it.

You may not have ever thought about it, but the eleven muscles of the lower leg are actually foot muscles. Anatomists call them *extrinsic* foot muscles, meaning they operate from outside the foot. The muscles in the foot itself are *intrinsic* foot muscles, meaning they work from inside the foot. The implication of these facts is that the pain in your feet may not be coming from your feet themselves. You can waste a lot of time rubbing and soaking your feet if the cause of your pain is trigger points in your calves and shins.

Trigger points in lower leg muscles also produce most ankle pain. Pain in the front of the ankle almost always comes from the shin muscles. Pain around the Achilles tendon in the back of the ankle is usually from the calf muscles. A "sprained" ankle is often nothing more serious than referred pain from trigger points in the peroneus muscles of the outer side of the lower leg. Many problems of the ankles and feet that get labeled "tendinitis," "heel spur," "plantar fasciitis," or a "strained ligament" can be fixed with simple massage of the muscles of the lower leg (Travell and Simons 1992, 355, 370, 427, 460).

Obviously, serious conditions resulting from physical trauma or congenital deformity do affect the ankles and feet of many people. Nevertheless, myofascial trigger points are always part of the picture even when other conditions exist. Knowing your trigger points will allow you to deal successfully and reliably with most kinds of pain in your lower legs, ankles, and feet.

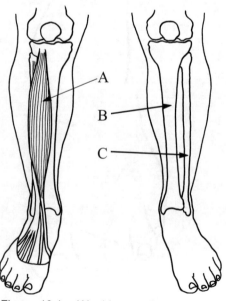

Figure 10.1   (A) shin muscles; (B) tibia; (C) fibula

Shin Muscles

There are three important muscles on the front of your lower leg (Figure 10.1). These three shin muscles act to *dorsiflex* (raise) the foot and toes. This is a vitally important function in keeping the toes from dragging when you walk. The shin muscles also help accommodate the foot to uneven ground and keep you balanced when you're on your feet. Shin muscles weakened by trigger points are a major cause of tripping and stumbling, which can result in physical injury, a special concern for older persons for whom a fall can mean broken bones and hospitalization (1992, 356, 361).

Pain from trigger points in the three shin muscles is sent to the front of the ankle and the top of the foot and toes. Myofascial pain in the big toe from the shin muscles is sometimes mistaken for gout. Other problems traceable to trigger points are ankle weakness, night cramps, hammertoe and claw toe, and numbness in the top of the foot and the front of the lower leg (1992, 478-480).

Chronic tension from trigger points in the shin muscles can result in shin splints, an extremely painful condition caused by stress on muscle attachments. Although the pain of shin splints is not the same as referred pain from trigger points, massage is the correct treatment, because it deactivates the trigger points and removes the chronic tension in the muscle (1992, 443-444).

Shin muscles that are chronically swollen from the effects of trigger points can eventually produce anterior compartment syndrome, a very serious condition in which circulation is impaired and muscle tissue may die. There are four muscle compartments in the lower leg. Each one contains several muscles and is separated from the other compartments by thick sheets of connective tissue, which can severely limit the space inside. A compartment syndrome is characterized by general tightness and tenderness over the whole compartment area; the internal pressure in a compartment can rise to a level that will rupture its fascial covering, constituting an emergency that must be relieved surgically. Compartment syndrome is less likely to occur if myofascial trigger points are taken care of in a timely way (1992, 361-362).

Tibialis Anterior

The word *tibialis* (tib-ee-AL-is) comes from *tibia*, the Latin word for "shinbone." The *tibialis anterior* muscle lies along the outer side of your shinbone. Interestingly, people in Roman times made flutes from the shinbone or tibia of certain animals. Such an instrument was naturally called a "tibia." If you've ever wondered why the flute stop on a pipe organ is called the "tibia," that's the ancient connection.

The tibialis anterior attaches to the top of the tibia and all along its upper half. Its long tendon descends parallel to the sharp edge of the shinbone. You can see this tendon stick out at the front of the ankle when you raise the front of your foot. The tendon crosses the top of the foot to its inner edge. It then wraps around to attach to bones on the underside of the foot.

The attachments of the tibialis anterior allow it to dorsiflex the foot and turn the bottom of the foot inward, an action called *inversion*. Dorsiflexion lets the foot clear the ground after you've taken a step and are bringing the foot forward for another. The actions of inversion and dorsiflexion are necessary for maintaining balance and adapting the foot to the surface beneath it. Understanding the effects of tibialis anterior trigger points may solve a number of otherwise very frustrating, unexplained problems in the feet and ankles, including weakness, stiffness, numbness, and pain. Consider that trigger points in tibialis anterior muscles are one of the chief causes of "growing pains" in the feet and ankles of children. They're no less common in adults. The two following cases illustrate typical problems originating in the tibialis anterior muscles (1992, 356; Bates and Grunwaldt 1958, 198-209).

Diane, age fifty-nine, arrived at her computer class with severe pain in the front of her right ankle and the top of her foot. She hadn't been able to sleep the night before and now could hardly walk. The tightness in her face displayed her agony. A massage therapist who was also taking the class showed her how to massage a horribly painful spot beside her shinbone. Within minutes, the intensity of the foot and ankle pain had subsided. To keep it from coming back, he showed her how to massage the spot herself with the heel of her opposite foot.

The cause of Diane's pain was her habit of sitting at her computer with her feet under her chair. This position, with her toes touching the floor and bent up as far as they would go, cramped the muscles in the fronts of her lower legs for hours.

Andy, age eighty, had chronic pain in his big toe. His toes also tended to catch on steps and the edge of carpets, causing him to trip unexpectedly. He had almost fallen several times. Falling and breaking a hip was his greatest fear. So for safety he had begun using a cane. The doctor prescribed medicine for gout, though the tests hadn't strictly confirmed that gout was the problem. The medicine didn't seem to help, however, and Andy's toe continued to hurt.

Trigger points were discovered in the muscles of the front of Andy's lower leg. Pressure on one particular spot reproduced the pain in his toe exactly. After massage, the pain was noticeably diminished. He found he was able to the massage the spot himself with the rubber tip of his cane. With continued self-applied massage as needed, Andy stopped tripping over his own feet and his "gout" soon disappeared.

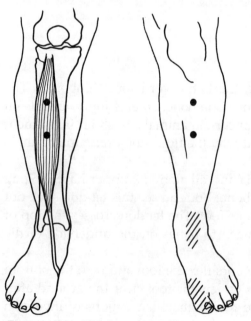

Figure 10.2   Tibialis anterior trigger points and referred pain pattern

Symptoms

Trigger points in the tibialis anterior send pain to the top and inner side of the big toe and to the front of the ankle (Figure 10.2). Walking makes the pain worse. Occasionally, pain may extend partway up the lower leg alongside the shinbone (not shown) (1992, 356).

"Gout" and "turf toe" are labels often applied to pain in the big toe. Pain in the big toe doesn't automatically mean you have gout. The referral pattern for trigger points in tibialis anterior and extensor hallucis longus muscles includes the big toe and the head of the first metatarsal bone, the place where the toe joins the foot. The pain can feel as though it's actually in the joint. Physicians who are unaware of these effects are likely to prescribe gout medications for this pain, even when tests fail to confirm the condition.

True gout, the deposit of urate crystals in the joints, is caused by uricemia, too much uric acid in your blood. A diet of too much meat and too little water is likely to promote uricemia. Gout and the trigger points that mimic gout often coexist, and uricemia can make your trigger points hard to get rid of. A vitamin C deficiency makes both conditions hard to get rid of.

Falls and presumed balance problems may actually be the result of the weakening effect that trigger points have on the tibialis anterior muscles. A weak tibialis anterior allows the foot to drop when it shouldn't. This can cause tripping and stubbing of toes on level ground and stumbling while climbing stairs. This effect can put the elderly in serious jeopardy, ending in broken bones or even worse injuries. No matter your age, if you tend to "fall over your own feet," you should check the fronts of your lower legs for trigger points (1992, 361, 363).

The pain patterns of several other muscles overlap that of the tibialis anterior. In seeking the cause of pain in the front of the ankle and the top of the foot and toes, troubleshoot all six muscles of the front of the lower leg and top of the foot. Besides the tibialis anterior, these include the peroneus tertius, extensor digitorum longus, extensor hallucis longus, extensor digitorum brevis, and extensor hallucis brevis (1992, 361).

Causes

The tibialis anterior muscles can be overloaded by strenuous running, walking, and climbing. Changing your running or walking style can also put the tibialis anterior muscles under stress. Walking on rough ground can strain all the muscles of the lower leg, including the tibialis anterior. Driving for long periods with the foot constantly on the accelerator is especially bad for this muscle (1992, 363).

Trigger points in the calf muscles make the muscles of the front of the lower leg work harder and cause them to tire very quickly. Conversely, trigger points in the front of the leg overtax the back of the leg. Such overburdening of the muscles continued over a length of time can predispose you to compartment syndromes in both areas, which can do permanent damage to the muscles. Chronic trigger points in the tibialis anterior itself are also a root cause of shin splints and stress fractures of the tibia (1992, 361-363).

Treatment

The tibialis anterior muscle is found just to the outside of the shinbone. Confirm its location by feeling it contract when you raise the front of your foot (Figure 10.3). Trigger points in the tibialis anterior occur approximately one-third of the way down the leg from the knee. They can be very deep in this thick muscle, seeming to be right at the bone. The difficulty in massaging them is in getting the leverage to exert adequate pressure. Supported fingers work well, provided you trim your nails right to the quick so you can employ the very tips (Figure 10.4). If you're reluctant to sacrifice your nails, try a

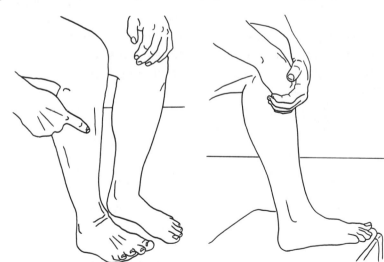

Figure 10.3 Locating tibialis anterior by isolated contraction

Figure 10.4 Tibialis anterior massage with supported fingers or Knobble

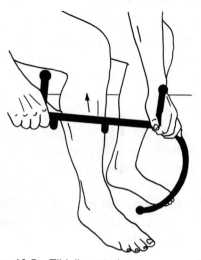

Figure 10.5   Tibialis anterior massage with Thera Cane

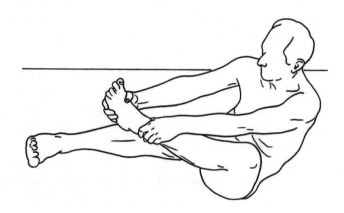

Figure 10.6   Tibialis anterior massage with the heel as the tool

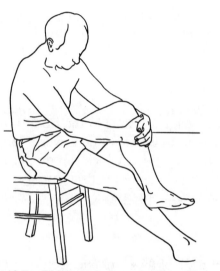

Figure 10.7   Tibialis anterior massage with heel

Knobble massage tool, applying pressure with both hands. The Thera Cane is excellent for this job if you employ the shaft instead of the knobs, which are a bit too hard for this sensitive area (Figure 10.5).

Possibly the best trick for working the tibialis anterior—if you're limber enough—is to use the heel of the opposite foot as a tool. While sitting on the floor or on the bed, hold the foot with both hands and drag it toward you over the muscle (Figure 10.6). You can also use the heel when you're sitting on the edge of the bed or in a chair (Figure 10.7). In this case, you'll be pushing your foot away from you, down your leg.

When you've had trouble with the tibialis anterior, check for trigger points in other muscles of the leg. The imbalances they cause can make it necessary for tibialis muscles to carry an extra load. View any small incident of tripping as a sign that latent trigger points may be limiting the actions of the shin muscles.

Extensor Digitorum Longus and Extensor Hallucis Longus

The *extensor digitorum longus* and *extensor hallucis* (HAL-uh-sis) *longus* muscles lie beneath the tibialis anterior. The extensor digitorum longus attaches to the top of the tibia and to nearly the entire length of the fibula. The other end of the muscle attaches by four separate tendons to the bones of the four smaller toes. The extensor hallucis longus also attaches to the fibula, beginning at that bone's midpoint. It then descends to attach to the bones of the big toe.

Both toe extensors help dorsiflex or raise the front of the foot. The extensor hallucis longus also aids in turning the sole of the foot inward (inversion). The extensor digitorum longus provides some of the force that turns the foot outward (eversion). All three actions—dorsiflexion, inversion, and eversion—adapt the foot to the ground and help you keep your balance when on your feet.

Trigger points in these long extensors of the toes are very common in both children and adults. The pain they cause in the ankles and feet is typically blamed on tendinitis. Conventional treatments such as exercise, stretching, and rest often fail to produce results. Ben's and Barbara's stories typify problems with the toe extensors (1992, 474-475).

Ben, age forty-six, had constant pain in the top of his left foot and the lower part of his shin. His ankle was so weak that he had difficulty raising his foot. Any attempt to do so greatly increased his pain. The immediate problem was that he was unable to pull up with his foot to shift gears on his motorcycle. As a consequence, he'd had to drop out early from a long-anticipated weekend tour with his motorcycle club.

Trigger points were found in the front of Ben's left lower leg, in muscles being overused in shifting gears. Tightness in the muscles caused pressure on the nerve that supplied motor impulses to the muscles, leaving them unable to make a strong voluntary contraction. Self-applied massage immediately stopped the pain in the top of his foot and over several weeks brought back the strength in the muscles.

Barbara, age seventy, was often awakened in the night by cramps in the fronts of her lower legs. The tops of her feet hurt most of the time and she couldn't straighten her toes, which stayed curled up like claws. She tended to walk flatfooted because of recurrent pain in the bottoms of her feet.

Horribly tender trigger points were found in the fronts of Barbara's lower legs. After professional treatment and instruction, she was able to stop the night cramps with self-applied massage to the fronts of her legs. Three weeks of an established routine of massage morning and night eliminated the pain in the tops of her feet. Eventually, her toes began to relax too. Deep massage to the soles of her feet brought additional relief.

Symptoms

Trigger points in the extensor digitorum longus send pain primarily to the top of the foot, though it may sometimes extend to the tips of the four smaller toes and up the front of the ankle (Figure 10.8). This distribution of pain overlaps that of the tibialis anterior, peroneus tertius, extensor digitorum brevis, and interosseous muscles. This makes it important to very accurately determine exactly where you feel the pain (1992, 479).

Tension in the extensor digitorum longus sometimes puts pressure on the deep peroneal nerve, which supplies motor impulses to all the muscles of the front of the lower leg. This impingement can cause severe weakness in these muscles and make it difficult to raise the foot. Compression of the deep peroneal

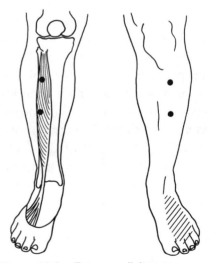

Figure 10.8 Extensor digitorum longus trigger points and referred pain pattern

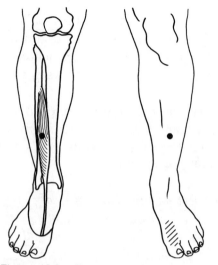

Figure 10.9   Extensor hallucis longus trigger point and referred pain pattern

nerve produces a distinctive patch of numbness in the top of the foot, at the base of the first and second toes (1992, 482).

Trigger points in the extensor hallucis longus cause pain in the big toe, centered on the head of the first metatarsal bone, the place where the toe joins the foot (Figure 10.9). Occasionally, pain may extend to the front of the ankle and can feel as though it's actually in the bone (not shown) (1992, 474-475).

Chronically tight toe extensor muscles contribute to the development of *hammertoe* and *claw toe*. These are conditions in which the toes are cramped and drawn up and can't be straightened either actively or passively. Permanent deformity of the foot can result if the muscles go untreated. Unrelieved tightness in the toe extensors also leads to recurrent night cramps (1992, 479-480).

Causes

The extensor muscles can be strained by the momentary overload that occurs when you stub your toes or kick a ball. The toe extensors are easily overworked by operating the gas and brake pedals if you do a lot of city driving. Pedaling a bike is another activity that may tire them excessively. Climbing long flights of stairs can exhaust the toe extensors, since they have to contract hard with each step in order for the toes to clear. Trigger points can also be set up by the inactivity imposed by a cast after a bone break (1992, 480-481).

Treatment

The toe extensors are buried under the edge of tibialis anterior, the thick mass of muscle that runs alongside the shinbone. They're hard to locate by isolated contraction, but not impossible. Search for the belly of the extensor digitorum longus about a hand's width below the lower edge of the kneecap. The extensor digitorum longus trigger point will be about an inch to the outside of the tibialis anterior trigger point, halfway between the front and the side of the leg. To contract the extensor digitorum longus by itself, raise the toes without raising the front of the foot (Figure 10.10).

Look for extensor hallucis longus trigger points halfway between the knee and the ankle, just to the outer side of the shinbone. Feel the muscle contract when you raise your big toe (Figure 10.11). When it does so, you can see its tendon stand out on the front of the ankle between the tendons for the tibialis anterior and extensor digitorum longus.

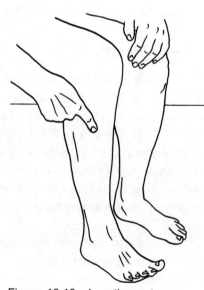

Figure 10.10   Locating extensor digitorum longus by isolated contraction

Since the toe extensor muscles are so deep, you'll probably find your heel ineffective as a massage tool. The Knobble, Thera Cane, or supported fingers will do better. If you can get the leverage to go deep enough, you'll experience almost immediate relief. Muscles of the lower leg respond exceptionally well to massage.

To be really good to your lower legs, give up wearing high-heeled shoes. They keep several lower leg muscles in a shortened state and put you at risk for overstretching or overcontracting muscles, should you lose your balance. Wear long pants in cool weather to keep the muscles from getting chilled, and put a throw of some kind over your legs when sitting around home in the wintertime. If you have recurrent trouble with your shin muscles, beware of too much running or walking, particularly up and down hills. When you're in the midst of trouble with them, take the elevator—stay off the stairs.

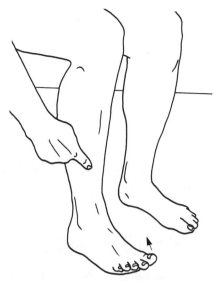

Figure 10.11   Locating extensor hallucis longus by isolated contraction

Peroneus Muscles

The three *peroneus* muscles are found on the outer side of the lower leg (Figure 10.12). The word *peroneus* (pair-uh-NEE-us) derives from the Greek word for "pin." The peroneus muscles all attach to the fibula, the thin, pinlike outer bone of the lower leg. The Latin word *fibula* also means "pin."

Trigger points in the peroneus muscles produce a great part of the pain that occurs on the outer side of the ankle. Many times, a presumed "sprain," particularly one with little or no swelling, is nothing more than referred pain from the peroneus muscles. If massage to the peroneus muscles gets rid of the pain, it's unlikely that you've suffered ligament injury (1992, 377).

The action of all three peroneus muscles is *eversion*—turning the bottom of the foot outward and the ankle inward. An extreme degree of the opposite action, *inversion*, turning the bottom of the foot inward and the ankle outward, is what causes most sprains. When this happens, the peroneus muscles are severely overstretched. Their typical response is to produce trigger points and tighten up in self-defense. When this overstretching is bad enough, ligaments and tendons can be torn. In such a case, the added pain and stiffness from peroneus trigger points help discourage you from moving your ankle, clearly a protective device (1992, 375-377).

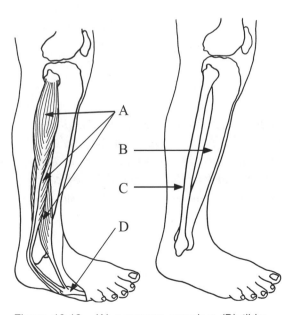

Figure 10.12   (A) peroneus muscles; (B) tibia; (C) fibula; (D) fifth metatarsal

Paradoxically, immobilization for an ankle injury tends to perpetuate trigger points in the peroneus muscles, causing them to long outlast the original injury. Persistent trigger points take the stretch out of the peroneus muscles and make new injuries almost inevitable. The ankle becomes weak and unstable, and sprains become more frequent and fractures more likely. Athletes are particularly vulnerable when trigger points handicap the peroneus muscles (1992, 379-380).

Under extreme conditions, the peroneus muscles can become so swollen and tight that they make the pressure intolerably high in the fibrous envelope that surrounds them. *Lateral compartment syndrome* can be the result, which, if it persists, may permanently damage the peroneal nerves unless you have surgery to relieve it.

Peroneus Longus

The longest and largest of the three peroneus muscles, the *peroneus* (pair-uh-NEE-us) *longus* is the one most often afflicted by trigger points. When you have ankle pain, think first of the peroneus longus.

The peroneus longus attaches to the head of the fibula and the upper two-thirds of its shaft. Its lower attachment is quite unusual: the tendon travels behind the *lateral malleolus* (the outer anklebone) and then crosses diagonally beneath the foot clear over to the inner side. There, it fastens to the underside of the base of the first *metatarsal* and one of the *tarsal* bones. (The tarsals and metatarsals are the bones in the front half of your foot, not including the toes.) These attachments enable the peroneus longus to point the foot downward and turn the sole outward (eversion). This is an action vital to walking, running, and climbing. You can feel the power of the peroneus longus under the ball of your foot as it helps impel you forward.

Many muscles, including the three peroneus muscles, automatically contract as they lengthen in order to balance and control the forces being applied by their antagonists, the muscles that work in the opposite direction. Peroneus muscles consequently do double duty, contracting while shortening and then again while lengthening. This can be very tiring for muscles that are constantly in use. The peroneus muscles, so important to all activities of the foot, are among the first to develop symptoms of overload, fatigue, and abuse.

Symptoms

Rachel, age twenty-seven, twisted her ankle and fell in her living room while dancing to Sesame Street *music with her small children. The severe pain took her right to the emergency room. A chipped bone in her ankle was discovered on X-ray, apparently torn loose by a strained ligament. Three weeks in a walking cast let the damaged bone heal, but pain and stiffness persisted for several months. She continued to have difficulty standing for any length of time, and walking brought immediate pain on the outside of her ankle.*

Trigger points were found in all the muscles of Rachel's lower leg. Pressure on a trigger point in her peroneus longus reproduced her ankle pain exactly. She learned to massage the outer side of her lower leg and was able to ease her ankle pain in just a few minutes whenever it started up. Within a month, pain ceased to be problem.

Trigger points in the peroneus muscle project pain to the outer side of the ankle (Figure 10.13). Pain focuses on and under the lateral malleolus, the outer anklebone or knobby end of the fibula that sticks out on the side of the ankle. *Malleolus* (mah-LEE-uh-lus) means "little hammer" in Latin. Pain occasionally occurs in the middle third of the outer lower leg and along the outer side of the foot (not shown). The ankle is usually diffusely tender to the touch, which differs from the sharply localized tenderness of a torn ligament. Symptoms of pain and tenderness in the ankle are often mistaken for signs of arthritis. Tendinitis is a common misdiagnosis (1992, 370-379).

Ankle weakness is characteristic of the effects of peroneus trigger points. In addition, nerve impingement by the tight peroneus longus

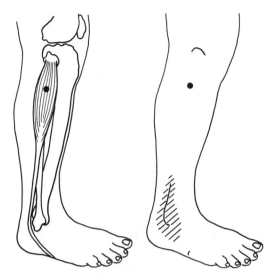

Figure 10.13   Peroneus longus trigger point and referred pain pattern

muscle can cause numbness in the lower leg, ankle, and top of the foot. Weakness in the muscles from nerve compression may make it hard to lift the front of your foot. When nerves are involved, weakness can occur with or without pain. These symptoms can be confusingly similar to those of nerve entrapment in the spine caused by a ruptured disk. Trigger points in peroneus muscles should be gotten rid of before conclusions are drawn about the spine. In some cases, however, the two conditions may coexist (1992, 377-385: Jeyaseelan 1989, 49-51).

Causes

Walking, running, and climbing, when done to excess, predictably create trigger points in the peroneus longus muscles. Walking is even worse for these muscles if you have a short leg, flat feet, or Morton's foot structure. (See the section on the feet for more information about Morton's foot.) Sleeping on your stomach or back with your toes pointed is bad for peroneus longus muscles because it keeps them in a shortened state. If you're not afflicted with too much compulsion for orderliness, try untucking the covers at the foot of the bed to give your feet and toes more freedom. Wearing high-heeled shoes puts shin muscles under increased stress by keeping them shortened and tight. In high heels, the weight of the body is thrown forward onto the toes, and peroneus muscles must stay contracted to maintain balance (1992, 377-380).

Therapeutic stockings or tight ankle socks put pressure on peroneus muscles and promote the formation of trigger points. Sitting with crossed legs can cause pressure on the peroneal nerves, which can lead to numbness and muscle weakness. Squatting compresses nerves and blood vessels alike, in addition to putting abnormal strain on a number of muscles, including the peroneal group. Trigger points are encouraged when you hold any extreme posture too long (1992, 379-380).

Treatment

Peroneus longus trigger points are found just below the head, or top knob, of the fibula. Confirm the location of the peroneus longus by feeling it contract when you turn the sole of

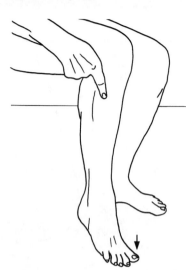

10.14 Locating peroneus longus by isolated

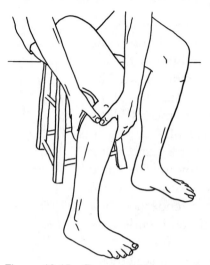

Figure 10.15   Peroneus longus massage with paired thumbs

your foot outward. You can make it contract harder by pointing your toes at the same time (Figure 10.14).

To gain greater access to all the peroneus muscles for massage, put your foot up on a chair. Another good position is sitting on the bed with the leg up on the bed with you. Massage the peroneus longus with paired thumbs using short, slow strokes (Figure 10.15). You may be able to use supported fingers also, but you'll see that the muscle tends to roll off the fibula

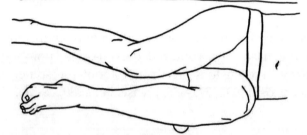

Figure 10.16   Peroneus longus massage lying on side with ball. Move the leg forward and back over the ball.

when you press on it. Paired thumbs let you trap it and hold it still. The Thera Cane works well if you employ the shaft instead of one of its knobs, just like with the tibialis anterior (see Figure 10.5). Massage lying on your side with a ball on the muscle works too (Figure 10.16). You'll easily find a trigger point centered on the bone, but note that the muscle wraps around the fibula: you'll often find a trigger point in the back edge of the muscle at the back edge of the bone.

You may not be able to keep from having trigger points in your peroneus muscles if you're an active person, but you should be aware that there's a special danger in ignoring chronic trigger points in these important muscles. Trigger point–sponsored weakness and inflexibility in the peroneus muscles leave you vulnerable to serious ankle injury, such as ruptured tendons, broken bones, and torn ligaments. To avoid these calamities, work on your trigger points at the first sign of pain in the outer side of your ankle. If your ankles seem weak and you're always suffering little sprains, it's a sign that latent peroneus trigger points are present and need to be attended to.

Peroneus Brevis

Trigger points are found less often in the *peroneus* (pair-uh-NEE-us) *brevis* than in the peroneus longus, but don't let this fact lull you into overlooking them. Pain from peroneus brevis trigger points occurs in a pattern similar to that of the longus but tends to extend further along the outer side of the foot since the muscle attaches there to the base of the fifth metatarsal (Figure 10.17). (The little knob you can feel in the middle of the outer edge of your foot is the end of the fifth metatarsal.)

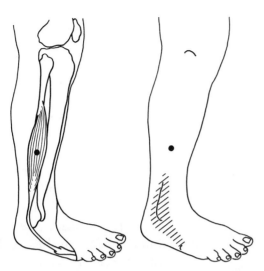

Figure 10.17 Peroneus brevis trigger point and referred pain pattern

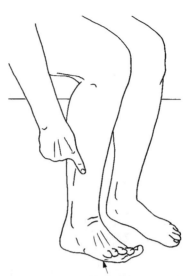

Figure 10.18 Locating peroneus brevis by isolated contraction

Locate the peroneus brevis by feeling it contract immediately in front of the peroneus longus tendon when you lift the outer edge of your foot at the same time you lift the front of your foot (Figure 10.18). This will be about a third of the way up the leg from the ankle. Massage the peroneus brevis at this point with the same tools you would use with the peroneus longus.

Peroneus Tertius

The *peroneus tertius* (pair-uh-NEE-us TER-shus) is a very special muscle simply because it is so well hidden. Peroneus tertius trigger points will make your ankle pain and weakness persist after everything else has been fixed.

The peroneus tertius attaches to the front of the lower half of the fibula bone. Its tendon passes in front of the lateral malleolus, or outer anklebone, to attach to the top of the base of the fourth and fifth metatarsals. This muscle's action is to turn the sole of the foot outward and to raise the front of the foot. The peroneus tertius can be a surprisingly large muscle, sometimes approaching the size of the extensor digitorum longus. The muscle is absent, however, in approximately 8 percent of the population. One person in seven has a fourth peroneus muscle, the *peroneus quartus*, located behind the lower end of the fibula. Its trigger points would be found between the fibula and the Achilles tendon and its pain pattern would be similar to that of the peroneus longus.

Trigger points in the peroneus tertius cause pain in front of the lateral malleolus and on the outer side of the heel (Figure 10.19). Characteristically, a surge of pain is felt with every step.

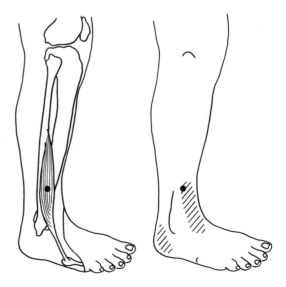

Figure 10.19 Peroneus tertius trigger point and referred pain pattern

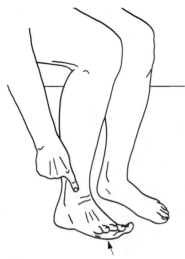

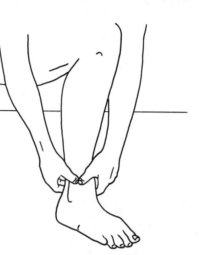

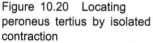

Figure 10.20 Locating peroneus tertius by isolated contraction

Figure 10.21 Peroneus tertius massage with paired thumbs

Ankle weakness usually accompanies the pain. These symptoms are commonly misinterpreted as a sign of ligament injury, tendinitis, or osteoarthritis (1992, 371, 377-379; Reynolds 1981, 111-114).

Locate the peroneus tertius above and just in front of the lateral malleolus. It lies just in front of the last three or four inches of the fibula. Feel it contract when you turn the sole of your foot outward at the same time you raise the front of your foot (Figure 10.20). Take note that this action also makes the extensor digitorum tendon stand out strongly on the front of the ankle. The peroneus tertius is behind this tendon. There's just room for a finger or two between this tendon and the fibula. Down deep in that spot lies the belly of the peroneus tertius.

Massage the peroneus tertius deeply with supported fingers or paired thumbs (Figure 10.21). A great way to massage the peroneus tertius and peroneus brevis at the same time is with a tennis ball on the edge of the bed (Figure 10.22). This position is particularly effective because you can use the weight of your leg to provide the force. This saves the fingers for work that only the fingers can do.

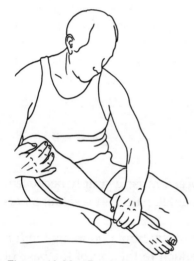

Figure 10.22 Peroneus tertius massage with ball on the edge of the bed

Calf Muscles

There are five muscles in the calf, separated as a unit into the *posterior compartment* by fibrous partitions. The muscles of the posterior compartment are strong and thick, even on slender individuals, and provide the major force for lifting the body to stand and propelling it forward to walk or run. They also participate in maintaining balance.

Trigger points in the calf muscles predictably foster calf cramps and cause pain in the ankles and the calves themselves. But you may be surprised to know that the calf muscles are also responsible for at least half of the pain felt on the bottoms of the feet and virtually all the pain felt around the Achilles tendon in the back of the ankle, pain that is so often blamed on the tendon itself (1992, 407–409, 440–442, 464–465, 492–494).

Gastrocnemius

The accepted pronunciation of *gastrocnemius* (gas-trock-NEE-me-us) is actually somewhat at odds with the word's derivation. It should probably be pronounced gas-tro-NEE-me-us. *Gastro* clearly comes from the Greek word for "stomach." *Cnemius* is from the Greek *kneme* (NEE-me) with a silent "k," which means "shank" or "lower leg." *Gastrocnemius* literally means "stomach of the lower leg." Take another look at your calves and you'll see why: it's the gastrocnemius muscles that give the calves their bellied contour.

The gastrocnemius muscle attaches to the lower end of the femur just above the back of the knee. Halfway down the back of the lower leg, the muscle joins the Achilles tendon, which then attaches to the heel bone. Because of the orientation of the muscle fibers in the gastrocnemius muscles' two heads, they have the power to lift the entire weight of the body. This power is needed for jumping, climbing, and the controlled descent of stairs and hillsides. Finer functions include stabilizing the ankle and knee joints and manipulating the feet for balance. Interestingly, the gastrocnemius muscles actually contribute very little to propelling the body forward, helping mostly in spurts of motion.

Ironically, signs of gastrocnemius trouble may only be felt in the feet. The logic of referred pain is evidently to make you hurt where you're most likely to pay attention and stop whatever activity is causing the muscle abuse. This is what one young woman experienced in the midst of a well-earned vacation.

April, age twenty-two, was to spend five marvelous weeks traveling around Europe after graduating from college. Unfortunately, during her first few days, she walked everywhere in shoes with two-inch platform heels and developed disabling pain in the arches of her feet. Every night in the hostels and hotels, she soaked her feet in hot water and gave them a good rub, but the next day, after walking only a short distance, the pain came back as bad as ever. She knew the high heels were bad for her feet, but it didn't seem to help much to change to low heels after the pain started. The pain actually seemed to get worse, and it was ruining her vacation.

A guidebook suggested massaging her calves to get rid of her foot pain. It made no sense to April, but she tried it anyway out of desperation. Amazingly, it worked. She made time at night and in the morning to massage the backs of her legs and then to carefully stretch them. Her feet, legs, and ankles responded by getting stronger with walking and climbing instead of reacting defensively by developing trigger points. Within a few days, pain ceased to be a problem.

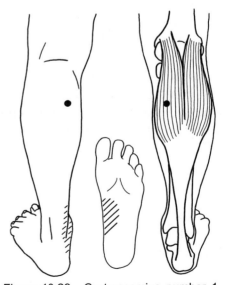

Symptoms

Pain in the long arch of the foot is the primary symptom of trouble in the gastrocnemius muscle (Figure 10.23). Pain from the number 1 trigger point may also sometimes extend to the back of the thigh, knee, and up the inner ankle (not shown). Trigger

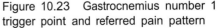
Figure 10.23   Gastrocnemius number 1 trigger point and referred pain pattern

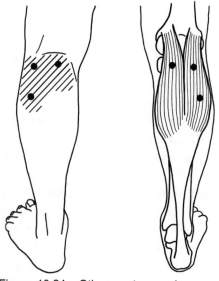

Figure 10.24   Other gastrocnemius trigger points and local pain pattern

points at other places in the gastrocnemius cause pain mainly in the muscle itself (Figure 10.24). The highest lateral trigger point, however, sometimes sends pain to the outer side of the heel (not shown). When trigger points shorten the muscle, it may be hard to straighten the knee with the heel on the floor. Children very often have these same symptoms from myofascial trigger points (1992, 398–399).

Trigger points toward the middle of the muscle are more likely to bring on night cramps in the calves than are those higher up. It's important to remember that nocturnal calf cramps can have many contributing causes, including vitamin deficiency, drug side effects, and poor circulation. Myofascial trigger points, however, head the list. Cramping can also occur while you're walking or running because of impeded circulation caused by muscle tightness (1992, 407–410).

Serious medical problems are often indicated by the same symptoms displayed by gastrocnemius trigger points. These include rupture of vertebral disks, tendon rupture, posterior compartment syndrome (which can cut off circulation), phlebitis, and cysts in the pocket behind the knee. Symptoms of gastrocnemius trigger points, however, can be misinterpreted as signs of any of these conditions when the practitioner is unaware of myofascial causes (1992, 406–407).

Causes

Climbing, walking uphill, or bike riding can overwork gastrocnemius muscles. On the job, leaning forward while standing for extended periods of time will wear them out and promote the formation of trigger points. Other causes include swimming with the toes pointed in the flutter kick, driving without cruise control, wearing high-heeled shoes, and sitting in chairs that restrict circulation by putting pressure on the backs of the thighs. Footstools or recliners that put pressure on the calves are a leading cause of trouble in calf muscles. Immobility from having the leg in a cast and poor conditioning from lack of exercise also lead to the establishment of trigger points. Viral illnesses often leave calf muscles tight and vulnerable to overuse. Chilling predisposes them to strain. Sleeping with the toes pointed keeps them in a shortened state and promotes cramping. You might curtail this hazard by not tucking the covers in at the foot of the bed (1992, 410–411).

Treatment

The location of the gastrocnemius on the upper half of the lower leg is usually well defined by the shape of the calf. You can also feel the belly of the muscle with your fingers as it bulges up when you point your toes.

For very focused, precise work on the gastrocnemius muscles, use supported fingers, the Knobble, or the Thera Cane. When using supported fingers, make it easy on your back by putting your foot up on the bed or a chair (Figure 10.25).

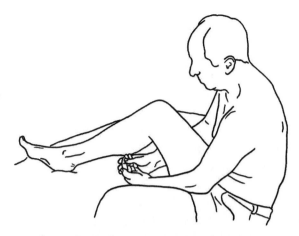

Figure 10.25   Gastrocnemius massage with supported fingers

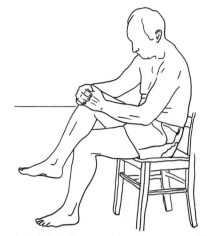

Figure 10.26   Gastrocnemius massage with opposite knee

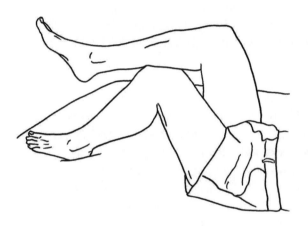

Figure 10.27   Gastrocnemius massage with opposite knee

Deep stroking massage with the opposite knee is particularly effective for the entire back of the lower leg and is very easy to do. This technique works well when you're either lying down or sitting up and is best done with bare legs (Figures 10.26 and 10.27). Simply move the leg down over the knee along three or four parallel lines, starting at the back of the ankle and going all the way to the back of the knee. When you encounter a trigger point, do extra work on that spot, going over it repeatedly with short strokes. Try massaging along the muscle and also across it. For concentrated work, move the skin of your calf with your knee instead of sliding over it.

Poor conditioning is probably the biggest reason for problems with the calf muscles. When they have become weak and inflexible, they are easily overworked or overstretched. Remember that even therapeutic stretching can be harmful when trigger points insist on keeping a muscle tight.

Soleus

The *soleus* (SO-lee-us) is a large, broad muscle that covers all of the back of the lower leg. Its lower half is immediately beneath the skin; its upper half is hidden by the gastrocnemius. The word *soleus* derives from the Latin word for "sandal." It has the same root as *sole*, the word for the bottom of the foot and for the popular flatfish that's also sometimes called "flounder." The soleus muscle is broad and flat, not unlike the flounder.

The soleus muscle attaches to the upper parts of both the tibia and fibula and to the strong membrane that connects them. The lower attachment is to the heel bone by means of the Achilles tendon, which is shared with the gastrocnemius and plantaris muscles. A small portion of the population have an additional head of soleus muscle immediately behind their Achilles tendons in the space ordinarily occupied by a pad of fat. This extra muscle can be quite large and is easily mistaken for a tumor (1992, 427).

Soleus attachments to the heel bone make it a primary plantar flexor of the ankle; this means it allows you to push down strongly with the front of your foot. Soleus muscles are very active during walking, running, cycling, jumping, and climbing, which are the activities that are most likely to promote trigger points in the soleus. Myofascial trigger points in poorly conditioned soleus muscles are the cause of the heel pain so common among week-end athletes. But people other than athletes very frequently have trouble with soleus muscles, as one man, who hadn't jumped or run in thirty years, could testify.

Jeffrey, age fifty, lived in a pleasant neighborhood near his job and enjoyed the walk to and from work, but he began to have sharp pain in his heels and had to go back to taking his car. The backs of his heels were extremely sensitive to touch, so much so that he had to hang his feet over the edge of the bed at night. At a medical clinic, he was told that bone spurs were the cause of his pain and that surgery was the only solution. Massage to Jeffrey's soleus muscles in his calves ended his heel pain. Subsequently, when the pain occasionally tried to come back while he was out walking, self-applied massage enabled him to get rid of it within minutes.

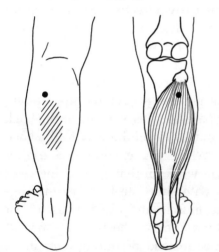

Figure 10.28   Soleus number 1 trigger point and referred pain paterrn

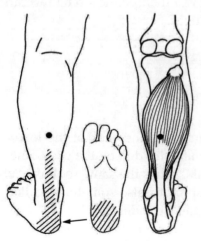

Figure 10.29   Soleus number 2 trigger point and referred pain pattern

An example of another kind of soleus trouble was Dorothy, age thirty-four, who had been an avid jogger. Running had kept her fit and feeling good about herself, but she hadn't been able to run in over a year. She couldn't even walk very far without terrible pain starting up in the backs of her ankles. She often had sharp pain in the bottoms of her heels and sometimes it was intolerable just to sit with her heels touching the floor. Lifting the front of her foot for any reason gave her a shot of pain in both places. She had been diagnosed as having Achilles tendinitis and was given a prescription for a painkiller and advised to stay off her feet as much as possible. A series of physical therapy sessions hadn't improved her situation. Massage of the backs of Dorothy's lower legs—much of which she was able to do herself—got rid of her "tendinitis" and heel pain. With continued self-treatment, walking gradually ceased to be a problem and she was eventually able to return to running.

Symptoms

Pain from soleus trigger points is referred primarily to the heel, calf, and back of the ankle (Figures 10.28 and 10.29). Surprisingly, soleus trigger points can cause deep pain in the sacroiliac area and maintain spasms in the muscles of the low back (Figure 10.30). Hypersensitivity to touch in the low back can sometimes be traced to soleus muscles. There are instances of pain even having been referred to the jaw. A trigger point in the inner edge of the soleus at the back edge of the tibia bone occasionally sends pain to the medial malleolus, which is the knob on the inner ankle (Figure 10.31) (1992, 428–430).

Several genuine medical problems exhibit symptoms similar to those caused by trigger points in soleus muscles and may cause confusion in diagnosis. Examples are thrombosis, phlebitis, stress fractures, and tendon or ligament tears. Myofascial pain can also be mistaken for shin splints or heel spurs. Heel spurs may actually be present and yet not be the cause of pain (1992, 440–442).

Achilles tendinitis is the typical diagnosis for pain in the backs of the ankles. "Plantar fasciitis" is a label often given to disabling heel pain. Conventional treatments for tendinitis and plantar fasciitis in the form of painkillers, steroid shots, physical therapy,

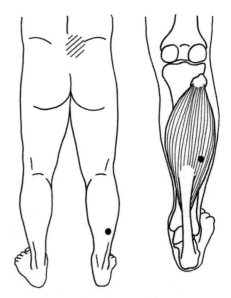

Figure 10.30   Soleus number 3 trigger point and referred pain pattern

and rest are often disappointing. This is understandable when you consider that none of these treatments would have a significant effect on trigger points. Most heel pain and most pain around the Achilles tendon come from trigger points in soleus, tibialis posterior, or quadratus plantae muscles (1992, 440–441).

Soleus trigger points can be an indirect cause of calf cramps when the tightness they cause in the soleus muscle impedes circulation. The soleus muscle is sometimes called the body's "second heart," because of its importance in helping pump the blood up from the feet and legs. In their normal functioning, soleus muscles contract when both shortening and lengthening, making them very efficient at pumping blood, just as long as they are active, healthy, and resilient. Myofascial trigger points, however, diminish their efficiency. Low blood pressure and unexpected fainting can be due to weak or poorly functioning soleus muscles (1992, 435-438).

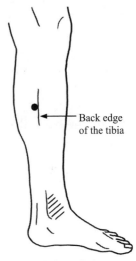

Back edge of the tibia

Figure 10.31   Soleus number 4 trigger point and referred pain pattern

Trigger points in soleus muscles may promote posterior compartment syndrome, which is increased intramuscular pressure that restricts circulation of the blood in the legs. Soleus trigger points can also contribute to the development of varicose veins, phlebitis and other manifestations of circulatory problems (1992, 442–444).

Causes

Overload of the soleus muscles can come from slipping as you walk or run on sand or gravel. The uncertain footing caused by hard leather soles can strain them. Trouble can come from stiff-soled shoes, from pressure on the backs of the legs by an ottoman or a recliner's footrest, or from skiing or skating without good ankle support. Aerobic dancing is an extremely common cause of soleus exhaustion. Wearing high heels keeps the soleus muscles shortened, which is a sure way to create and perpetuate trigger points. The ankle instability typically caused by high heels also strains the soleus muscles with each step (1992, 444–445).

Treatment

Locate the soleus muscle by feeling it contract below the lower border of the gastrocnemius when you point your toes. Use the same massage techniques for the soleus muscles as for the gastrocnemius; massage with the opposite knee works especially well for the soleus (see Figures 10.26 and 10.27). Be sure to cover the whole width of the back of the lower leg with several parallel vertical strokes.

If you tend to get light-headed when you get up from a seated position, try shifting your weight from foot to foot for a few seconds as soon as you're on your feet, at about the speed of your normal walking rhythm. This gets your soleus blood pumps going and moves oxygen to your brain at a faster rate. After sporting events or exercise, quick recovery of breath and energy can be accomplished by this same means: indeed, after any strong exertion, alternately contracting the calf muscles keeps the blood flowing strongly up from the legs and through the whole system at the very time the tissues need that extra boost. Soldiers standing at attention for long periods have been known to pass out because of the prolonged inactivity in their soleus muscles. When they've had good training, they know how to prevent this by rhythmically contracting and relaxing their calves.

The soleus muscles need exercise to maintain their strength for propelling the body forward and for their duties as blood pumps. At the same time, they should not be abused by overuse or unnecessary strain. A suddenly increased level of activity in the form of a new program of exercise, a spurt of weekend sports activity, or unaccustomed yard work can play havoc with the soleus and other muscles of the calf as well.

Preventative maintenance is especially important for the calf muscles. A good habit is to take a few moments in the morning to sit on the edge of the bed and massage your calves with your knees. As an added benefit, this can often clear up morning soreness and stiffness in the lower back if soleus trigger points are involved.

Tibialis Posterior

The *tibialis* (tib-ee-AL-iss) *posterior* lies under the soleus and gastrocnemius between the tibia and the fibula. It attaches to both bones and to the fibrous interosseous membrane that fastens them together. The muscle's long tendon wraps around the inner side of the heel and goes forward to attach to several bones in the middle of the foot's arch. The function of the tibialis posterior is to help flex the foot downward. Its action also maintains the long arch of the foot and keeps weight properly distributed to the outer side of the foot. Trigger point–sponsored weakness in the tibialis posterior muscles allows the ankles to bend inward, giving the appearance of fallen arches.

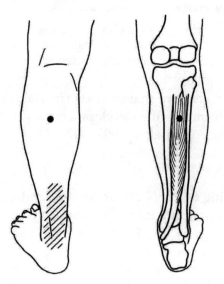

Figure 10.32   Tibialis posterior trigger point and referred pain pattern

Symptoms

Pain from tibialis posterior trigger points concentrates primarily in the Achilles tendon (Figure 10.32), especially while you're walking or running. Pain may sometimes extend to the calf, heel, and entire sole of the foot (not shown). Myofascial pain caused by tibialis posterior trigger points can be mistaken for evidence of shin splints, posterior compartment syndrome, and tendinitis. In fact, so-called "Achilles tendinitis" is a mistaken notion in most cases. This is indisputable when deep massage of the tibialis posterior takes the pain away, which it may begin to do almost immediately (1992, 460–461, 464–465).

Causes

Walking or running on rough, uneven ground stresses the tibialis posterior. Badly worn shoes or any surface that causes rocking of the foot does the same. Morton's foot, in causing you to walk on the inner edges of the foot, can overwork the tibialis posterior and bring about pain in the back of the ankle (1992, 465–466).

Treatment

You won't be able to locate the tibialis posterior muscle by isolated contraction, because all the calf muscles tend to contract at the same time, no matter what movement you make with your foot. To find tibialis posterior trigger points, feel for exquisite tenderness along a vertical line between the two heads of the gastrocnemius. Do the massage with a tool that will go deep, such as the Thera Cane, a Knobble, or supported fingers. The opposite knee, although it might seem too broad a tool, will also work just fine. The weight of the leg will project the force through the thick overlying muscles. Move your leg across your knee so that the tibialis posterior is repeatedly squeezed against the back of the fibula. Remember that the fibula is the outer bone in the lower leg.

Flexor Digitorum Longus and Flexor Hallucis Longus

The *flexor digitorum* (dih-jih-TAW-rum) *longus* and the *flexor hallucis* (HAL-uh-sis) *longus* are the long flexors of the toes. They are companions to the tibialis posterior and lie with it beneath the larger muscles of the calf—the soleus and gastrocnemius. These long flexors operate in conjunction with the short flexors, which reside in the underside of the foot.

The flexor digitorum longus is located along the back of the tibia, the flexor hallucis longus along the back of the fibula a little lower down. These positions are opposite what you would expect when you see where their tendons attach. The tendons of both muscles wrap around the inner side of the heel and then cross one another, digitorum going to the four smaller toes and hallucis to the big toe. This crossed arrangement gives a mechanical advantage to the toes, allowing them to press more powerfully against the ground. The two long toe flexors, along with the short flexors in the bottom of the foot, are important for maintaining balance. They also help propel the body forward.

Symptoms

Trigger points in the long toe flexors make the soles of your feet hurt when you walk. Flexor digitorum longus trigger points send pain to the metatarsal arch and to the undersides of the toes (Figure 10.33). The metatarsal arch is the slightly upward curved line formed by the heads of the metatarsals, the five long bones in the front of the foot. Pain from the flexor hallucis longus is felt under the big toe and the head of the adjoining first

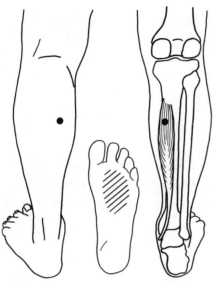

Figure 10.33   Flexor digitorum longus
trigger point and referred pain pattern

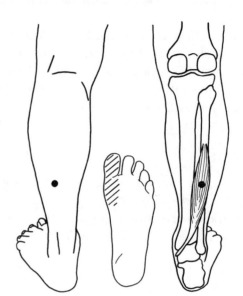

Figure 10.34   Flexor hallucis longus
trigger point and referred pain pattern

metatarsal (Figure 10.34) Numbness in the underside of the big toe is a classic symptom of flexor hallucis longus trigger points.

Pain on the underside of the front of the foot is typically blamed on bad shoes, flat feet, and gout. Few people imagine that it could be coming from muscles in the calf. Trigger points in the long toe flexors are also capable of sponsoring cramps in the smaller muscles of the bottoms of the foot and contributing to the development of hammertoe and claw toe, in which the toes stay cramped in distorted positions (1992, 488-494).

Causes

Trigger points in the long toe flexors come about when the toes are worked to the point of exhaustion by the activities of the foot and lower leg. An example is when you run or walk barefoot on soft beach sand or a rocky hillside. Walking on uneven ground behind a lawn mower can be very tiring for the toe flexors. Trigger points in the soleus and gastrocnemius muscles that weaken them can make more work for the long toe flexors. All five muscles of the calf are likely to harbor trigger points when running or walking has been done to excess (1992, 494).

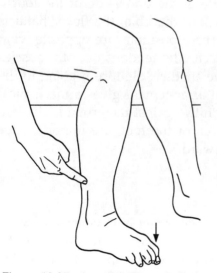

Figure 10.35   Locating flexor hallucis
longus by isolated contraction

Treatment

Flexor digitorum longus trigger points are buried deep beneath the soleus and gastrocnemius muscles right beside those in the tibialis posterior and like them can be massaged with the opposite knee. With the flexor digitorum longus, you will make the knee go in the other direction and repeatedly squeeze the muscle against the tibia. You can visualize this area more accurately if you understand that the fibula is not only parallel to the tibia but slightly to the rear.

Flexor hallucis longus trigger points are a third of the way up from the ankle on the back of the lower leg, a little toward the outer side. Locate the flexor hallucis longus by feeling it contract when you curl your big toe under (Figure 10.35). To keep from contracting the overlying soleus at the same time, avoid pushing down with the foot. An easy way to massage the flexor hallucis longus is to press the muscle against the fibula with the opposite knee. This technique is shown in Figures 10.26 and 10.27. Move the leg repeatedly across the kneecap with short strokes, taking care to move the skin, not to slide along it.

Foot Muscles

You probably don't usually give much thought to your feet until they start to hurt. This is unfortunate, because your feet are literally the foundation for every vertical activity of the body. They don't get that much of a break even when you're sitting down. When the feet hurt, they're capable of sponsoring pain in a lot of other places, all the way to the top of your head. When the feet don't function well, nothing else is likely to function well. Foot pain can truly undermine the quality of every aspect of your life.

The feet are extraordinarily complex, each containing nine separate, individually named muscles. Add to this the seven interosseous muscles—the tiny muscles between the long metatarsal bones in the front of the foot. Then there are the four even smaller lumbricals, which are left over from the days when our ancestors' toes were longer and were used for grasping. This makes twenty muscles in each foot, which sounds like a lot of muscles to come to terms with. Fortunately, success in getting rid of foot pain doesn't require being on a first-name basis with every one of them. It does help, however, to understand the nine major foot muscles individually because they all have different pain referral patterns. The interosseous and lumbrical muscles cause only local pain and can be treated as a group. Interestingly, there are only two muscles on the top of the foot. The other seven are on the underside. The bottom of the foot is called the *plantar surface*, the word *plantar* coming from another Latin word for "sole." The word is easy to remember if you think of plantar warts.

Many things beside myofascial trigger points can cause foot pain, including bunions, bursitis, arthritis, plantar warts, calluses, ingrown toenails, infections, gout, broken bones, ligament tears, and certain structural abnormalities like Morton's foot. You may need help with medical and structural problems such as these, but you won't need help with Morton's foot. You can take care of Morton's foot yourself.

Morton's Foot

In a correctly structured foot, the length of the first metatarsal bone should be equal to or greater than that of the second metatarsal. If you have Morton's foot, your second metatarsals are longer than the first metatarsals (Figure 10.36). (This doesn't necessarily make your second toes longer than your first toes.) A long second metatarsal causes instabilities and inefficiencies in the operation of the foot and ankle that frequently lead to the development of trigger points and chronic pain. Morton's foot in itself is not painful.

One person in four has Morton's foot, also called "Morton's foot structure" or "Morton's toe." Another commonly used term is "classic Greek toe." In Greek statuary, the heroes

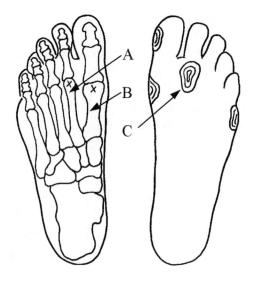

Figure 10.36   Morton's foot: (A) second metatarsal; (B) first metatarsal; (C) calluses

were always given a beautifully long second toe. Real heroes with feet like that would've walked splayfooted.

The problem caused by a long second metatarsal is poor distribution of the body weight on the bottoms of the feet. For good balance and stability, the foot should contact the ground like a tripod, with the weight evenly spread between the heads of the first and fifth metatarsals and the heel. When the second metatarsal is too long, its head contacts the ground first and takes the full weight meant for both points at the front of the foot. This gives you a two-point support instead of a three-point support. It's like walking on ice skates: your ankles become unstable, too easily bending in and out.

The natural adjustment to Morton's foot is to turn your toes outward so that the weight is thrown back onto the first metatarsal. This makes the ankle more stable, but also causes it to be bent unnaturally inward and places undue strain on numerous muscles, including those of the foot, lower leg, thigh, buttocks, back. The effects of Morton's foot are often manifested in chronic muscle tension and pain even in the upper back, neck, and head (1992, 381–383).

Figure 10.36 shows the interior of Morton's foot, as well as exterior evidence of the condition. In the skeletal view, the Xs mark the heads of the first and second metatarsals. Note that the length of the second toe has no relationship to the length of the second metatarsal. You may have a long second toe and a normal metatarsal, or you may have a long metatarsal that doesn't show up in any lengthening of the second toe. In some cases, both may be extra long. You can check your feet for Morton's foot by simply bending your toes back so that you can see the heads of the first two metatarsals and gauge their relative length (Figure 10.37). As you pull down on your toes, push up on the heads of the metatarsals from underneath to make them stand out under the skin.

The other foot illustrated in Figure 10.36 shows the positions of four unnaturally heavy calluses typically associated with Morton's foot. The heaviest one appears right under the head of the second metatarsal. The other three are found along the edge of the big toe and the edges of the heads of the first and fifth metatarsals. Another distinctive sign of Morton's foot is a longer than normal web between the second and third toes. Directly gauging the relative length of the metatarsal bones, however, is the best way to tell.

The simplest way to deal with Morton's foot is to place a thin pad under the head of the first

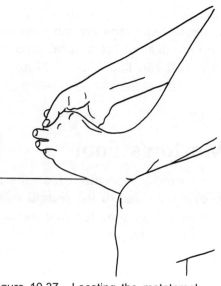

Figure 10.37   Locating the metatarsal heads

metatarsal, a point sometimes called the "ball of the foot." Cut a circle the size of a quarter to a half dollar (depending on the size of your feet) out of Dr. Scholl's Molefoam Padding. Trim off any sharp edges with scissors. You'll probably need a pad for each foot. Keep the pads in place by sticking them on the bottoms of a pair of Dr. Scholl's Work Comfort Insoles or something similar (Figures 10.38). Take care that the pads don't extend under the second metatarsal.

Professional practitioners of foot care often err in placing a pad under the second metatarsal and the middle of the metatarsal arch. This is done in an attempt to give local relief to pain in that area. The effect, unfortunately, is to create a condition of Morton's foot where none may exist, adding all the

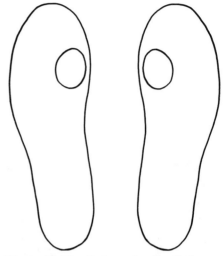

Figure 10.38 Pads under the first metatarsal heads

symptoms of Morton's foot to foot pain that may already be intolerable.

Morton's foot is not a problem that you should ignore. Put pads in all your shoes and don't forget your house slippers. You'll be astounded at the difference it will make. You'll find that when you walk your feet will point forward instead of out to the side. Proper function of the foot returns immediately and pain in the foot and other parts of the body becomes much easier to resolve. The author can personally testify to this, having suffered from boyhood with all the problems that characterize Morton's foot. Most of the problems with his ankles and feet ended when his first massage therapist gave him this incredibly simple solution.

Dorsal Foot Muscles

The dorsal foot muscles are found on the top of the foot (Figure 10.39). The interosseous muscles, which occupy the spaces between the metatarsal bones, are also thought of as dorsal muscles, because they're most easily approached from the top of the foot (not shown). Treatment of the dorsal and interosseous muscles is quite straightforward. Pain from their trigger points is generally local and is not referred away to any other site.

Extensor Digitorum Brevis, Extensor Hallucis Brevis, and Interosseous Muscles

The *extensor digitorum* (dih-jih-TAW-rum) *brevis* and *extensor hallucis* (HAL-uh-sis) *brevis* are short toe extensors. They lie beneath the tendons of the long toe extensors on the top of the foot. Both short and long extensors work together in raising the toes so they can clear the ground with every step you take.

There are actually two sets of *interosseous muscles* between the metatarsal bones of the foot: the *dorsal interosseous* and the *plantar interosseous*. A third set of small muscles, the *lumbricals*, are parallel to the metatarsals on the bottom side of the foot but aren't between them. The interosseous muscles move the toes from side to side and help with flexion and extension. This confusing mass of tiny muscles may seem annoyingly insignificant, but they

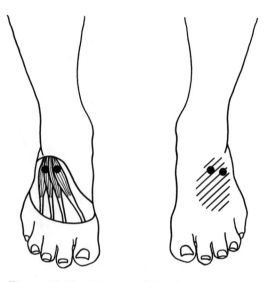

Figure 10.39   Extensor digitorum brevis and extensor hallucis brevis trigger points and referred pain pattern

contribute mightily to balance and to adaptation of the foot to the ground. Their actions are also vital for countering excesses in the actions of the larger but less sensitive muscles of the foot.

Symptoms

Pain from trigger points in the short extensors occurs right around the muscles, which are located on the outer side of the top of the foot (Figure 10.39). In the illustration, the extensor digitorum brevis is made up of the three heads of muscle attaching to the smaller toes. The extensor hallucis brevis is the single muscle leading to the big toe. Their combined pain pattern overlaps that of the long toe extensors, the tibialis anterior, and the peroneus tertius. It's sometimes necessary to troubleshoot all these muscles to find the trigger points that are causing the pain. One woman would've gone to her grave with her foot trouble if she hadn't stumbled onto some new information.

Peggy, age fifty-six, was awakened nearly every night by cramps in the tops of her feet and toes. Her toes had been curled up for years, a condition she'd been told was called "hammertoe." Her feet hurt most of the time. A massage therapist stopped her nighttime foot cramps with massage to the fronts of her legs and the tops of her feet. He then showed her how to massage her own legs and feet and suggested that she work on them every night before going to bed. Peggy continued doing her bedtime massage even after she stopped getting foot cramps because it helped her wind down and go to sleep. Several months later, she happened to notice that her toes weren't curling up as much as they used to.

Pain from the interosseous trigger points is felt at the base of the toes, often extending to the ends of the toes (Figure 10.40). Pain may occasionally cover the entire front of the foot and move up the front of the shin (not shown). Trigger points in the interosseous muscles often cause cramping and swelling of the front of the foot. A dull aching in the top of the foot may come from any of the dorsal foot muscles. Trigger points in the first dorsal interosseous can make the big toe tingle. Numbness rather than pain can be present in any of the referral areas (1992, 524).

Danny, age thirty-seven, an auto mechanic, had developed chronic pain in the ends of his toes from working on the concrete floor in the shop. His feet felt cramped in shoes that had previously fit well. Soaking his feet after work helped them, but

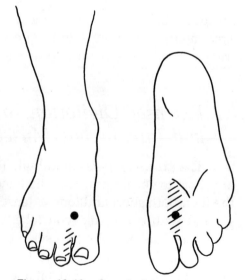

Figure 10.40   Sample interosseous trigger point and referred pain pattern

sometimes he was too tired to go to the trouble. A shoe clerk told him that people's feet tended to get wider as they got older, so he bought a new pair of shoes. The bigger shoes solved the tightness problem across the front of his feet but they didn't stop the pain in his toes.

A friend at church showed him a trick for massaging between the bones in the front of his feet with his thumb. It was extremely painful but he was surprised that it had an immediate effect on his toe pain. It also seemed to reduce the width of his feet. Encouraged, he worked on his feet morning and night. Toe pain after work became less and less and his new shoes began to feel loose on his feet. Trying on his old shoes, he found they didn't feel tight anymore.

Causes

Too much walking, running, or climbing can set up trigger points in any of the extensor and interosseous muscles. It's not unusual for all of them to be involved, since each depends on the others for proper functioning in the foot's delicately balanced system of operation.

Be wary of shoes that are too tight across the front of the foot. Tightness there restricts circulation and movement and encourages problems with the interosseous and short toe extensor muscles. To favor these much-abused muscles, it would be a good idea to put your high-heeled shoes away. They cause your feet to slide down into the toes of your shoes, crowding the muscles in the front of the foot. At the other extreme, going without shoes if you're not used to it can also put unaccustomed strain on the muscles of the foot.

Treatment

Locate the extensor digitorum brevis and extensor hallucis brevis by feeling them contract when you raise your toes (Figure 10.41). Use only the tips of the fingers or the supported thumb to massage the dorsal foot muscles. They're generally small and thin and don't require a lot of pressure.

To massage the interosseous muscles, dig the tips of two fingers or a supported thumb in between the metatarsals from either above or below (Figure 10.42). Two other methods for interosseous massage are shown in Figures 10.43 and 10.44. When interosseous trigger points are bad, this can be excruciatingly painful and can even cause cramping if you massage too vigorously. Stretching the bottom of the foot in an effort to cope with a cramp in the arch can also set off cramps in the interosseous muscles and in the short extensors in the top of the foot. If you like stretching, reduce the risks with some preliminary massage.

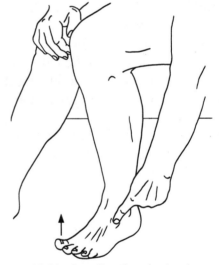

Figure 10.41   Locating the short extensors by isolated contraction

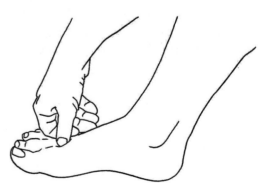

Figure 10.42   Interosseous massage with supported thumb

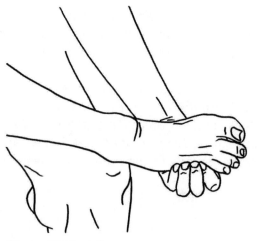

Figure 10.43   Interosseous massage with fingers wrapped around the foot (from either side)

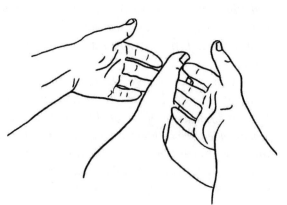

Figure 10.44   Interosseous massage from both sides, working the dorsal and plantar interosseous muscles at the same time

Plantar Foot Muscles

A good foot rub can feel really great and yet do absolutely nothing to get rid of chronic foot pain. If you want to massage your feet effectively, it's essential to try to visualize and understand what's inside. There are seven muscles in the bottom, or plantar surface, of the foot. Each muscle has a specific job to do and causes its own special kind of pain when afflicted with trigger points. The following three case histories show some of the many ways people can experience problems with the plantar foot muscles.

Cliff, age twenty-eight, an assistant manager in a supermarket, was on his feet with hardly a break all day long. It didn't help a bit to stop and rest. The bottoms of his feet hurt even when he was sitting down. Betty, his boss, showed him how to massage his feet by rolling them across a little rubber ball. It hurt so bad the first time he tried it, he didn't think he'd be able to stand it. But he kept the ball in his pocket and worked on his feet whenever he had a chance. A couple of days later when Betty asked how his feet were doing, he suddenly realized they didn't hurt anymore.

Dorothy, age sixty-three, liked to go walking at the mall in the morning before it opened, but she thought she would have to stop. She'd started getting a sharp pain on the bottom of one foot right behind her toes. It felt as though she had bruised her foot stepping on a stone. She found herself walking on her heel to avoid the pain. She put a pad in her shoe at the place that hurt but it only made the pain worse. At the doctor's office, she was told she had "plantar fasciitis," a problem that usually required surgery. A friend said she could get rid of the pain by rolling her foot on a golf ball. It worked.

Raymond, age seventy-seven, often had cramps in the bottoms of his feet and his toes were numb most of the time. The doctor thought the numbness might come from the chemotherapy Ray had had for lymphoma. His daughter had been reading about trigger points and began rubbing his feet whenever she came to visit, which she did two or three times a week. Some of the places on the bottoms of his feet hurt terribly when she rubbed them, but she tried to use only the pressure he could stand. After a few weeks,

Ray noticed that he rarely got cramps anymore and that the numbness in his toes was almost gone.

Abductor Hallucis

The *abductor hallucis* (ab-DUK-ter HAL-uh-sis) is one of several muscles that move the big toe. It lies along the inner edge of the bottom of the foot near the heel, attaching to the heel and to one of the bones of the big toe. Its job is to bend the big toe downward and move it away from the other toes. This action contributes to propulsion and helps keep the foot and ankle from rocking inward. The workload of the abductor hallucis is increased when trigger points in other muscles of the lower leg and foot make the ankles weak and unstable. Instability caused by Morton's foot also puts an extra load on the abductor hallucis.

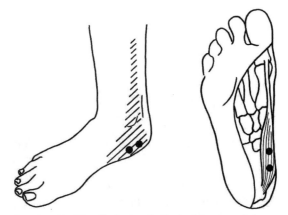

Figure 10.45   Abductor hallucis trigger points and referred pain pattern

Trigger points in the abductor hallucis cause pain primarily on the inner side of the heel and a short way up the inner ankle (Figure 10.45). When trigger points are active enough, pain is felt under the first metatarsal (not shown). Abductor hallucis trigger points occasionally cause nerve entrapment, resulting in numbness in the foot and toes (1992, 502, 512).

Locate the abductor hallucis at the inner edge of the heel by feeling it contract when you press the big toe against the floor (Figure 10.46). The abductor hallucis is very easy to get to, but it can be a thick muscle and you'll need to get some leverage to penetrate it. The best massage tool for this muscle is the supported thumb (Figure 10.47), although supported fingers also work. The Thera Cane, the Knobble, or a 35 mm high bounce ball against the floor are all very useful tools for the abductor hallucis and other muscles of the bottom of the foot (Figures 10.48, 10.49, and 10.50). A golf ball is the traditional tool for working the bottom of the foot, but it is less effective than these other tools because it's too large to go deep enough. It's also too slick and too hard. Everything considered, the little high bounce ball may be the most effective and practical tool. Although the illustrations show bare feet for the sake of clarity, you'll probably find massage of the feet more comfortable with your socks on no matter what tool you use.

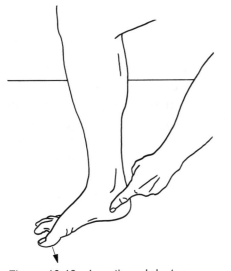

Figure 10.46   Locating abductor hallucis by isolated contraction

When one of the muscles on the bottom of the foot is in trouble, they're all bound to be in trouble. You'll usually be working on all of them at the same time with one tool or another. Massaging the bottoms of your feet can be so horribly painful that you may not want to do it. Just remember that if the muscles were healthy, pressure on them wouldn't hurt at all. Lighten up to the point where the pressure feels therapeutic. Trigger point massage should "hurt good." It should induce a pleasant kind of pain.

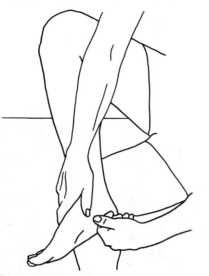

Figure 10.47   Abductor hallucis massage with supported thumb

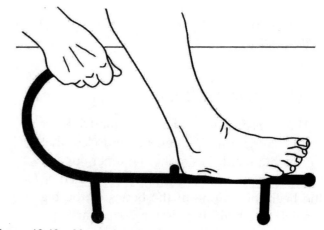

Figure 10.48   Massaging the bottom of the foot with small nipple on the Thera Cane

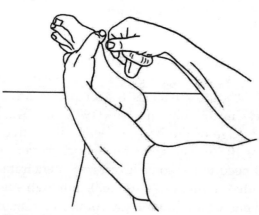

Figure 10.49   Massaging the bottom of the foot with the Knobble

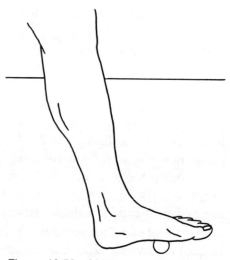

Figure 10.50   Massaging the bottom of the foot with a small hard rubber ball on the floor

Abductor Digiti Minimi

Digiti minimi means "little toe." The function of the *abductor digiti minimi* (ab-DUK-ter DIH-jih-tee MIH-nih-me) is to move the little toe away from the other toes. This action (abduction) helps control side-to-side rocking of the foot when the body is in motion. Because of its importance, the abductor digiti minimi can be a relatively large muscle. Walking or running on rough, uneven ground makes hard work for toe abductors and promotes trigger points. High-heeled shoes and shoes or sandals with stiff, inflexible soles are bad for them, too.

Trigger points in the abductor digiti minimi cause pain primarily in the muscle itself along the outer edge of the foot near the heel and sometimes a short way up the outer side of the ankle (Figure 10.51). When sufficiently active, trigger points will also cause pain in the little toe and under the head of the fifth metatarsal right behind the toe (not shown). Pain in the outer side of the foot and ankle that feels like a sprain can be coming from the abductor digiti minimi (1992, 502).

Locate the abductor digiti minimi by feeling it tighten when you spread your toes (Figure 10.52). Massage the muscle with a small hard rubber ball on the floor. Note that a ball with a diameter greater than one inch will not penetrate deeply enough. The Thera Cane can be used for this, although it's a little awkward to use this tool

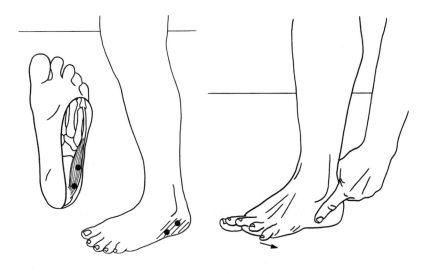

Figure 10.51 Abductor digiti minimi trigger points and referred pain pattern

Figure 10.52 Locating abductor digiti minimi by isolated contraction

along the edge of the foot. You may find the worst trigger point just above the edge of the sole on the outer side of the heel.

Flexor Digitorum Brevis

The *flexor digitorum brevis* attaches to the heel bone and the toe bones and lies squarely in the middle of the long arch. The flexor digitorum brevis assists the flexor digitorum longus of the calf in plantar flexing the four smaller toes (curling them under). Trigger points in both muscles send pain to the front of the foot under the heads of the metatarsals just behind the toes (Figure 10.53). This pain can be like walking on sharp rocks and is one of the most common manifestations of "sore feet" (1992, 503).

Arch supports or other orthotic devices are often used to treat pain in the sole of the foot in the mistaken assumption that it's being caused by weak or fallen arches. When the pressure from arch supports increases the pain under the front of your foot, look for trigger points in the flexor digitorum brevis (1992, 517).

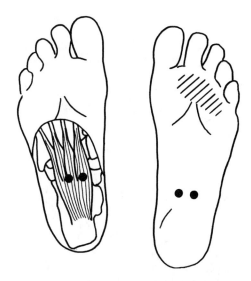

Figure 10.53 Flexor digitorum brevis trigger points and referred pain pattern

In trying to fix sore arches, it's natural to massage the arch itself, but don't forget that most pain in the long arch actually comes from trigger points in the gastrocnemius muscle in the calf. Although the flexor digitorum brevis occupies the arch, it does not cause pain in the arch.

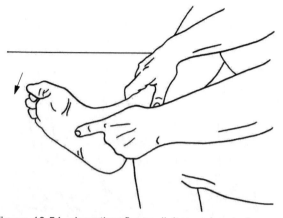

Figure 10.54   Locating flexor digitorum brevis by isolated contraction

Locate the flexor digitorum brevis by feeling it contract when you curl your toes under (Figure 10.54). The two best tools for working this short toe flexor are the Thera Cane and the small hard rubber ball against the floor.

Plantar fasciitis is currently an extremely popular diagnosis for foot and heel pain. The medical explanation would seem to make sense if you knew nothing about trigger points and myofascial pain. The defining test used in the diagnosis is to press into the arch and see if it hurts. This is where you find the plantar fascia, the thick tendinous tissue that supports the arch. Pain at this spot supposedly indicates that the fascia is "inflamed." The problem with this view is that the flexor digitorum brevis and quadratus plantae muscles immediately underlie the plantar fascia, and their trigger points quite naturally hurt when pressed. Self-applied massage to these exquisitely tender spots can dramatically improve even longstanding "plantar fasciitis" in just a few days. When dealing with this mysterious affliction, don't forget the soleus muscles in the calf, whose trigger points are probably the major cause of heel pain.

Quadratus Plantae

The *quadratus plantae* (quad-DRAY-tus PLAN-tee) attaches to the heel bone near the attachment for the flexor digitorum brevis. At its other end, it attaches to the tendons of the flexor digitorum longus, allowing it to assist with flexion of the toes. This action gives the quadratus plantae its alternate name, *flexor accessorius*. This important and often troublesome muscle lies very deep in the foot just in front of the heel and is completely hidden by the flexor digitorum brevis.

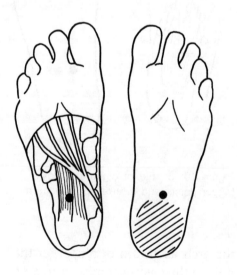

Figure 10.55   Quadratus plantae trigger point and referred pain pattern

Quadratus plantae trigger points cause sharp pain in the heel that feels like you've bruised it stepping on a stone (Figure 10.55). When you step down, it can feel like a nail is being driven in. Sometimes it's impossible to put your weight on your heel, leaving you to walk on your toes. This pain is often mislabeled "plantar fasciitis" or falsely blamed on a heel spur. Heel spurs can be present and actually not be the cause of the pain: indisputable evidence of the harmlessness of a heel spur is when massage stops the pain. Of course, genuinely painful heel spurs and myofascial trigger points can coexist (1992, 441, 509–510).

It's not possible to locate the quadratus plantae by isolated contraction because it contracts together with the flexor digitorum brevis, which overlies it. The trigger points for both muscles are approximately in the same spot, except that those for the quadratus are a bit closer to the heel and much deeper. In fact, you won't be able to go deep enough with your fingers or thumb to massage the quadratus plantae. To get to it, you will need to put some weight on a small hard ball or one of the small nipples on the Thera Cane.

Adductor Hallucis and Flexor Hallucis Brevis

It helps to keep trying to remember what all these Latin words mean. *Hallucis* is the big toe. An *adductor* pulls the big toe toward the midline of the foot. A *flexor* bends the big toe downward. *Brevis* means "short."

These two muscles can't be distinguished from one another by isolated contraction, since they contract at the same time when you push down with the big toe. They do have different pain patterns, however. Trigger points in the *adductor hallucis* (ad-DUK-ter HAL-uh-sis) cause pain under the heads of the metatarsals just behind the four smaller toes (Figure 10.56). Sometimes they cause numbness in the same area. Pain from *flexor hallucis brevis* (FLEX-er HAL-uh-sis BREH-vis) trigger points focuses under the head of the first metatarsal (the ball of the foot) and on the inner side of the foot near the big toe (Figure 10.57).

Trigger points in the adductor hallucis and flexor hallucis brevis are among the most common causes of pain felt in the front of the foot while you're walking. They cause much less pain when you're not on your feet. These muscles of the big toe are overworked when you must compensate for foot imbalance caused by a long second metatarsal. For this reason, chronic pain in the metatarsal arch can often be traced to a Morton's foot structure. (The metatarsal arch is formed across the front of the foot by the heads of the metatarsal bones.)

Locate the adductor hallucis and flexor hallucis brevis muscles by feeling them contract when you flex the big toe downward (Figure 10.58). Search for trigger points in the metatarsal arch and behind the head of the first metatarsal. One of the best tools for massage in this area is the supported thumb (Figure 10.59). Supported fingers also work, as does the Thera Cane or a 35 mm high bounce ball against the floor. Some trigger points in these muscles can be quite deep since the muscles themselves are very deeply placed under everything else.

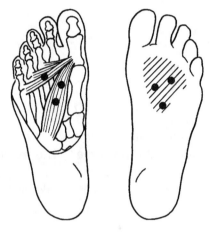

Figure 10.56 Adductor hallucis trigger points and referred pain pattern

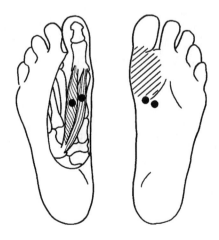

Figure 10.57 Flexor hallucis brevis trigger points and referred pain pattern

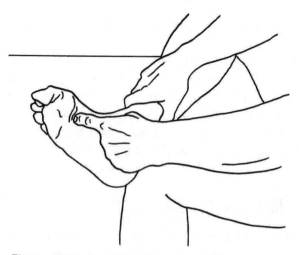

Figure 10.58   Locating adductor hallucis and flexor hallucis brevis by isolated contraction

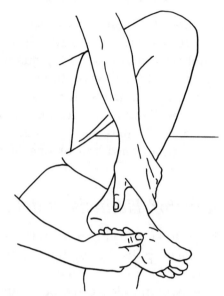

Figure 10.59   Adductor hallucis and flexor hallucis brevis massage with supported thumb

Flexor Digiti Minimi Brevis

Flexor digiti minimi brevis (FLEX-ur DIH-jih-tee MIH-nih-mee BREH-vis) means "short flexor of the little toe." The muscle is actually bigger and stronger than you would think, judging from its association with the little toe. But it plays a very important role in maintaining balance when you walk, run, or simply shift your weight. Try pushing against the floor with the little toe by itself and feel the muscle contract all along the underside of the fifth metatarsal. This action keeps the ankle from turning too far to the outside when you walk or run. It helps keep your body centered over your feet.

Unstable ankles can overload the flexor digiti minimi brevis muscles. You can also abuse them by carrying heavy objects or just by carrying too much weight of your own. Walking or running on uneven ground puts a strain on the flexor digiti minimi brevis muscles because they have to work so hard keeping your balance.

Trigger points in the flexor digiti minimi brevis cause pain at the outer edge of the foot just behind the little toe (Figure 10.60). Massage it with the Thera Cane or the little ball against the floor.

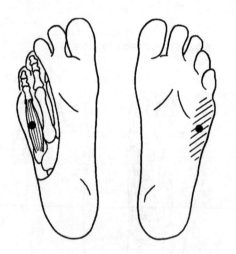

Figure 10.60   Flexor digiti minimi brevis trigger point and referred pain pattern

Chapter 11

Clinical Trigger Point Massage

by Clair and Amber Davies

This chapter is intended primarily for massage therapists, but it can be a useful study for anyone who wants to help someone else deal with pain. We hope those who find it useful will include physicians, physical therapists, occupational therapists, nurses, and others in the field of health care.

The Massage Therapist's Role

In presenting this new method for the clinical treatment of pain, we conceive of a new, expanded role for massage therapists. Beyond their traditional function of providing direct, hands-on treatment, therapists will become self-treatment coaches, helping their clients learn to treat their own pain where possible. This valuable new role for the therapist will foster self-care, self-reliance, and self-empowerment, which are some of our clients' deepest needs.

In the time since this book was first published in 2001, we have worked with more than eight-hundred massage therapists from thirty-nine states in our Trigger Point Therapy Workshops. The workshops encompassed both the self-treatment and the clinical treatment of pain. Massage therapists everywhere told us that trigger points had been covered only briefly in their massage schools—if at all! Very few therapists had a clear understanding of trigger points and referred pain. Few could identify common trigger point sites, even though they regularly treated many of those places intuitively. Consistently, however, our work-shops participants were well aware of their deficiencies. A common theme in their class evaluations was the suggestion that something like this chapter be written.

We feel that massage therapists need to take a much more clinical approach to the treatment of pain. Unfortunately, the requisite skills will have to be mainly self-taught at present. Weekend workshops can only give you a start. And true clinical therapy requires a much greater facility in finding and treating trigger points than is currently attainable in most massage schools.

In general, too many modalities are lumped into clinical massage therapy programs and trigger point therapy is given no emphasis. Trigger point massage is presented as just one of a dozen or more other treatment systems supposedly of equal value in the treatment of pain. This suggests that schools lack a clear sense of what actually works and are giving the student every weapon in the arsenal in the brave hope that something will hit the target. The integrated "whole person" approach to pain therapy so much in vogue in the wider health-care community has much the same flavor. It does make sense to target improved health for the whole of the body, mind, and spirit, but we've found that trigger point massage does the job of getting rid of pain quite well by itself.

We believe that trigger point massage is the most appropriate treatment for most kinds of common pain and should be taught to student practitioners in all fields of health care, including the field of medicine. Self-treatment, in particular, should be taught in massage schools as the best foundation for understanding and successfully treating trigger points. If therapists can find and treat the causes of their own pain, the pain problems of their clients will hold few mysteries. Our clinical method derives directly from what we've learned from treating ourselves.

New Approach to Therapeutic Massage

Trigger point massage is a profoundly practical and versatile approach to pain therapy. As a stand-alone therapy, it can be done anywhere, not necessarily requiring a massage table or massage chair. If need be, it can even be done through the clothing. Trigger point massage can be the sole therapy employed in the massage studio, or it can be integrated into other massage modalities, greatly increasing their effectiveness. As a purely clinical modality, trigger point massage can be limited to specific problems and specific muscles and doesn't have to be part of a full-body treatment. We hope that physicians and health insurance companies will see the potential in this.

A single, exceedingly simple therapeutic treatment stroke is used for trigger point massage everywhere in the body. It's exactly the same deep, repeated stroke that is used for self-treatment. Different hand positions are used in clinical work, however, with even greater attention to ergonomics and safety, because of the extraordinary physical demands made on the professional therapist. Some of the traditional ways of using the hands for massage are actually quite damaging to the hands when overused. Petrissage, specifically, (kneading with unsupported thumbs) is a technique that can very quickly lead to overuse injuries. Many massage therapists graduate from school with hands and forearms already hurting. The techniques shown in this chapter are not only safer for the hands than generic massage techniques but are greatly more effective in treating trigger points and the pain they cause. The techniques are very specific and efficient and require much less effort than the usual strokes. We reserve kneading with unsupported thumbs to the few places where nothing else will do.

The advantage in our therapy for clients and patients is that their pain problems can be solved expeditiously and with only a minimal amount of pain from the treatment. Treatment of the "hot" spots is relatively brief. Pressure is focused and relatively light. Trigger point massage can be as pleasant and as deeply relaxing as "feel-good" massage, when done correctly.

Preliminary Considerations

In our attempt to bring a higher level of objectivitiy into the practice of clinical massage therapy, we dispense with background music, at least while we are involved in locating and treating specific trigger points. Music makes it hard to talk without raising our voices. Music also encourages clients to sleep, which is not what we want. We need to know what the client is experiencing from moment to moment. This calls for a continuing flow of information from the beginning of the session to the end.

Assessment

It's wise to have the client fill out a pictorial pain chart as a record of where you began. A chart of the client's various kinds of pain will also insure that you don't forget anything in subsequent treatments. Have the client fill out a new chart periodically to keep track of progress. Clients sometimes complain that they still have pain and don't seem to be improving. A glance at earlier pain charts can be reassuring. We use a form containing simple line drawings of the whole body. The client uses a red pencil to color the places where pain is felt.

Clients never get it all told in the first interview. Predictably, they forget to tell about some of their lesser pain problems. They may consider some of their symptoms too trivial or unimportant to share. But everything ties together, and small clues can be important in tracking down the source of major symptoms. Keep asking questions. Inquire about pain in other areas. Probe their memory for falls or auto accidents that may be all but forgotten. Check the client's posture and the range of motion in pertinent joints. Observe the client's state of general tension. Determine whether the client is a chest breather, which can be a critical factor in creating and perpetuating trigger points in any of the auxiliary breathing muscles, such as the serratus anterior, sternocleidomastoid, and scalenes. Ask whether there are joints that pop. Ask about joints that are stiff.

Communication

More communication is needed during a trigger point massage than in a general relaxation massage session. It's important to initiate the conversation and to continue to check in with the client throughout the treatment. Some clients may endure an amazing amount of pain just to avoid hurting your feelings or to "get their money's worth." They may be giving too much credit to the notion of "no pain, no gain." Clients shouldn't dread trigger point massage. They should look forward to it.

Since you don't have the advantage of being able to feel the pain yourself when working on someone else's trigger points, you must rely on the client to tell you when you're on a trigger point. Some therapists have the ability to find trigger point nodules with their fingers. But even those who have this facility can still have difficulty feeling trigger points when they're deep in large muscles or when the client is overweight. When you're within the target area, ask the client to guide you to the most tender spot.

You will need an efficient means to get feedback from the client, not only about the precise location of trigger points, but most especially in regard to level of pain. It's important not to make trigger point massage so painful that the client tenses the muscles you're working on. The pain should be a pleasant kind of pain that can still be relaxed into. We define this as a number seven on a scale of one to ten (one is no pain; ten is intolerable). Oftentimes this level can be felt by your fingers as the place where your pressure meets resistance. But don't rely only on your hands. You need to constantly ask for numbers and watch body language so you can always know what the client is feeling. It's not enough to ask, "How does this feel?" or "Is this too much pressure?" Answers to such questions will not give you objective information about pain, whereas a number will.

Watching the client's face when supine can tell you if you're using too much pressure even before you get a verbal indication. When the client is prone and you can't see her face, you can still see when she is holding herself tight or is guarding against you. Even so, verify your impressions by asking for numbers. After working with a client a couple of times, the number system will give you a better sense of the right therapeutic pressure to use with that individual. Your hands will begin to know.

It pays to be conservative with a new client. Many fibromyalgia sufferers respond very well to trigger point massage if done at an individually appropriate level, but it's very easy to overtreat people with that condition. With fibromyalgia, it's better to risk undertreating. Limit the time spent working trigger points to no more than thirty minutes during the first couple of sessions.

In learning about how much pressure to use on someone else's trigger points, it will be of great benefit to have thoroughly explored your own. When you have mastered self-treatment of trigger points, you will have gained a fundamental intuition about them that you can't get any other way.

Clinical Massage Guidelines

Four new ideas distinguish our therapy from other modalities of trigger point massage:

1. It incorporates self-treatment.

2. It employs a short, repeated stroke in place of pressing and holding.

3. It works very well without stretching.

4. It doesn't seek an immediate "release."

The rationale behind these four ideas is that the therapist can only create conditions that foster healing. It's foolish to think that we have a significant degree of direct control as "healers." It's the body itself that does the healing. You can accomplish quite a lot, however, if you can stimulate the process. In creating the conditions that foster healing, it's helpful to get the client involved in providing part of the therapy, because the body responds much sooner and more completely with multiple daily treatments. Realistically, this kind of frequent attention can only be provided by the client.

The therapy is achieved by the repeated short, deep stroke, which very efficiently flushes the trigger point and specifically stretches the tissue that needs to be stretched. Conventional stretching can very easily irritate trigger points and make the problem worse. We've also found it counterproductive in trying to force a release in trigger points. That mindset makes overtreatment a great danger. We believe that if we can just get the healing process started, we can trust trigger points to release in their own time after the appropriate level of treatment. An optimum treatment of an individual trigger point is actually quite brief, requiring no more than a dozen strokes. Then you need to let it alone and let the body do its work.

Troubleshooting

Use the Trigger Point Guides in chapters 4 through 10 to narrow down the search for trigger points. Then you will need to consult the drawings of the muscles and their referred pain patterns in the appropriate chapters. Remember that pain anywhere in the body can be a composite of the referred pain from trigger points in more than one muscle.

Although trigger point massage can be a stand-alone therapy, ordinarily you will be integrating it into your familiar routine. The difference is that you will be thinking now in terms of specific muscles and their specific patterns of referred pain. The information clients give you about their present pain problems will be of primary interest. But you will want to check all muscles as you go, not just the ones that directly relate to the problems they tell you about. Clients almost always have latent trigger points that activate from time to time to make trouble. It's often a great surprise to the client when you find these points and can quickly clear up long-standing mysteries regarding recurrent problems.

There is a common misconception that it's not a trigger point unless it reproduces its pain pattern when pressed on. Sometimes it does and sometimes it doesn't. If pressure on a trigger point does reproduce the client's pain, take it as a fortuitous confirmation that you've found the culprit, but don't depend on it happening. The thing you must grasp is that trigger points occur at predictable sites. In general, if it hurts to press one of those spots, it's a trigger point virtually by definition. In fact, our main criterion for finding trigger points is their exquisite tenderness when pressed. The ultimate test, of course, is whether massage reduces both the tenderness and the referred pain.

When pressed directly against bone, some trigger points feel like bruises. Others, in such muscles as the piriformis, scalenes, and levator scapulae, produce an electrical sensation, as though you were pressing on a nerve. Some clients may be able to give you valuable information if you ask about referred sensations, such as burning, numbness, or tingling, rather than pain.

In our workshops, therapists often ask how to determine the right pressure to use for trigger point massage. The basic sense of this can be acquired by practicing trigger point massage on yourself. Naturally, although self-treatment does give a valid frame of reference, the pressure that you use for yourself may have to be increased somewhat for certain clients or decreased for others. It's a good idea to begin with the trapezius muscles when working with a new client. The client's response to your pressure in treating these muscles is a good gauge of the requirement throughout. If you inadvertently evoke a pain level of eight or above, simply remove pressure from the trigger point and allow ten to fifteen seconds for the client's painkilling endorphins to kick in. You can often resume massage with nearly the same pressure but with much less pain. Even so, resume cautiously.

Using Your Best Tools

Make it your mantra to "find the easy way" to do massage. For the safest use of the hands, pair them whenever possible. This divides the labor between them and makes overuse less likely. Minimize use of the unsupported opposing thumb (the free thumb). Keep your elbows straight when you can, so that you can lean into the stroke, using your body weight instead of your muscles for applying pressure. This minimizes the effort expended by the shoulder, arm, and hand muscles. Various ways of using the hands ergonomically are illustrated throughout this chapter when the specific muscles are discussed. Three kinds of strokes are used in trigger point massage, each for its specific purpose.

Warming Stroke

This is a good beginning stroke for calming and connecting with the client. Massage therapists everywhere recognize this as *effleurage*, or "flowing" strokes. No matter which muscles you're working on, do a few strokes of effleurage before and after addressing a muscle. You'll note that in self-treatment warming strokes are not used, nor are they called for. It may be more a warming of the spirit than a warming of the muscles that is needed. Look at warming strokes as a structured way of connecting with the client and helping to bring calm. Trigger point massage causes a certain amount of pain, which, even when pleasant, can tend to cause the client to defensively tense the muscles. The long, soothing effleurage strokes help offset this.

Searching Stroke

This is a shorter stroke, only three to six inches long, and confined to the target area or the "ballpark" in the belly of the muscle. Be aware of fiber arrangement in a given muscle. Fibers don't always run the length of a muscle from attachment to attachment. Unipennate and bipennate muscles have multiple bellies, as do muscles like the rectus abdominis that are divided into sections. Trigger points aren't found everywhere in a muscle, so it's not necessary to search everywhere. The illustrations will get you in the ballpark, most of the time near the center of the muscle fibers. Search a baseball-sized area, feeling for increased resistance in the tissue. Sometimes you will be able to feel the trigger point nodule. Usually, the taut band of muscle fibers associated with the trigger point will be quite obvious.

Treatment Stroke

This is the heart of trigger point massage—a very short, repeated stroke, no more than an inch or two in length. This is exactly the same stroke as described in the Massage Guidelines for self-treatment (see chapter 3). An efficient treatment requires only that you stroke from one side of the trigger point to the other. Think of it as a "milking" stroke, a squeegee action, repeatedly squeezing the blood out. Relax the hands between strokes. Do six to twelve strokes and then move on to the next trigger point or next area. Move the skin with the tool if you can, instead of sliding over it, as this helps free the fascia.

The exact use of the hands varies depending on what muscle is being addressed. As a rule, we position the fingers nearly vertical to the skin, using their ends to make a sharper tool (see Figures 3.3, 3.5, and 3.6). The flats of the fingers make a dull tool and tire the hands very quickly. When the tool penetrates easily, it calls for less effort. The therapist should be constantly aware of ergonomics, using body weight instead of muscle to apply pressure wherever possible.

Reasonable Expectations

After a well-executed trigger point massage, you can expect the client to get off the table feeling better. Sometimes the improvement is quite profound after a single treatment and the primary pain problem may be gone entirely. More often, of course, multiple treatments will be needed to completely remove the problem. Also, the areas that received massage can sometimes be a little sore to the touch for a couple of days. When treatment is successful, symptoms may not return for several days or weeks. They may not come back at all. Unfortunately, in such felicitous cases, the client may not come back either and may neglect to let you know that you were successful. When clients don't call for another appointment, call and see how they are doing. Don't assume that you failed. Then again, don't assume that you succeeded.

When Massage Fails to Deliver

Negative outcomes can include increased pain, all-over soreness and fatigue, new symptoms, bruising, or increased stiffness and decreased range of motion. Sometimes the client reacts favorably to the level of pressure during the session, but begins to feel worse over the next twenty-four hours. This may indicate that you used too much pressure, worked a trigger point too long, or worked the entire body too long. Clients may have nausea for a short while after treatment of abdominal or psoas muscles. After overtreatment of the sternocleidomastoid muscles, clients may have both nausea and dizziness.

A number of things can conspire to ruin a good massage or cause it to fall short of expectations. It's easy to get caught up in treating satellite trigger points and overlook primary trigger points that have created the satellites in the first place. In this case, the primary trigger point will reactivate the satellites, sometimes rather quickly, and there may seem to be no improvement. Symptoms may return in full force within hours. It's very important to keep in mind that the main reason for a failure of trigger point massage is that you've simply treated the wrong spots or have missed a trigger point somewhere.

When massage seems to have failed, it may not be your fault. The client may be involved in an ongoing activity that is unusually taxing or requires repetitive motion. If this is the activity that created the problem in the first place, it's unreasonable to think it could do anything but bring the problem back and perpetuate it. Remember that chest breathing, nervous tension, and bad posture are significant factors in perpetuating trigger points, as are structural abnormalities such as Morton's Foot (see chapters 2 and 10).

If clients complain that massage didn't help or made their pain worse, you may have used stretching too soon or too aggressively. Most therapists (particularly physical therapists) need to be a great deal more circumspect about the use of stretching. A great number of people can't be stretched at all without exacerbating their problem. The safe approach is to leave stretching until you have deactivated all the trigger points. Even then, overly ambitious stretching can reactivate trigger points. Stretching enthusiasts may find it hard to believe that properly executed trigger point massage works without stretching. They should remember that, even with clients who benefit from stretching, it's trigger points that keep muscles shortened. When trigger points are gone, muscles lengthen naturally and range of motion returns with normal activity.

If massage seems to have created new symptoms, these may only be pain problems that were hidden from awareness by the client's preoccupation with the main problem, which massage may have reduced or removed. In this case, nobody is at fault and the "new" symptoms actually may be a sign of progress.

When You Make a Trigger Point Worse

Too much massage can irritate a trigger point and make it worse. Overtreatment may even cause a muscle to go into spasm. When this occurs, first calm yourself down and get centered. It's a temporary problem, and you should be able to fix it simply with the information you find in this book.

Do a few strokes of calming effleurage and then leave the muscle alone for a period of time and work on other areas. If you choose to come back to the troublesome area later in the session, begin gently and cautiously, as if you were massaging a baby. Icing an over-stimulated muscle at the end of the session may help some clients. The application of moist heat may be more helpful for others. It may be enough just to give it a rest. When you make a trigger point worse, it's usually because you're too intent on getting a result. Remember that you must trust the body to do its own healing. Your job is to give the trigger point a few strokes to flush the tissue and to accomplish the very specific microstretch, simply creating the conditions that foster healing. It's counterproductive to seek too much control.

Keep an Open Mind

It doesn't make sense to fall into the habit of applying exactly the same routine to everybody. Everyone's body is different to some degree and requires a carefully considered, specific treatment. If your therapy is less than successful with a particular client, don't waste time defending the rightness of your approach. If the client says it isn't working, the client is right. It's the client's body and the client's pain.

Janet Travell believed that our patients are our best teachers. When things don't go the way you thought they should, look at it as an opportunity to learn. Keep consulting this book. Consult Travell and Simons's *Trigger Point Manual*. Bounce the problem off other therapists that you respect. Take workshops where you can rub elbows with other highly motivated learners. Take it even further and form a study group, using this book as your text. Have faith that with trigger points and referred pain, there's always an answer. It's only a matter of persisting until you find it.

Treating the Client (Prone)

Some massage therapists still work primarily with the client facedown, concentrating on the neck, back, arms, calves, and feet. In our society, we tend to avoid touching the front of someone else's body unless we know them extremely well. The same is true for the zone between the waist and the knees.

Fortunately, the vast majority of professionally trained massage therapists feel far less squeamish about massage in these "forbidden" areas than the general public does. Modern massage schools are doing a very good job of instilling an ethic of "safe touch" in their students. That's good, because trigger point therapy requires treatment of abdominal, buttock, and inner thigh muscles if you expect to deal effectively with pain. Nevertheless, discretion dictates that you start in the very safest of places—the upper back. The muscles are discussed here in the order used in Amber's protocol. For each muscle, treatment of only one side is shown, but we treat the corresponding muscle on the other side before moving on.

Trapezius

Since virtually everyone's trapezius muscles have trigger points, we believe the trapezius is a good place to explore the client's levels of pain in relation to your pressure.

Upper trapezius. Use the thumb and index finger to massage trigger point number 1 in the tiny roll of trapezius muscle in the angle of the neck (Figure 11.1). As described in chapter 4, this trigger point is just under the skin in a strand of muscle no thicker than a knitting needle. Since this little bit of muscle is hard to hold on to, work on it before applying lotion.

To treat trapezius number 2 trigger point, stand at the client's elbow facing the head of the table (Figure 11.2). Use both hands together to massage the muscle on the near side, grasping it with your fingers underneath and your thumbs on top, as shown. If this position is not comfortable, move to the head of the table and reposition your hands with the palms up. In either position, stroke along the muscle fibers with both thumbs, from the angle of the neck toward the outer shoulder. It also works well to massage the muscle across the fibers. You can increase the pressure slightly with each stroke. Be aware that there may be two trigger points in this thick roll of muscle, one in the central part and another an inch or two toward the outer shoulder. Take note also that the central trigger point is usually nearer the front of the muscle, in closer contact with the fingers than with the thumbs.

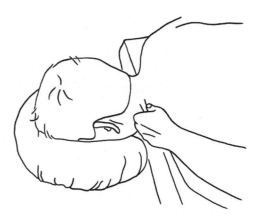

Figure 11.1 Trapezius number 1 kneaded between fingers and thumb. Feel for the "knitting needle" just under the skin.

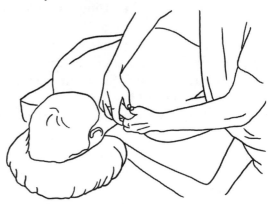

Figure 11.2 Trapezius number 2 massage with paired hands. Stroke with the thumbs either cross-fiber or with the fibers laterally.

Lower trapezius. Position yourself at the upper corner of the table and locate the inferior and superior angles of the scapula. Trapezius number 3 trigger point is halfway between these two bony landmarks, where the lower edge of the trapezius crosses the medial border of the scapula. This lower edge of the muscle feels like a speed bump as you rub your fingers along the medial border. Keep the muscle from moving by placing one thumb just below its lower edge, just off the scapula (Figure 11.3). Using the other

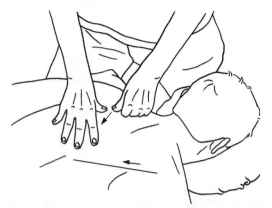

Figure 11.3   Trapezius number 3 massage with supported thumb while the other thumb keeps the muscle's lower border from moving.

thumb, stroke along the edge of the muscle in a diagonal direction toward vertebra T12. In the drawing, the therapist is massaging with her left thumb (supported) and trapping the muscle with the right one. The long, diagonal line on the right side of the client's back indicates the lower edge of the lower trapezius on that side.

There may be other trigger points in the lower edge of the trapezius, an inch or so further down toward the spine and further up where it travels across the scapula. Remember that lower trapezius trigger points can keep trigger points in the upper trapezius and posterior neck activated and make neck pain and headaches hard to get rid of. They can also be the source of an obstinate mid back ache.

Levator Scapulae and Splenius Cervicis

Trace the levator from the base of the neck to the superior angle of the scapula. This is just two or three inches, depending on the size of the client. Notice how the levator makes an "X" with the thick roll of upper trapezius muscle as it goes underneath it. For treatment of the lower trigger point of the levator scapulae, use paired supported thumbs (Figure 11.4). Dig under the trapezius from its anterior aspect with your thumbs and feel for the superior angle of the scapula, stroking all around its contour. To make it easier on your hands, brace your elbow against your hip as you lean into this stroke, using your weight for the pressure. You can also massage this trigger point with supported fingers, working through the trapezius instead of under it. In this case, stand at the client's elbow and stroke toward yourself (the hand positioning for this is shown in Figure 11.13).

For the levator scapulae's middle trigger point, use one supported thumb to stroke the muscle against the ends of the transverse processes of the sixth and seventh cervical vertebrae very low on the neck (Figure 11.5). The lower splenius cervicis trigger point can be treated with this same stroke by following the transverse processes an inch or two down to the first and second thoracic vertebrae. The levator scapulae's third trigger point

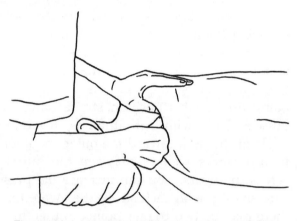

Figure 11.4   Levator scapulae number 1 trigger point massage with access under the front edge of the upper trapezius

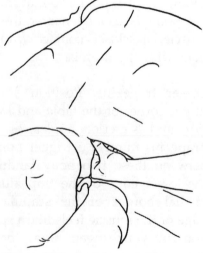

Figure 11.5   Levator scapulae number 2 trigger point massage with supported thumb against the transverse processes of vertebras C6 and C7

is halfway up the side of the neck, immediately behind the sternocleidomastoid. The muscle is very thin at this spot, and a single thumb is an adequate tool.

Posterior Neck

Warm and relax the neck with two-handed petrissage. Then, starting right next to the spinous processes, stroke from the base of neck to the occiput and onto the skull with either supported fingers or paired thumbs (Figures 11.6 and 11.7). With supported fingers, pull toward yourself. With paired thumbs, push away. Supported fingers feel especially good at the occiput and are a better tool for more sensitive clients. Do several parallel strokes until the entire back and side of the neck are covered.

When you find a trigger point, give it six to twelve slow, short strokes, and then move on. To avoid using too much pressure, continue asking for numbers to gauge the client's level of pain. Be sure you can locate and trace all the posterior neck muscles, including the splenius capitis, the splenius cervicis, semispinalis, deep spinals, and suboccipitals. It's helpful to be able to locate the individual suboccipitals, especially the lowest one, the obliquus capitis inferior, which is a primary rotator of the head. Remember that the more skill you acquire in treating your own neck, the better you'll understand the anatomy of your client's neck.

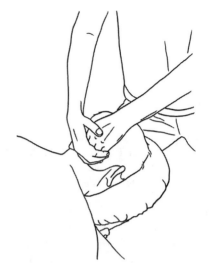

Figure 11.6 Posterior neck massage from the base of the neck to the occiput with supported fingers

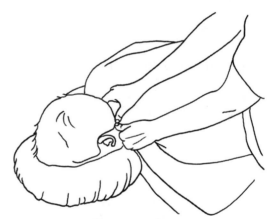

Figure 11.7 Posterior neck massage with paired thumbs stroking toward the occiput

Superficial Spinal Muscles

Supported fingers, the heel of the hand, or your forearm can be used interchangeably for treating trigger points in the superficial spinal muscles. Middle trapezius and rhomboid trigger points can also be treated with any of these tools. When using your forearm or elbow, avoid pressing on spinous processes of the vertebrae. Notice in the drawing that the therapist's right thumb is keeping track of the spinal column and guiding the forearm (Figure 11.8). Begin with a preliminary series of long parallel strokes down the back, from the base of the neck to the pelvis, and then lateral strokes along the top of the hip bone. Cover the same lines again more slowly with deeper pressure and begin searching for trigger points. When you find one, use the very short treatment stroke, repeated six to a dozen times.

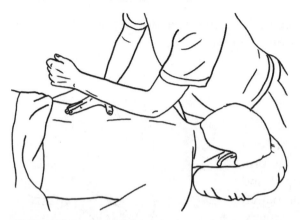

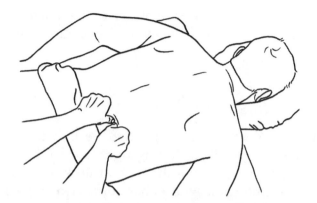

Figure 11.8   Superficial spinal muscles massage with the elbow or the blade of the ulna. The thumb of the opposite hand serves as a guide to keep the elbow off the spinous processes.

Figure 11.9   Longissimus lumborum massage with paired supported thumbs stroking up against the lowest rib

To treat trigger points in the lower part of the longissimus and iliocostalis muscles, use supported fingers or paired supported thumbs and stroke upward against the lowest rib (Figure 11.9). Review the diverse pain patterns of trigger points in the superficial spinal muscles. They can be the primary cause of low back or sacroiliac pain.

Deep Spinal Muscles

Paired supported thumbs work extremely well for treating trigger points in the deep multifidi and rotatores muscles along the spine (Figure 11.10). It's likely that you will find taut and tender diagonal fibers in the deep spinal muscles at the same vertebral level where you found trigger points in the superficial spinal muscles.

Work your way down the back, starting just below the seventh cervical vertebra. Reach across the body and press both thumbs into the *lamina groove*, the narrow trough between the spinous and transverse processes. Stroke away from yourself with

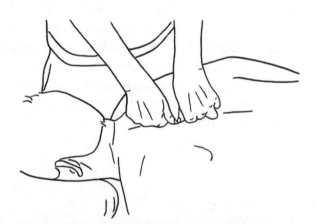

Figure 11.10   Deep spinal muscles massage with paired supported thumbs working cross-body in the narrow groove between the spinous and transverse processes of the vertebrae

tiny scoops of your thumbs (the thumbs can work together or alternately). This stroke is extremely short and should not cross the fibers of the spinalis thoracis, because the effect can be quite irritating to the client and may even provoke a spasm. You'll feel the spinalis as a strong vertical band, separated from the spinous processes by no more than half an inch. Treat trigger points in spinalis muscles with strokes along the fibers.

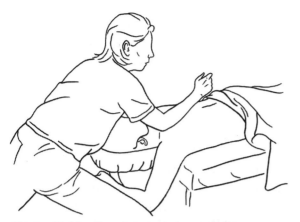

Figure 11.11 Serratus posterior superior massage with the blade of the ulna. The therapist is grasping the client's left hand and pulling the arm cross-body to help move the shoulder blade out of the way.

Serratus Posterior Superior

To reach trigger points in the serratus posterior superior muscle, you must move the scapula to the side. Notice that the client's arm is hanging over the end of the massage table (Figure 11.11). Under the face cradle, the therapist is pulling the client's wrist toward the opposite side, which helps move the scapula even farther away from the spine. Search for trigger points right next to the medial border of the scapula, very close to the superior angle.

A gentle forearm or supported thumb is a good tool to use here, always employing short, repeated strokes from one side of the trigger point to the other. Supported fingers are good, too, if the client can use an arm support that attaches to the table (or simply have the client grasp the underside of the face cradle). Alternatively, you can treat the serratus posterior superior in the supine position at the same time you treat the subscapularis. Remember that the serratus posterior superior is an accessory breathing muscle and habitual chest breathing tends to perpetuate its trigger points. The client may need to know this.

Supraspinatus

Treat supraspinatus trigger points with double supported thumbs from the head of the table (Figure 11.12). The thumbs should be facing one another with the nails touching. This makes a very sharp tool that is capable of penetrating through the trapezius, which can be very thick and muscular where it overlies the supraspinatus. Keep your wrists and elbows straight, and then simply lean in, using your weight for the pressure. Focus on the small triangular space between the superior angle and the spine of the scapula. Use short strokes toward the outer shoulder to treat this deep central trigger point, and then move a short distance farther out to where the muscle dives under the

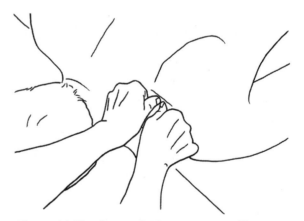

Figure 11.12 Supraspinatus massage with paired supported thumbs. The thumbnails face one another and the stroke follows the scapular spine laterally. Keep the elbows straight and lean in.

acromion. If this outer trigger point is present, it will feel highly sensitive, very much like a bruise. Treat this thin part of the muscle gently.

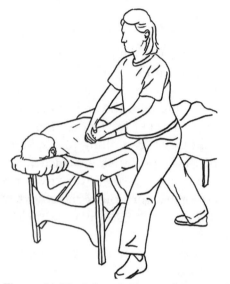

Figure 11.13   Infraspinatus and teres minor: The edge of the right hand is on the body and does most of the work in moving the fingertips of the left hand. Relax the left hand and move the skin with the tool.

Infraspinatus and Teres Minor

Use supported fingers or paired supported thumbs to treat the infraspinatus (Figure 11.13). Infraspinatus trigger points can be present in several places below the scapular spine between the medial and lateral borders. The infraspinatus often needs multiple deep strokes before trigger points "wake up" and begin to produce the familiar sense of exquisite tenderness. It may take ten or fifteen seconds before the client can give you a number high enough to indicate the need for treatment. Notice that the therapist is showing good body mechanics in keeping her neck and spine straight and in using her body weight instead of muscle action to exert pressure.

Use supported fingers also for the teres minor, searching along the lateral border of the scapula, about an inch above the crease of the armpit. Paired supported thumbs can also be used. This muscle is about the size and thickness of an index finger. When it's tight, you may be able to feel it crossing high on the lateral border toward the head of the humerus.

Latissimus Dorsi and Teres Major

The latissimus dorsi and teres major can be treated by kneading with fingers and thumb, reaching across the body (Figure 11.14). You can differentiate the two muscles by feeling for the narrow trough between them. Teres major is the deeper muscle. The teres major can also be pressed against the bone with supported fingers, halfway down the scapula's lateral border (not shown). The outer edge of the lower part of the latissimus dorsi can be treated by grasping and kneading it with both hands (Figure 11.15). You can also use supported fingers on these muscles on the side nearest you.

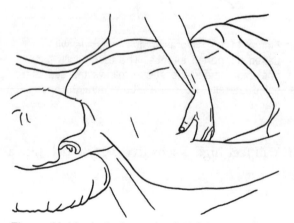

Figure 11.14   Latissimus dorsi and teres major kneaded between fingers and thumb cross-body. This can also be done from the head of the table.

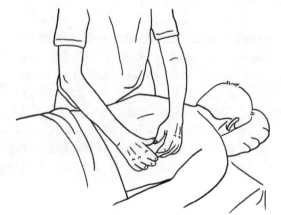

Figure 11.15   Latissimus dorsi massage by kneading between fingers and thumb of both hands cross-body, using very specific, short strokes

Serratus Anterior

Serratus anterior trigger points can be treated by reaching across the body with supported fingers, as shown (Figure 11.16). Alternately, you can treat the side nearest you, using supported fingers with the palms up (this position of the hands is used in self-treating the gastrocnemius, as shown in Figure 10.25.) The primary trigger point in the serratus anterior lies on the most prominent rib about three finger widths down the rib cage from the armpit. If you find this primary trigger point, search the entire side of the rib cage under the arm for trigger points in other bellies of the muscle.

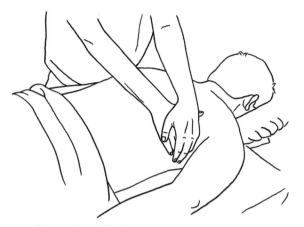

Figure 11.16   Serratus anterior massage with paired hands cross-body, about three finger widths straight down from the armpit

Deltoids, Triceps, and Flexors

Massage the deltoids first with the heel of your hand to warm them. Then use either the knuckles of an open fist or a supported thumb for specific trigger points (not shown). Deltoid trigger points can be treated when the client is either prone or supine.

For treating the triceps, let the client's arm hang over of the side of the table (Figure 11.17). Offset the supported thumbs from one another. This will bring your hands a little closer together and let you use the knuckles of your fingers to keep the arm in position. You can treat all five triceps trigger points with this tool. You may want to try working the medial trigger point near the elbow by kneading it between fingers and thumb (not shown).

To massage the flexors, place the arm back on the table with the palm up. Use double supported thumbs for specific trigger points (Figure 11.18). Supported fingers or a gentle forearm are also valuable tools. Most of the trigger points in the inner forearm will be in an oval-shaped area that extends three or four inches just below the crease of the elbow.

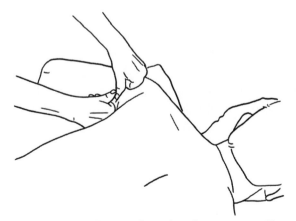

Figure 11.17   Triceps (long head) massage with offset, paired supported thumbs stroking away from the therapist

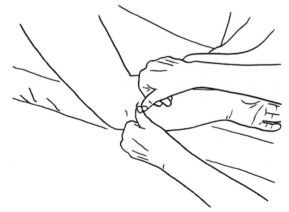

Figure 11.18   Flexors massage with offset, paired supported thumbs stroking toward the medial epicondyle of the elbow. This can also be done with the knuckles of an open fist or the blade of the ulna.

Remember that the large flexor pollicis muscle of the thumb occupies the middle third of the inner forearm. Its trigger points not only cause thumb pain, but are also the cause of locking or catching in the last thumb joint.

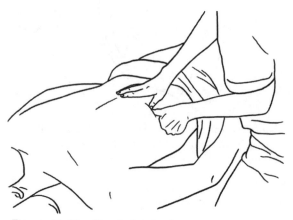

Figure 11.19   Quadratus lumborum massage with paired thumbs at the lowest rib and transverse processes of the vertebrae. The pressure is toward the opposite shoulder.

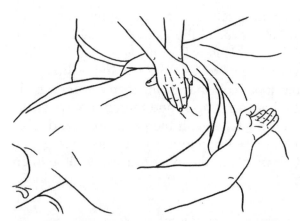

Figure 11.20   Quadratus lumborum massage cross-body with paired hands stroking at the lateral border of the muscle. Lean back and pull.

Quadratus Lumborum

Use paired thumbs or paired hands for treatment of quadratus lumborum trigger points (Figures 11.19 and 11.20). To differentiate the muscle from the spinal muscles, have the client hike the hip several times to make the quadratus lumborum contract in isolation. The inner edge of the quadratus lumborum is at the outer edge of the thick spinal muscles, two to four inches to the side of the spinous processes, depending on the size of the client.

When working with supported thumbs on the side nearest you, first face slightly toward the head of the table (Figure 11.19). Treat the upper two trigger points by searching the spot where the outer edge of the muscle attaches to the lowest rib, and then the angle the rib makes with the transverse processes. Start on the body of the muscle and stroke into this angle. Quadratus lumborum trigger points can feel like sore bruises when pressed against these bony surfaces.

For the lower pair of trigger points, reposition your body to face the gluteal area. In this case, search for trigger points at the spot where the outer edge of the muscle attaches to the top of the hip bone, and then the angle the pelvis makes with the transverse processes. Stroke into these places. As an alternative to your thumbs, you can reach across the body and treat these same four places with paired hands (Figure 11.20). Start all the way across at the abdominal obliques and then lean back, using your weight to pull your fingertips toward you. Stop when you reach the spinal muscles. Shorten this stroke to treat specific trigger points.

Piriformis and Gluteus Muscles

Massage of the gluteal area can be on the bare skin, through a sheet, or even through thin shorts or slacks. Tools include your choice of a gentle elbow, supported fingers, supported knuckles, or supported thumbs. Your elbow may be the most ergonomic tool because you can support yourself with one hand and use your weight to apply pressure (Figure 11.21). Begin by verifying the location of the top of the hip bone, sacrum, greater trochanter, and ischial tuberosity (sit bone). These bony landmarks are vital in guiding you to specific trigger points in this otherwise ill-defined area.

Search the gluteus medius for its first trigger point high along the edge of the sacrum. You may find the second gluteus medius trigger point halfway along a line crossing just below the top of the hip bone toward the side of the buttocks. Search for the third trigger point two to three inches above the greater trochanter.

Move down an inch to search back across towards the sacrum. You may find gluteus minimus trigger points along this line and in a third line another inch down, just above the greater

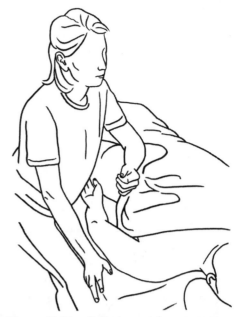

Figure 11.21 Buttock muscles massage with the elbow. This can also be done with supported fingers.

trochanter. Piriformis trigger points lie on a line approximately level with the greater trochanter, just posterior of the trochanter and at about the center of the edge of the sacrum. Approach this second piriformis trigger point with caution because it overlies the sciatic nerve and can be extremely tender.

The upper trigger point in the gluteus maximus may be found at the edge of the sacrum, just above the second piriformis trigger point. For the lower trigger point in the maximus, press straight down on the ischial tuberosity or sit bone. As always, use short, repeated strokes. You may find other maximus trigger points against both the medial and lateral sides of both ischial tuberosities. Ask the client's permission before checking the maximus trigger point in the gluteal fold next to the tail bone. You may prefer to instruct the client in self-treatment for this one.

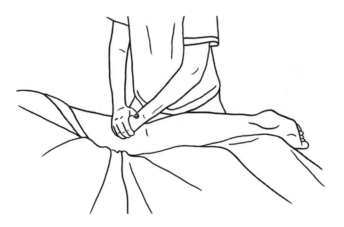

Figure 11.22 Hamstrings massage with supported fingers. This can also be done with supported knuckles or the knuckles of an open fist, palm up.

Hamstrings

Use supported knuckles, supported fingers, or your forearm for treating trigger points in the hamstrings (Figure 11.22). Starting just above the knee, use long searching strokes all the way to the ischial tuberosity. One stroke will follow the semimembranosus and semitendinosus. The other stroke will follow the biceps femoris. Notice that these two lines begin on opposite sides of the knee and make an inverted "V" ending at the sit bone. Trigger points may be found anywhere along the semimembranosus and semitendinosus muscles, but only in the middle third of the biceps femoris. Make your stroke very short to treat individual trigger points.

Calf Muscles

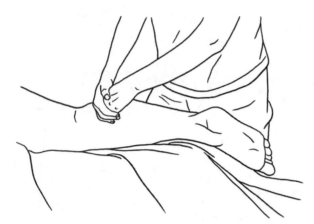

Figure 11.23   Calf massage: The edge of the right hand contacts the skin and moves the fingertips of the left hand. Relax both hands.

The safest and most ergonomic tools for the calves are supported fingers or supported thumbs, which penetrate with minimal effort for treating specific trigger points (Figure 11.23). To save your hands, don't use petrissage (kneading) for massage of calf muscles. Very often, trigger points in calf muscles have never been treated specifically, especially in the three deep muscles. The calf is a very tender area on most people. It's wise to progress slowly with successively deeper strokes.

Begin by defining the lower edge of the gastrocnemius by mentally drawing a line across the back of the lower leg about halfway down. If the muscle is well shaped, its lower edge will be somewhat irregular, with the medial head coming a little lower than the lateral head. Next, draw an imaginary line down the middle of the calf to mentally separate not only the heads of the gastrocnemius but the two bones of the lower leg, the tibia and fibula. It's very important to be able to visualize what's hidden beneath the skin.

In each of the heads of the gastrocnemius, look for a trigger point in the center of the muscle belly and also close to the crease of the knee. You may find a deep soleus trigger point between the two lateral gastrocnemius trigger points. The two lower soleus trigger points are just below the edge of the gastrocnemius, barely over the midline on either side.

You will access the tibialis posterior and flexor digitorum longus between the heads of the gastrocnemius, pushing the gastrocnemius to one side or the other as required. To treat the tibialis posterior, press down between the heads of the gastrocnemius at its very center and then move the entire muscle toward the fibula (toward the outer side of the leg). Don't let your fingers slide onto the thick belly of the gastrocnemius or you will have to treat the underlying tibialis posterior through it. Stay between the heads of the gastrocnemius and use short, repeated strokes to massage the tibialis against the fibula.

The flexor digitorum longus can be massaged in the same way, only this time pushing the gastrocnemius toward the tibia (toward the inner side of the leg). Massage the muscle against the tibia with short repeated strokes. The flexor hallucis longus trigger point is just below the midline of the calf, near the lateral soleus trigger point. You will be working through the soleus, pressing the flexor hallucis longus against the inner side of the fibula, just as you did with the tibialis posterior higher up.

Morton's Foot

To check for Morton's Foot, compare the relative lengths of the first and second metatarsal bones to see if the second is longer (Figure 11.24). Press the toes back with your thumb while pushing up on the heads of the first and second metatarsals with your fingers. This will make the heads of the two metatarsals stick out enough to see or feel them. Look for a heavy callus under the head of the second metatarsal, which is a strong indicator that the bone is too long (see Figure 10.36). An extra long web between the second and third toes is another indicator of Morton's Foot.

If the toes won't bend back to expose the heads of the metatarsals, it's very likely that you'll find that the extensor digitorum longus and interosseous muscles are being kept shortened by trigger points. The simple treatment for Morton's Foot is just to put pads under the heads of the *first* metatarsals, which will let them make more immediate contact with the ground. Don't make the mistake of putting a pad under a second metatarsal just because pain is felt at that spot.

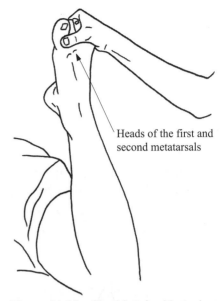

Heads of the first and second metatarsals

Figure 11.24   Checking for Morton's Foot. Pull back with the thumb and push up with the fingers.

Plantar Foot Muscles

To address the seven muscles in the bottom of the foot, use paired hands so that several fingers can share the load (Figure 11.25). A supported thumb also works well, especially for the deep quadratus plantae muscle (Figure 11.26). With this tool and your hands at waist level, you can lock your elbow against your side and use your body weight to apply the pressure. Use a supported thumb to search between the metatarsals for interosseous trigger points (not shown).

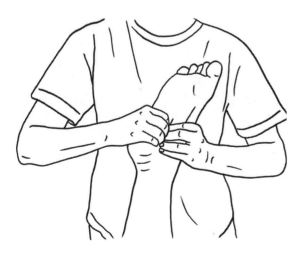

Figure 11.25   Plantar foot muscles massage with paired hands

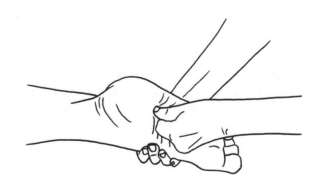

Figure 11.26   Quadratus plantae massage with supported thumb stroking laterally, immediately in front of the heel bone

Deep trigger point massage to the plantar side of the foot is hard work for the therapist. It's enough to simply locate and only briefly treat the trigger points. Show the client how to use a 35-mm high bounce ball for self-treatment.

Treating the Client (Supine)

To maintain continuity, finish with the leg after turning the client over. Be aware that two muscles with opposing functions very often have trigger points in both. Look for indications of this in the client's pain symptoms. As an example, pain in both the top and the bottom of the forefoot tells you to look for trigger points in both the flexors and extensors of the toes.

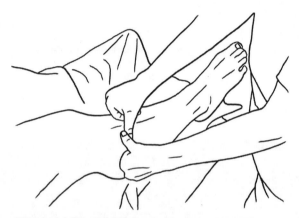

Figure 11.27   Tibialis anterior massage with paired supported thumbs, a hand's width down from the knee, immediately beside the shinbone

Shin Muscles

Address trigger points in the tibialis anterior and extensor digitorum longus muscles with supported thumbs about a hand's width below the knee (Figure 11.27). The tibialis anterior is right next to the tibia. The extensor digitorum longus is only about a finger's width further to the outer side of the leg. There may be more than one trigger point along the three- or four-inch length of each muscle's belly. Trigger points in the extensor hallucis longus may be found about a third of the way up from the ankle, roughly on a line with the extensor digitorum longus.

Peroneus Muscles

Treat trigger points overlying the fibula in the peroneus longus about a hand's width down from the knee with a supported thumb or the large knuckles of a loose open fist (Figure 11.28). Stabilize the leg with your opposite hand. Use the same tool for the peroneus brevis trigger points, also overlying the fibula, about a third of the way up from the ankle. Use a supported thumb to search for peroneus tertius trigger points just in front of the fibula, two to four inches up from the lateral malleolus (not shown).

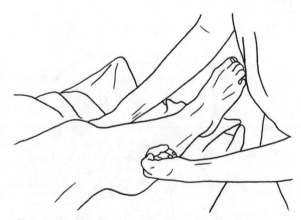

Figure 11.28   Peroneus longus massage with the big knuckles of an open fist, palm up. Support the leg with the opposite hand.

Quadriceps, Sartorius, and Tensor Fasciae Latae

Search for tensor fasciae latae trigger points just below the anterior superior iliac spine (the front of the hip bone). To be certain of the muscle's location, have the client rotate the knee inward several times for isolated contraction. For treatment, use paired, supported thumbs or supported fingers (not shown). The same tools can be used for the upper trigger point in the rectus femoris, just an inch medial to the tensor fasciae latae trigger point and perhaps an inch lower. To verify the location of the rectus femoris, have the client raise the leg repeatedly with a straight knee. Use supported fingers, supported knuckles, or paired supported thumbs to massage trigger points in the vastus intermedius, vastus medialis, and sartorius muscles (Figure 11.29)

Search for multiple trigger points in the vastus lateralis from the knee to the greater trochanter with a loose, open fist with the palm up (Figure 11.30). To keep the leg from rolling away, support it at the knee with the opposite hand. It may be necessary to use this technique in both the supine and prone positions since the very broad vastus lateralis wraps all the way around the side of the thigh from front to back. Tightness in the vastus lateralis caused by trigger points may be misinterpreted as tightness in the iliotibial band. Tension in the iliotibial band comes from shortening of gluteus maximus and tensor fasciae latae muscles due to trigger points.

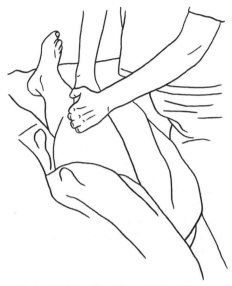

Figure 11.29 Vastus medialis: The edge of the left hand is on the skin and moves the fingertips of the right hand. Move the skin with the tool.

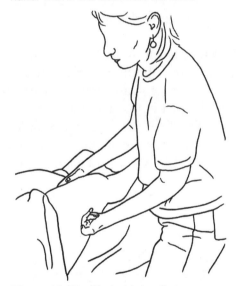

Figure 11.30 Vastus lateralis massage with the knuckles of an open fist, palm up, stroking toward the hip. Support the thigh at the knee.

Inner Thigh Muscles

For treatment of inner thigh trigger points, the client's knee should be rotated outward and supported with your knee (Figure 11.31). A pillow or rolled-up towel can be used instead. To locate the adductor longus, place one hand on the client's inner knee and the other hand high on the inner thigh (not shown). The adductor longus will contract prominently against your hand if you have the client press against the hand at the knee. Differentiate the adductor longus and the more posterior adductor magnus by feeling for the narrow trough between them. It may be helpful to think of the adductor magnus as a fourth hamstring. It's very close to being on the back of the thigh.

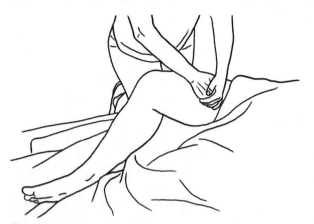

Figure 11.31   Inner thigh massage with supported fingers stroking from side to side, not toward the groin.

Massage the trigger points in the adductors with a side-to-side stroke with supported fingers (Figure 11.31). This side-to-side stroke feels less invasive than stroking up and down the inner thigh. The gracilis and adductor magnus trigger points can also be massaged by grasping and kneading them between the fingers and thumb. The upper adductor magnus trigger point just below the ischial tuberosity can be treated less invasively in the prone position or by self-treatment. The pectineus muscle near the groin may also require self-treatment.

Abdominal Muscles

To foster a better understanding of abdominal trigger point locations, it's helpful to separate the muscles into four groups.

Upper abdominals. The first stroke will be along the attachments of the abdominal oblique and rectus abdominis muscles on the lowest three ribs. Reach across the client's body and pull slowly toward yourself with the searching stroke, using paired hands. The next stroke will be just below the lowest rib (Figure 11.32). Press the tissue up against the underside of the rib all the way across to the center. When you encounter a trigger point, switch to the very short treatment stroke with supported fingers and give it six to twelve repetitions (Figure 11.33). Take care to avoid the xiphoid process.

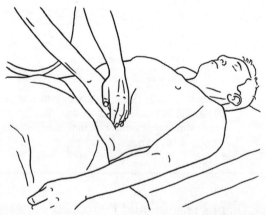

Figure 11.32   Abdominal obliques massage with paired hands cross-body. Lean back with straight elbows and pull.

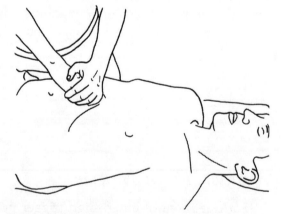

Figure 11.33   Rectus abdominis massage: The supporting hand moves the fingertips of the tool hand. Avoid the xiphoid process.

Mid abdominals. The same cross-body strokes are used in the midsection. Remember that the obliques wrap all the way around to the latissimus dorsi at the edge of the back. Trigger points may be found anywhere in the mid abdominals, but the worst are often in the rectus abdominis on either side of the belly button. Keep in mind that the rectus abdominis is divided into eight to ten sections, each with its own "muscle belly." The two sections just below the belly button are also apt to have very active trigger points. In the area between the belly button and the pubic bone, your pressure on a trigger point may reproduce the client's referred pain in any of the internal organs, genitals, or rectum. This is a clear indication that trigger points are producing at least part of any chronic pain in those areas.

Lower abdominals. Use the same searching stroke, beginning all the way across at the edge of the quadratus lumborum. Pull toward the center, following the top of the hip bone around to the inguinal ligament and then on across to the midline, pressing the muscle against the top of the pubic bone. There can be multiple trigger points along this path. Give each one several short treatment strokes. Since the pubic area remains draped, you may want the client to touch the pubic bone to identify its location. To ease potential embarrassment, therapy can actually be done in this area with the client's hand as the massage tool or by teaching the client how to self-treat. Trigger points can also be found on the front of the pubic bone on either side of the midline. The thin muscle at these places can feel like little bruises when pressed against the bone.

Psoas and iliacus. Put the client in the same position as illustrated for self-treatment in Figure 7.31. The client's bent knees should fall to the side away from you (Figure 11.34). This should turn the pelvis and raise the near hip slightly off the table. This helps move the intestines out of the way to the opposite side. A pillow or a bolster under the knees may be used to prevent any excessive twisting in the low back. Once in position, take a moment to get centered. Have the client take a slow deep breath, and you do the same. It may help both parties avoid self-consciousness if you keep a conversation going, but without too much convulsing humor.

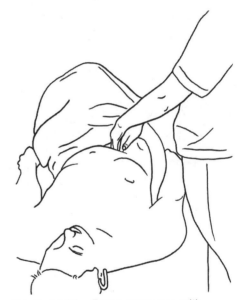

Figure 11.34 Psoas massage with paired hands. The fingers are perpendicular to the table and the client's knees are to the opposite side.

Find the midpoint between the hip bone and the belly button. Use paired hands with the fingers nearly vertical to sink very slowly into the belly, aiming straight down toward the spine (Figure 11.34). The psoas muscle is almost parallel to the spine, and it may feel like it's just under the skin in this position. As you work, watch the client's face for indications that you're using too much pressure. Be aware that you may elicit a pain response before actually coming in contact with the psoas. Use short, very gentle cross-fiber strokes to locate the firm, sausagelike roundness of the muscle. If you can't find this rounded firmness, the psoas on that side may not have trigger points that are active enough to make the muscle tight and firm. Search for exquisitely tender spots, repositioning your fingers an inch at a time up and down the muscle, above and below the belly button and all the way down to the inguinal ligament. The iliacus can be massaged against the front of the hip bone.

Treat each trigger point with the usual short, repeated strokes. The stroke direction can be either with the muscle fibers or across them. In treating the left psoas, be alert for the heavy pulse of the descending aorta under your fingers. If you feel the pulse, move your fingers away from the midline just enough to get off it. You may have to angle in behind the aorta to get to the psoas. Finish the abdominal treatment with several long, circling strokes, following the colon in a clockwise manner.

Pectoral muscles

Use supported fingers to find and treat trigger points in the pectoralis major, sternalis, subclavius, and pectoralis minor (not shown). The pectoral muscles can be addressed through the sheet if necessary. Pectoralis minor trigger points can be treated directly through the pectoralis major. Another approach is to use a supported thumb under the outer edge of the pectoralis major to press the pectoralis minor obliquely against the ribs (Figure 11.35). Raising the arm can help clear the way. Trigger points in the outer border of the pectoralis major can be kneaded between your fingers and thumb (Figure 11.36).

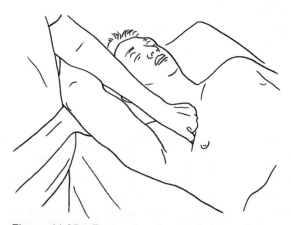

Figure 11.35   Pectoralis minor massage with supported thumb under the lateral border of the pectoralis major

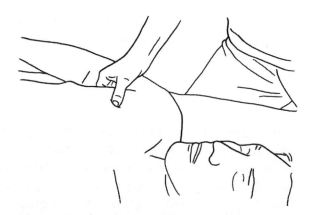

Figure 11.36   Pectoralis major (lateral border) massage by kneading between fingers and thumb

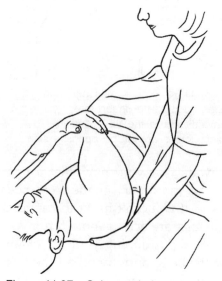

Figure 11.37   Subscapularis massage with the ends of the fingers stroking toward the therapist. Start with the backs of the nails tight against the ribs.

Subscapularis

Place the client's hand on the opposite shoulder to move the shoulder blade toward you. The client should use the other hand to press the elbow gently down against the chest (Figure 11.37). This creates a larger space for your treatment hand. To avoid abrading the client's skin, use plenty of lotion in the armpit and make sure your fingernails are very short.

Reach under the client's shoulder with one hand and curl your fingertips around the medial border of the scapula and gently pull it toward you. (With your hand in this position, you can massage the serratus posterior superior with a few strokes just medial to the superior angle of the scapula.) Place your other hand into the armpit with the palm toward you. In the correct position, your fingers will be in the slot between the scapula and the chest wall, and the blunt ends of your fingers will be touching the subscapularis muscle. The backs of your nails should be firmly against the client's ribs. Exert pressure down toward the hand that is underneath the scapula (Figure 11.38). Proceed slowly and with caution. Even light pressure on active subscapularis trigger points can be quite intolerable. Keep asking for numbers on the level of pain.

Two directions are possible for the treatment stroke. You can stroke with the fibers of the muscle down along the edge of the scapula, or you can stroke in a very short, cross-fiber scooping motion toward you. When you use the cross-fiber stroke, you can readily feel the tendon-like tautness of the muscle. Work your way up toward the head of the humerus where the subscapularis attaches, and then down to the inferior angle of the scapula. Although treatment would ordinarily call for six to twelve strokes for each trigger point, it's wise to use many fewer strokes with the subscapularis and undertreat it the first couple of sessions. Be aware that in this position you can inadvertently exert pressure on the serratus anterior with the back of your fingers. Pain evoked in this way from active serratus anterior trigger points can easily be mistaken as a subscapularis problem.

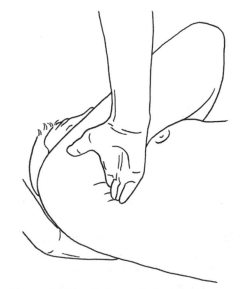

Figure 11.38 Subscapularis massage with the fingers in the slot between the shoulder blade and ribs. The opposite hand pulls the scapula toward the therapist.

Biceps, Brachialis, and Extensor Muscles

Find and treat biceps trigger points with a supported thumb or with the knuckles in an open fist, the same tool that is used for self-treatment (see Figure 5.38). A supported thumb can also be used to locate and treat brachialis trigger points just above the lateral epicondyle and under the outer edge of the biceps (Figure 11.39). Slacken the biceps and brachialis by keeping the elbow slightly flexed.

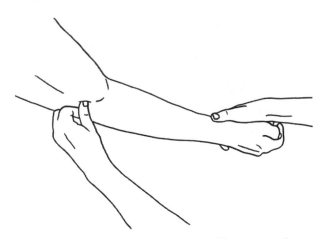

Figure 11.39 Brachialis massage with supported thumb under the edge of the biceps, just above the crease in the elbow

Massage the extensors with the forearm (Figure 11.40). Offset, paired supported thumbs also make an excellent tool for individual trigger points. This is the same tool that you use on the flexors (Figure 11.18). Make a special search all around the head of the radius for specific trigger points in the extensor carpi radialis longus, supinator, and brachioradialis. As you work, facilitate the search by rotating the forearm through pronation and supination. Keep studying the anatomy of the forearm. You should aim at acquiring the ability to find and treat any of these muscles individually.

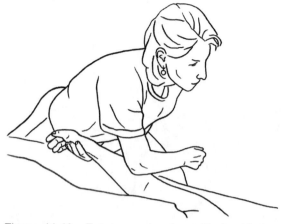

Figure 11.40   Extensors massage with the blade of the ulna stroking toward the elbow. Paired supported thumbs also work well.

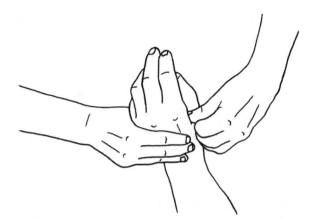

Figure 11.41   First dorsal interosseous massage with supported thumb stroking the muscle against the metacarpal

The muscles at the base of the thumb can be treated with a supported thumb (not shown). Treat the first dorsal interosseous also with the supported thumb (Figure 11.41). The other interosseous muscles are best left for careful self-treatment by the client with the tip of a supported thumb or the clamp-and-eraser tool (see Figure 6.48).

Sternocleidomastoid

Treat trigger points in the sternocleidomastoid muscles by kneading one side at a time with your fingers and thumb (Figure 11.42). Differentiate the sternal and clavicular branches of this muscle by feeling for the narrow trough between them. Remember that the clavicular branch is deeper than the sternal branch. To reach the clavicular branch, you must take all of the soft tissue on the side of the neck into your hand. Beginning just below the ear, slowly search the muscle along its entire length, treating trigger points in both branches as you come to them. Use the flat pads of your fingers and thumb rather than the tips. The action of the treatment stroke should be like rolling a pea repeatedly between your fingers and thumb. Note that you will have more control of the sternocleidomastoids if you treat them without lotion.

When the muscle is rigid with tension, the clavicular branch can be very difficult to grasp, particularly low on the neck where the two branches separate. To make a tight sternocleidomastoid easier to treat, slacken it by bending the neck slightly toward that side. Unless the muscle has been injured, any pain caused by massage can be considered an indication of trigger points. Squeezing a healthy sternocleidomastoid doesn't hurt.

There should be little danger of inadvertently abusing the carotid arteries if you treat the sternocleidomastoids and scalenes as described. It's wise, however, to know

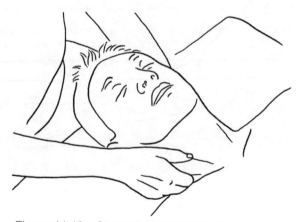

Figure 11.42   Sternocleidomastoid massage by kneading between the fingers and thumb. Stroke with the thumb following the fibers.

exactly where the carotid arteries are. They're what makes the pulse just above the Adam's apple on either side of the windpipe. This is the place where they would be the most vulnerable to direct pressure. When addressing any of the anterior neck muscles, simply move away from any pulsing that you feel under your fingers. We believe that the carotids are in very little danger from trigger point massage, and that it's unfortunate that so many therapists have been taught to stay away from the front of the neck. Your understanding of this area will be greatly increased by mastering self-treatment.

Scalenes

To effectively treat the scalene muscles, you must have a clear mental picture of their location relative to the sternocleidomastoid muscles. The anterior scalene may be the most difficult to treat, since it is entirely hidden behind the sternocleidomastoid. Address the anterior scalene by moving the sternocleidomastoid firmly toward the windpipe with the backs of the index and middle fingers (Figure 11.43). In the correct position, the fingers will be partly covered by the sternocleidomastoid.

Press the anterior scalene downward toward the table and against the vertebrae, searching its length all the way down to the clavicle. Treat each trigger point with the usual short, repeated treatment stroke, moving the fingers cross-fiber away from the windpipe. Scalene massage often reproduces the client's particular referred pain or numbness pattern. Pressure on scalene trigger points can also produce an unpleasant electrical sensation in them that feels like you're pressing on a nerve. This doesn't happen after trigger points have been deactivated.

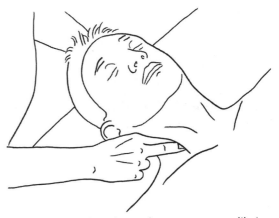

Figure 11.43 Anterior scalene massage with two fingers under the sternocleidomastoid and pushing it aside toward the windpipe

The middle scalene covers the side of the neck just behind the sternocleidomastoid. With two fingers or your thumb, stroke with the fibers or across them all the way down to the clavicle. The posterior scalene can be found just above the clavicle at the angle it makes with the thick roll of trapezius muscle on top of the shoulder. Pressure for the treatment stroke should be toward the client's feet. Use a short stroke with the middle finger (supported by the index finger) along the top of the clavicle toward the throat (Figure 11.44). With a deep chest inhalation, you may feel the posterior scalene contracting and the first rib rising against your fingers. Don't be concerned about the scalenus minimus, a fourth scalene muscle present in part of the population. Anterior scalene massage projects through to any scalenus minimus trigger points that may be present.

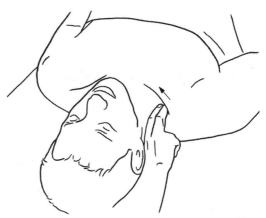

Figure 11.44 Posterior scalene massage with middle finger pressing toward the client's feet and stroking along the top of the collarbone

If you're unsure of the location of the individual scalene muscles, palpate them while having the client repeatedly sniff through the nose while taking air into the chest (as opposed to abdominal breathing). This causes the scalenes to contract more strongly so they can be felt more clearly.

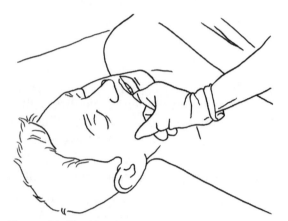

Figure 11.45   Masseter massage between the index finger and thumb

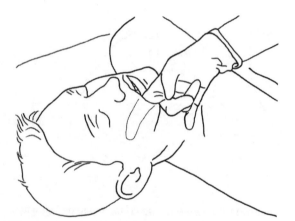

Figure 11.46   Lateral pterygoid massage with the index finger. Follow the outside of the upper gum all the way back, then press upward and stroke forward with tiny scoops.

Masseter and Pterygoid Muscles

Treatment of masseter trigger points is simple and straightforward. Insert a gloved index finger inside the client's cheek. Find trigger points by kneading the muscle between the index finger and the thumb (Figure 11.45). Massage medial pterygoid trigger points with your fingers or thumb against the inside of the lower jaw, just in front of the angle of the jaw. This is quite similar to the self-treatment technique (see Figure 4.34).

Treat the lower border of the lateral pterygoid muscle with a gloved index finger inserted into the small pocket behind and above the upper gum (Figure 11.46). This place is between the gum and cheek. Press upward toward the top of the head and stroke forward toward the front of the face. This stroke is only about a quarter of an inch long. When the lateral pterygoid is in trouble, pain from the slightest pressure from your finger can be intolerable. Watch the client's face and work very cautiously. If your state regulations prohibit therapeutic massage inside the oral cavity, simply teach your clients the self-treatment techniques.

The End of the Session

Trigger points in all of these muscles can be treated appropriately and adequately in a single session in seventy-five minutes, or less on some clients. However, don't feel you have to do a full-body treatment. It may be of more benefit to take a slower approach and focus on the places where most of the trouble lies. Take enough to time to ensure the client a pleasant experience.

Leave time at the end of the session to coach clients in the self-treatment of two or three muscles. They'll forget everything you say if you try to teach them more. Teaching your clients self-treatment will speed their recovery and increase their confidence in you. Naturally, not everyone will want to self-treat or have the capacity to do it. Nonetheless, encourage clients to give themselves some kind of treatment several times a day, even if it's only a gentle rubbing. Their abilities and interest in self-care are bound to grow.

Although this book has been widely praised for its readability and clear presentation of self-treatment, many, many people have found the process overwhelming because of their unfamiliarity with the muscle system. Accordingly, there is an enormous need for experts who can guide the general public in learning to deal effectively with trigger points. Massage therapists are ideally suited for this role. Therapists should not fear that they will give away their business and starve if they teach their clients how to self-treat. To the contrary, you'll find it brings more people to you. Sharing your knowledge and expertise demonstrates that you care more about helping people than for harvesting an income through their distress and disability. This is an ethic sorely needed everywhere in the field of health care today.

Be assured that if you teach self-care in addition to providing direct therapy, your reputation will benefit and you will be sought out by people who wouldn't be drawn to you otherwise. We should all look forward to the day when everyone will know about trigger points and massage therapists will be regarded with the respect they deserve as inspired and compassionate healers.

Chapter 12

Muscle Tension and Chronic Pain

Chronic excessive muscle tension can promote and perpetuate trigger points, thereby undermining the effectiveness of trigger point therapy. The release of habitual muscle tension can be an important part of the therapy for chronic pain (Simons and Travell 1999, 221).

Millions of people use some form of systematic relaxation to cope with stress. I'm one of those people. I learned Jacobson's progressive relaxation thirty-five years ago as a part of treatment for nervous tension, and I've used it practically every day since. I've refined the method quite a bit over that time into two distinct parts, which I've named *passive tension flooding* and *active tension release*. I believe these techniques are an improvement on progressive relaxation. You may want to give them a try, particularly if you've had trouble getting your tensions under control with other methods.

My active tension release procedures have grown out of Jacobson's progressive relaxation, in which you release the tension from your body in an systematic manner, part by part. With active tension release, however, it isn't necessary to contract muscles before relaxing them. When you've acquired enough skill, it's possible to relax your whole person instantly upon the first perception of a state of tension.

Passive tension flooding is an approach directly opposite of active tension release. Instead of attempting systematic relaxation, which can be very difficult when you're right in the midst of stress, you passively immerse yourself in your tension until it peaks and disperses on its own. Passive tension flooding is related to the various methods of desensitization that ask you to face your fears and fully experience the associated feelings. With passive tension flooding, however, you center your consciousness exclusively on the tension in your muscles. It bypasses the cognitive aspects of emotion and deals in a very direct and practical way with muscle tension, emotion's chief physical symptom.

Passive tension flooding facilitates a deeper level of active tension release and is perhaps the most powerful part of the method. In my own quite extended experience with it, passive tension flooding can quickly cut through the most intense states of anger and emotional distress, while diffusing high levels of otherwise unmanageable muscle tension. Without the stimulus of excessive and habitual muscle tension, muscles are less apt to develop trigger points and most pain problems can be resolved much more easily.

Anecdotal Evidence

In chapter 1, I wrote in the first person in order to give a more intimate report of my personal experience with trigger points. I did this to gain a conditional suspension of your disbelief so that you might give self-applied trigger point massage a try. In this chapter, I'm switching to first person again for the sake of another personal narrative. I have no imposing academic credentials that would supposedly qualify me to talk about the therapeutic use of relaxation, but I think I do have the right to claim the provisional authority of my own experience. The academics may get a little huffy about what I have to say, but I think you can make up your own mind whether I know what I'm talking about.

Personal experience is derisively called "anecdotal evidence" by academics. But what better science is there than to check something out for yourself and see if it works? The innovative psychologist Carl Rogers fervently believed in personal experience. He said that whatever is most personal is most general—in other words, most true, most in touch with reality. Carl Rogers was better known a generation ago as the author of *Client-Centered Therapy* (1951), a groundbreaking text for psychologists. He proposed that therapists should trust clients to find their own way and should help them do so by giving full attention to understanding and accepting them as they are. He believed it was vitally important that people come to trust the wisdom that grew out of their own experience.

In a later book, *On Becoming a Person* (1961), Dr. Rogers went even further in suggesting that perhaps all science is given too much credit for objectivity, when in reality it is based at every turn on decisions and subjective choices made by the scientist. It appeared to him that personal experience was ultimately the sole source of knowledge. In Rogers's opinion, personal trial and error was the heart of the experimental method and scientific evidence existed only as reports of firsthand observations by individuals. Stripped to its essentials, science could be viewed fundamentally as a collection of personal experiences, ideally limited in scope and described in enough objective detail to be replicated and validated by others (Rogers 1961, 215-224).

Back When I Was an Actor

Subscribing completely to Carl Rogers's views, I believe it's necessary to tell you about my own experience with systematic relaxation. First, I have to tell you that my move from New York City to Kentucky, as reported in chapter 1, wasn't as smooth as I made it seem. I was joking when I said I was just looking for a place to park my new car. It was a bit more complicated than that.

Lexington, Kentucky, was supposed to be a temporary stop on my road to success. I was a piano tuner who wanted to be an actor. Or a playwright. Or a professional guitarist. Or something! I loved working on pianos, but I wanted to do something more important in the world. The truth is that at the age of thirty-one I didn't know *what* I wanted. I was a pretty mixed-up lad.

For three years, I had been trying to break into theater, finally abandoning a successful piano business in New York in pursuit of a career as an actor. In the fall of 1968, I had just finished a season of summer theater in Harrodsburg, which is about thirty miles from Lexington. Afterward, an audition for a couple of other regional theaters hadn't impressed anyone and, not knowing what else to do, I started back for New York City. If you know that I didn't get the theater bug until about the time I had gotten fed up with the city, you'll understand that I wasn't in a hurry to get there.

On a drizzly early autumn day somewhere in the Blue Ridge Mountains, I abruptly pulled off the road at the top of a rise and stopped. I couldn't go any further. Who was I kidding? I was done with New York! I had had enough of the dirt and the tension and the frenzy. But what in the world was I supposed to do? I wanted to be an actor! Sitting in the car and staring through the dripping trees at the gray horizon, I turned the question over and over again. I couldn't answer it. I began to see how screwed up I really was. I had a sense that nothing was going to work in the shape I was in. Despite the good feeling I'd had about the show in Harrodsburg, it hadn't been a good year.

It had actually been my second season in Harrodsburg. After the first season, I had spent the intervening year wandering about the country in the midst of a classic existential crisis. I had given Hollywood a trial run but didn't like it and had fled back to my family home in Illinois just in time to participate in an existential crisis my dad was having. His chick hatchery had finally gone bust. He was physically broken down, in debt, and thoroughly demoralized. Mom told me he'd had a dream in which he had fallen down the basement stairs. He couldn't get up and lay there calling for her, but couldn't get her to hear him.

I wasn't much help to my dad that year, considering that I was lying at the bottom of my own flight of basement stairs. After several months of getting in each other's way, I took flight again back to Kentucky for another summer as an actor. There's no need to go into detail about that summer, except to say that it was as unsettling in its way as the whole year had been. Anyone who has been in a theater company knows how nutty a bunch of actors can be. Relationships get too intense and tangled, just like among other people—except more so. It's very much like being part of a big neurotic, dysfunctional family. Even so, though it had been a very turbulent three months, when the show ended I left Harrodsburg feeling like an orphan.

Sitting beside the highway in Virginia on that foggy, damp day, I puzzled through all these things, trying to see where it was all supposed to lead me. Somehow, the gentle rain and the simple beauty of the glistening roadside greenery finally began to clear my mind. Sometimes just stopping and sitting still is exactly the right thing to do. I realized I really didn't want to trade the greenness of the country for the bricks and asphalt of the city. Why couldn't I simply turn the car around and go back to Lexington for a while? It was a beautiful place to be when the leaves were turning. It was also big enough to have a good psychiatrist somewhere in it. I would find that guy, whoever he was, and stay in Kentucky until I knew what I wanted to do with myself. As I wheeled back out onto the highway and headed west, I felt halfway relaxed for the first time in weeks. This felt right.

In Lexington, I continued to be confused, of course. The failure of Dad's hatchery haunted me, and I felt deep guilt for not being a better son, for not going home and helping him. But the obsession with acting haunted me, too. I yearned to be on stage in costume and makeup, doing my lines. It was too late to audition for the current show at Lexington's community theater, Studio Players, but I hung around there, filling in for people who were late or couldn't make rehearsals. I got a furnished room in the neighborhood and began to feel at home. If only I could just stay in Lexington and make my living as an actor! I didn't want to go back to a regular life again. Every thought of having to tune pianos again made me angry.

I went on with my plan, however. I found that good psychiatrist, Dr. Hugh Storrow, a professor in the University of Kentucky Medical School who had a private practice in the community. I had confidence in Dr. Storrow at first sight and my trust in him grew as we talked. He was calm and in control. I told him of my unstable, unsettled, directionless life, and how I seemed to run from one thing to another, not trusting myself to stick to anything, to resist the "greener grass." I also touched on my uncertain relationships with people, my tendency to get angry and shut out even my best friends when things got sticky. I also told Dr. Storrow I needed help with noises. I had always been horribly irritated by eating sounds—forks on teeth and the grinding and smacking of lips. I said I wanted a wife and children, and I could foresee my problem with noises being an obstacle. In a way, the noise problem seemed central to all my other difficulties.

Dr. Storrow told me he had recently published a book on his methods and that I could probably find a copy in the library. I was so fired up with enthusiasm for the man that I read his entire book, *Introduction to Scientific Psychiatry* (1967), before our next appointment.

Sounds and Noises

At my second meeting with Dr. Storrow, he asked me to outline a little more of my history. I told him I had grown up a very tense, nervous boy, tormented by my hypersensitivity to sound. Even a slight whistle in someone's nose could throw me into a state of extreme distress. My mother had been like that. She'd told me once that she almost died when she realized I was going to be like her.

I told him it wasn't unusual for Mom to get so upset about eating noises at meals that she would have to run to the bathroom and throw up. She made my dad so self-consciousness and awkward about his eating that he made even more noise. Then his nose would begin to run, and he'd sniff all through the meal. I suspected him sometimes of doing it on purpose. I suspected everybody of doing it on purpose.

Mom constantly tried to relax, but only succeeded in becoming as motionless and still as a statue. I could feel her tension when she was in the room, and it made me tense too. It made me nervous to see her chest moving when she breathed. It made me try not to move my own chest. I was careful not to make any breathing sounds. I hardly breathed at all. That was family life for me.

When I was about twelve, I stopped eating at the table and began taking my plate to my room. After that, I never ate a meal with the family unless we had company or it was a holiday and I had to act normal. In boy scout camp, I slept with my fingers in my ears. I couldn't escape eating with the troop, but it made my stomach a mass of knots. I always had a bad stomach when I was a kid. The doctor said I should eat less fried food. He didn't say anything about my "nerves." What do you say to a nervous parent who has a nervous kid? There weren't any psychologists to send me to in Vandalia, Illinois, the little town we lived in.

Naturally, I had trouble in school with other kids' gum chewing and nose noise. I could detect a whistling nose clear across the room. My solution was to surreptitiously keep a finger in one ear. When I went away to college, the snoring of my roommates drove me crazy and I stopped talking to them. Later, after I had dropped out of college to join the Coast Guard, I slept with rolled up Kleenex in my ears and a pillow over my head. After leaving the Coast Guard, something led me to piano tuning, which was a fitting use of my hypersensitivity to sound, but it just brought me more trouble with noise. It's the tiny harmonics that you listen to when tuning a piano, and it doesn't take much to drown them out. It was an unending battle with barking dogs, washing machines, lawn mowers, television sets, and noisy children.

I finished my short biography by telling Dr. Storrow about the trouble I'd recently had with eating sounds in a restaurant, about getting so upset and angry that I left without finishing my meal. He listened and asked a few more questions. Then he said he would like to start reducing my anxiety with relaxation exercises. He also wanted to begin conditioning me for hypnosis, with which he hoped to extinguish needless nervous tension and bring to light repressed feelings regarding situations and people. Storrow said his techniques were based largely on *systematic desensitization*, a therapy developed by a South African psychiatrist named Joseph Wolpe.

He told me to begin observing my feelings in social situations and to start working with the relaxation exercises in a little blue pamphlet he gave me. I was eager to start doing the relaxation procedure, and I was delighted when I discovered how well it worked right away. Some sessions were so good that I'd go to sleep right in the middle of the exercise.

Desensitization

I kept a journal all the while I was going to Dr. Storrow. I still have it—seven spiral notebooks full. On September 26, 1968, after my third session with him, I made this entry about a remarkable event, every detail of which still remains a crystal clear memory:

I have had a day! Storrow hypnotized me, much to my surprise. A truly amazing experience! Seemed to remain fully conscious—not asleep or in a trance, as hypnosis is described. I would say I could have stopped any time I wanted, especially through the induction. He said that whether it worked was dependent on how well I concentrated. It really seemed to be a matter of responsiveness and cooperation. It worked because I wanted to be hypnotized.

First, he told me to put my attention on a spiral figure printed on a card. While I looked at the card, he told me to begin relaxing. We commenced with the fingertips of my right hand, then bit by bit up to the shoulder. Then we worked with my left arm segment by segment and then the right leg, relaxing each bit in turn. All the while, he was telling me my eyes would soon close from sleepiness. Very shortly my eyelids drooped and then did close. He immediately went to work on my body as a whole—telling me that with each breath I would get heavier and more relaxed. I got very relaxed, to say the least, much more so than I had been able to achieve on my own.

Then he had me visualize going into the restaurant where I had had the trouble with eating sounds. He said the object was to recreate the scene as vividly as possible. He told me to sit at the counter and try to imagine how everything looked. He said that as I begin studying the menu, someone starts slurping coffee. I immediately sensed tension start up in several areas. He said to keep my attention on the sounds, creating all the detail I could. As we continued with the "dream," tension increased dramatically in my wrists, forearms, and fingers. The fronts of my thighs got so tight they went numb and began to tingle. The greatest tension imaginable built up in my lower chest, stomach, face, arms, and upper legs. I couldn't believe how quickly it all came on.

Then he said to imagine that I hear someone just one stool away smacking their lips as they chew. Then I hear someone else behind me scraping their teeth on their fork with every bite. I felt an immediate increase in tension that quickly turned into pain in my left wrist and left leg. I cried out "No! No!" I didn't want any more tension and pain, but he kept me in the dream. The tension was incredible, but at one point I began to laugh. He asked why I laughed. I said it was because I didn't believe this could happen to me. I'd seriously doubted that I could even be hypnotized. He told me to stay with the picture and to continue observing the physical sensations very closely.

After a few minutes, the most amazing thing happened. The tension suddenly subsided to about half—all on its own. After I sat in the state of half tension for several minutes more, it occurred to me that I could make the rest go away. And I did! He asked me to indicate when it all went to zero. He said the scene in the restaurant was fading now and the sounds were dying away. I was again as heavy as a chunk of lead. I gave the signal that I was relaxed again. Then he told me I would feel better than I had in months and woke me on the count of five.

When I left Storrow's office that day, I felt like my feet weren't touching the floor. I was so relaxed all the rest of the day it was like still being in the dream. I had a surprisingly productive day calling on churches and getting piano work, actually doing what I hadn't thought I wanted to do. The deep relaxation wore off, of course, and I went to bed extremely tense that night. I tried tension control but couldn't get it to work. Then I had diarrhea and vomiting all night. It felt like I was purging everything in my life that had come before.

Back to Reality

During the eighteen months I worked with Dr. Storrow, we had many similar sessions of hypnosis and systematic desensitization, and I learned that nervous tension was no big deal. I began feeling that I could handle it, and I began finding my way. During that time, I acted in several plays at Studio Players. And I met a girl in one of the shows. Half-Sicilian and half-Scandinavian, she was the most beautiful girl I'd ever seen. She really turned things around for me, and in no time we were married. I still didn't know exactly who I wanted to be, so just to make good use of the time, I went back to school. I finally got a degree, with a double major this time—psychology and theater arts!

Not long after my therapy ended, our first daughter was born, and it hit me that I was going to have to get serious and get some money rolling in. I committed myself anew to my profession as a piano technician, but with much less conflict than before. My obsession with acting died after I got the theater degree, but by then I was acting a far more fitting role, that of husband, father, and provider.

I began to understand that I'd always tried too hard at the piano work. I'd tried to be too good, tried to be better than I needed to be. I don't think I'd ever seen the enormous tension this created in me. With my increased awareness of muscle tension, I also woke up to the fact that piano tuning, or any piano work, required a lot of bracing and holding of tense positions. I was overdoing that too, bracing tighter than was necessary and adding to my excess tension. Maybe that had been why I kept trying to get out of the tuning business. I think acting attracted me because it gave me a chance to blow off some of that tension. But now, my growing skill at systematic relaxation was making the piano work less taxing. I began to enjoy its satisfactions, not the least of which was some very good money.

After my first successes with progressive relaxation, I realized that my hypersensitivity to noises could be used as an index of my general state of nervous tension. When I noticed that a noise was bothering me, I would immediately check my muscles for tension. I was always surprised at just how tight I was, without even knowing it. Noise annoyance became a signal to use my techniques.

Systematic relaxation has effectively solved my noise problem and has made me better at coping with things in general. I'm much calmer about everything than I used to be and more productive in much more meaningful ways. I want to make it clear, however, that it took years, not just weeks or months, to make systematic relaxation a consistently effective habit. Even now, when I'm worn out by stress or overwork, noises can get to me. Still, if I have the presence of mind to use what I know, the problem never lasts longer than it takes me to do a quick tension release.

Habitual Muscle Tension

It is well-known that nervous tension, or anxiety, causes overactivity of the autonomic nervous system, increasing your heart rate, blood pressure, respiration, muscle tension, and metabolism to levels far beyond reasonable needs. Muscle tension is a primary expression of nervous tension, but unlike all these other reactions, it's subject to virtually complete direct control. This fact holds enormous promise, because a reduction of muscle tension can have a strikingly immediate effect in reducing anxiety. In fact, tension release can be your most powerful and direct means of moderating anxiety. When nervous tension or anxiety get out of bounds, an ability to relax your muscles can very quickly return you to a calmer state. If you don't have this ability, you are liable to be victimized by your emotions, which can lead to chronic states of both emotional and physical pain (Jacobson 1964, 14–47).

Muscles that are habitually tense because of nervous tension are in a continuous state of nervous preparedness, braced for action. They never get a break, never get a chance to rest. Over time, this unnecessary overuse of your muscles can be a significant factor in the persistence of trigger points. The release of excess muscle tension can make trigger points more responsive to treatment and less likely to come back. Unfortunately, relaxing your muscles will not get rid of trigger points directly. Massage remains the correct treatment for trigger points themselves.

Many people have little awareness of tension in their muscles and too often have no idea how to obtain a sense of calm without drugs, tobacco, alcohol, or mind-numbing distractions like television. Supposedly relaxing activities like gardening, sports, or hobbies are very often anything but relaxing and can actually leave people with even more tension in their muscles due to overuse, strain, or excessive concern.

Obviously, some muscle tension is necessary in order to function. Movement, and indeed life itself, isn't possible without the contraction of muscles. But stress and strain and nervous concern tend to leave residual muscle tension in their wake. If this tension becomes excessive and habitual, it not only can contribute to a deadly cycle of mounting nervous tension and anxiety but also can seriously undermine your physical health. Among other things, habitual excess tension in skeletal (external) muscles keeps your blood pressure high, fosters disease-producing tension in your internal organs, and weakens the immune system (Jacobson 1967, 70).

Active Tension Release

My method of systematic relaxation is based on the procedure that Hugh Storrow taught me thirty-five years ago. Day after day of practical use, however, has allowed me to continually refine it. Active tension release should be learned before you try passive tension flooding, which requires considerable skill in detecting tension in muscles. You will acquire that skill by practicing active tension release. A lack of awareness of muscle tension is the biggest obstacle to deep relaxation. You may think you're relaxed, when in reality you're only partially or superficially relaxed at best.

Active tension release is derived from Jacobson's original progressive relaxation system, but is much simplified and has more options. Active tension release can be a long detailed festival of relaxation, or it can be shortened to varying degrees for varying needs. To get a high degree of skill at relaxation, you need to patiently practice the long routine for quite a long while. Many people have tried to simplify Jacobson's method, which has unfortunately resulted in codifying the technique as *contract/relax*, an oversimplification that is very different from what Jacobson intended.

Progressive Relaxation

Edmund Jacobson (1885–1976) is widely recognized today as the originator of progressive relaxation, his highly structured method for releasing needless tension in principal muscle groups, one after the other. His discovery occurred in 1908, when he was finishing work on his third doctorate at Harvard. (He ultimately had doctorates in medicine, physiology, and law.) Unfortunately, he was afflicted with a very common problem. His mind was still going so fast at the end of the day that he had great difficulty sleeping.

One night, as he lay restlessly in the dark, he began to wonder how the extreme tension he felt in his body might relate to his insomnia. Perhaps if he could relax his body he might also be able to relax his mind and finally get to sleep. He tried relaxing his body part by part, starting with his arms, and then his legs, stomach, back, and so on, progressing through to his jaws, mouth, and eyes. He found that as long as he was thinking about his muscles he was not thinking about anything else, certainly not his worries! And when he was finally able to get his eyes, mouth, and jaws relaxed, he would stop thinking and drift off.

Relaxing the body's muscles in a systematic way was one of those personal discoveries that is so simple, so intuitive, and so obvious that you have to marvel that nobody had ever written about it before. It's a perfect illustration of subjective personal experience being at the very heart of science. Jacobson spent the next several years scientifically validating his intuitive discovery with controlled measurements of tension under various conditions. He was particularly interested in verifying that his system of methodical relaxation truly succeeded in quieting the autonomic nervous system and diminishing nervous tension. To gain maximum objectivity, Jacobson devised ways to measure the tiny electric currents generated in muscles when they were tense and then again when they were relaxed. His innovations became the foundation for biofeedback and electromyography, which are widely used today in many kinds of treatment and research.

In his book *Progressive Relaxation*, first published in 1929, Jacobson offered the medical world his procedure for systematically relaxing the skeletal muscles. He promoted his method as "scientific relaxation" because he had proven it could not only alleviate anxiety and other psychological problems, but could also help prevent serious medical problems like heart attacks, ulcers, chronic fatigue, irritable colon, and high blood pressure. His physiological measurements had shown that the smooth muscle of the internal organs becomes overly tense along with the skeletal muscles. He intended that this "reeducation" of the neuromuscular system could be prescribed by physicians as an alternative to sedative drugs (Jacobson 1938, 6-27).

As a physician, Jacobson did prescribe sedative drugs from time to time, although he generally preferred to avoid them. He would be disappointed in today's practice of medicine with its overreliance on psychoactive drugs. The movement towards drug therapy and away from counseling is based on the unproven assertion that emotional problems are caused by "chemical imbalances" in the brain. Nonconforming psychiatrist Peter Breggin says that "biochemical imbalances are the only diseases spread by word of mouth!" Breggin believes there is ample evidence that psychoactive drugs cause more problems than they cure. Sadly, writing a prescription is much more profitable and convenient than taking the time to help someone in a truly compassionate and interested way (Breggin 1999, 6).

Jacobson's more humanistic system of therapy, as presented in his first book, required a long series of lessons, because he didn't believe that "scientific" relaxation could be learned without professional help. Later, he changed his mind about that and wrote several books designed to introduce progressive relaxation to the layman in a form that could be self-taught. He hoped that progressive relaxation would ultimately be taught to children in the schools.

It's Not Contract/Relax

In the second edition of *Progressive Relaxation* (1939, 43), Jacobson says that as soon as patients have developed a clear awareness of muscle tension, they should no longer contract before relaxing. In *Self-Operations Control* (1964, 6), a little manual for the patient that accompanied *Anxiety and Tension Control*, another book for physicians, Jacobson specifically advised against developing a habit of contracting before relaxing. In *You Must Relax* (1970, 180), his final word was that you should use the rule of "diminishing tensions," contracting less and less until you don't need to contract at all. Unfortunately, in all cases this instruction is buried in the text and cast as something just said in passing. In some of his books, Jacobson neglected to mention it at all, leading to the widespread misunderstanding today that contraction is an intrinsic element of the method and is always required. As a consequence, writers of current books on relaxation consistently present Jacobson's progressive relaxation as "contract/relax," which is actually the opposite of what he intended.

The problem with contract/relax is that you can't contract a muscle without making the rest of your body contract to some degree at the same time—even the muscles that you've already relaxed! This can slow the process of reaching a state of deep relaxation or keep you from attaining it altogether. In my view, most people have an instinct for relaxation and can do it even under stress if it occurs to them to try. As a massage therapist, I frequently find it helpful to have the client consciously relax the muscle I'm working on. No one ever has difficulty with this.

All of this having been said, if you're occasionally unsure whether you sense tension in a muscle, go on and tighten it slightly to give yourself a point of reference. But it should be just a *shadow* of tightness and held only briefly. As Dr. Jacobson says, you shouldn't make a habit of it.

Tension Release Procedures

In the beginning, when you're first learning active tension release, you should give all your attention to it. No other activity should distract you from the sensations in your muscles and the single task at hand. To attain the deepest state of relaxation, you should plan on sessions of thirty minutes to an hour, alone in some quiet place so you can really get focused. If you want to make the process work well for you, put it on your calendar and make a regular date with yourself. Routine is everything.

Jacobson referred to relaxation as your "built-in tranquillizer" (1970, p. x). It works better than a pill and is entirely without side effects. You will tend to fall asleep in the middle of doing active tension release whether you're sitting or lying down. It's just a sign that you're doing well at releasing tension. If you find your mind wandering while doing active tension release, simply keep bringing your attention back to your muscles and pick up where you left off. You may have to do this repeatedly.

If you're human and not some rarified extraterrestrial being, I'll guarantee that you have unnecessary tension in your muscles. Many people, however, have very little awareness of this state. You may not believe that you're particularly tense. You may not be able to detect tightness in some of the specified places. Have faith that your awareness and skill will grow with practice. With each step, just focus on letting the specified place get softer and looser than it already is. You'll catch on very quickly to what localized tension feels like in all the various places. Experience will be your teacher.

Sixteen-Step Release

Each step of this full procedure can be divided into smaller ones. In step one, for instance, it's best to do one forearm at a time. You can also relax each forearm in two steps instead of one, doing first the back of the forearm and then the front. You can even go so far as to relax individual muscles. People who have learned their muscles well by doing self-applied trigger point therapy can become quite good at this. You will use your mind's eye to visualize the part you're relaxing. Take plenty of time, several minutes at least for each step, savoring the experience. Change the sequence if you like, but you should relax the eyes last, since they are working as monitors throughout the process. You may feel your eyes slightly cross and go out of focus when you release their tensions.

1. Forearms

2. Hands

3. Upper arms and shoulders

4. Lower legs

5. Feet

6. Thighs

7. Buttocks and hips

8. Abdomen and chest

9. Lower back

10. Mid and upper back

11. Top of shoulders

12. Back of neck

13. Scalp and temples

14. Jaws and front of neck

15. Mouth and tongue

16. Forehead and eyes

Eight-Step Release

This little procedure should take no more than thirty or forty seconds, but you won't have much luck with it until you're quite skilled with the long version. In each of the eight steps, release the tension as you exhale. You can go through the entire procedure in just eight breaths. If you'd like to take a bit more time, allow yourself a few breaths between the tension release exhalations.

1. Shoulders, arms, and hands
2. Legs and feet
3. Buttocks and hips
4. Abdomen and chest

5. Back
6. Back of the neck
7. Jaws, temples, and mouth
8. Eyes

Four-Step Rapid Release

You will be more successful doing this four-step routine after you've become fully experienced with the previous two procedures. But you can try it at any time. You will be releasing the tension in all your body in one exhalation. This routine takes only fifteen or twenty seconds. You can use it in virtually any situation frequently throughout the day. You can't do it too often.

1. Turn your eyes upward without moving your head.

2. Tune in to your general tension for a few seconds.

3. Inhale deeply as you count slowly to five.

4. On five, lower and close your eyes, exhaling as you do so and letting yourself go limp all over. That's all there is to it.

Take two or three more calm breaths, going even more limp and heavy with each successive exhalation, and then go on with whatever you were doing. Hypnotists use this short routine for quick inductions. It's great for getting your attention calmly back on task.

One-Step Instant Release

In time, you will become so adept at dealing with excess muscle tension that mere awareness of tension will trigger the response to let it go. This is the One-Step Instant Release, the true "relaxation response," a purely physical response requiring no verbal affirmations, meditation, repeated mantra, or cognition of any kind. I experience this simplest form of tension release dozens of times a day. It's my secret. Nobody ever knows I'm doing it, but it has become an integral part of who I am. You already possess a degree of this inborn ability to let go of tension at will. Practice at systematic relaxation will hone this natural ability and take you places you never thought you could go.

Passive Tension Flooding

Edmund Jacobson believed that once you've learned to detect tension there's never any need to contract a muscle before relaxing it. It may seem a contradiction now to propose that you should *encourage* muscle tension by the process of passive tension flooding. I believe Jacobson would've liked the idea of tension flooding, but there's no indication in his writing that it ever occurred to him. That's too bad because I think he also failed to see that there were limits to direct tension control.

When nervous tension is very high, an attempt to use active tension release can be highly frustrating, actually resulting in increased tension. Muscles sometimes seem to have minds of their own. Trying to force them to relax can be like trying to keep the lid on a pot of boiling water. You're able to relax to a certain level, but then you reach a tension barrier that you can't break through. The tension you've gotten rid of seems to want to come right back. Keeping the lid on it becomes a continuous battle. Many people simply quit trying and take up drinking again, or whatever.

Passive tension flooding is a procedure to be used when active tension release fails. With passive tension flooding, instead of trying to relax, you stop resisting the tension or trying to suppress it. When you're in a state of anxiety, it's actually the excessive muscle tension that creates the extreme sense of discomfort that you're motivated so strongly to escape. Facing and accepting this discomfort is profoundly therapeutic. If you say to your muscles in effect, "Okay, get it out of your system," the tension will consume itself very quickly and the sense of anxiety will be diminished to a very marked degree. Muscle tension and nervous tension are so intimately linked that the relief of muscle tension alone can free your mind and facilitate your taking action to resolve whatever issue is generating your anxiety (Wolpe 1958, 135–138).

Before trying passive tension flooding, you should develop considerable skill with active tension release to hone your awareness of tension and gain some skill in the objective control of it. After you've learned passive tension flooding, you will use it before active tension release when coping with stress. With passive tension flooding, you'll be able to break through the tension barrier that active tension release can't penetrate. Going on then with active tension release will take you even further into the relaxed state. The procedures complement one another. Together, they work far better than either one alone.

The Flooding Experience

First, simply take a tension inventory. With your mind's eye, scan all the muscle groups that you normally relax in the sixteen-step tension release procedure. Tune in to the sense of muscle tension everywhere you find it. Don't be surprised if it's worse than you thought. It almost always is. Take note of the places where the tension is greatest—the stomach, jaws, and posterior neck being the places where you probably hold your worst tensions.

Don't try to relax. Allow the tension to be. Give it permission to exist. Don't fight it. Don't resist. If the tension wants to dramatically increase like it did in my hypnosis session with Dr. Storrow, let it do so. It may not increase at all, but if it does, let it gain full expression. Think of it as an adventure. Be curious to see how far will it go.

Take special note of your mouth, tongue, face, and eyes, where tension is amplified by thinking and worrying. You will probably notice that you're breathing very shallowly, tending to hold your breath. As the tension rises toward a peak, you may feel like you're going to explode, especially the first time you try this. You may begin to wonder how much of this you can take, but stay with it. Experience the tension as fully as you can. Immerse yourself in it.

Your knotted-up muscles may be hurting by this time, but continue monitoring. Keep watching and observing. You may feel now that you want to let the tension go, that you can barely hang on to it, but hang on a little longer. There will come a point at which you simply can't support the tension any longer and it will quite suddenly flood away all in a moment. As the tension goes, you'll let go of the air you've been holding in, your chest collapsing with an enormous sense of relief. But then, as you take in a big refreshing breath of air, the tension will come rushing back, everything tense like before, all in a knot. Don't be afraid or discouraged. This is good.

Don't try to relax yet. Let the tension return. Let it happen. Don't fight it. Much more quickly this time, the tension will rise to a peak. But you'll see that this level of tension isn't as high as before, hardly more than half. Don't seek control over it. Simply keep watching. Soon it will flood away again, just like before, all in a moment. Are you done now? No, here it comes once more. But it's a smaller peak yet. It goes to maximum right away and then rapidly fades, just like before.

Expect three or four more tension peaks, each one less than the one before it. You'll get one last small surge of tension, hardly worth the name. At this point, take control and begin one of the active tension release procedures. You'll immediately see that you've penetrated the barrier, and you'll be surprised at how extraordinarily easy it is to relax now. You've broken the big knot, the big logjam. Active tension release will work much better now than before, and you'll go to a state of deep relaxation that was unattainable before the flooding. The whole process of passive tension flooding typically takes between ten and fifteen minutes in the beginning. After you've gained sufficient skill, the flooding experience can be gone through in less than thirty seconds.

It's very important to understand that passive tension flooding is the direct opposite of the contract/relax method, in that you don't contract muscles intentionally. It might seem that you could compound the effect by tightening your muscles on purpose and giving them a real workout, but it doesn't work that way. Intentional contraction tends to leave more residual tension than if you let the muscles tighten, peak, and release on their own. You may fear that you risk cramping by indulging the tension in muscles. This may be true occasionally for some people, but in thirty-five years I've never had a muscle cramp doing passive flooding. Ironically, even though the experience can feel quite dramatic, the amount of tension the muscles undergo is actually much less than during many ordinary kinds of work or play.

In focusing solely on muscle tension, passive tension flooding gives you an objective handle on nervous tension, leaving emotional issues to take care of themselves as a natural consequence of the lessened tension. Dealing cognitively with emotional issues may or may not be necessary. Passive tension flooding seems to work even without a clear understanding of your emotional responses or their history. The effectiveness of this simple idea is explained by *paradoxical intention*, a therapeutic model introduced by Viktor Frankl, the Viennese psychiatrist famed for surviving the Nazi death camps by making use of this distinctly proactive mindset.

Paradoxical Intention

Dr. Frankl used the term "paradoxical intention" to describe the age-old ethic of gaining victories over your fears by doing the last thing in the world you would ordinarily want to do. The object is to intentionally confront the thing you're afraid of. You not only deliberately expose yourself to your fears, you come to desire that exposure (1984, 126–127).

Failure to face your fears tends to perpetuate them. Avoidance of the hated object increases your fear of it, because you never give yourself a chance to learn to cope with it. As an example, it's a mistake to use earplugs when irritated by noises. Escaping noise in this way too quickly relieves your anxiety and teaches you that escape is the correct response. Further, it reinforces your conviction that annoying noises should be avoided because you "can't stand them." It becomes more and more true that indeed you really can't stand them. My job in learning to cope with noises was, paradoxically, to cultivate a desire to hear them and to learn not to fear the muscle tension they provoke.

Fundamentally, any flight from anxiety-provoking situations undermines the habit of coping. The relief granted by escape reinforces the flight response. You never get the chance to strengthen yourself in the face of adversity. To be truly successful in coping, you must not give yourself the option of running away (Frankl 1988, 102–103).

We supposedly have just two choices when faced with a threat: either fight or flight. But a third response may have fundamentally greater clout, at least in its potential for facilitating change. That third response to threat or fear is neither fighting or fleeing, but simple *acceptance*. This is the core of paradoxical intention. It is also the core of passive tension flooding.

Beyond Tension Control

Muscle tension is the common theme in anxiety, anger, phobia, depression, fear, and physical pain. Habitual muscle tension can compound these problems by predisposing you to becoming even more tense and inappropriately emotional at any provocation. Muscle tension then feeds on itself, snowballing, magnifying the sense of anxiety, and perpetuating not just physical pain but emotional pain. According to Edmund Jacobson, your feeling of nervous tension or anxiety consists largely of the physical sensations caused by uncontrollable tension that exists in your muscles and internal organs. In essence, nervous tension may be very little more than this acutely uncomfortable sense of muscle tension (Jacobson 1938, 79).

The interaction between emotional disturbances and muscle tension can constitute a feedback loop of mutual reinforcement and perpetuation. Passive tension flooding and active tension release can be used to break this vicious circle and overcome overly emotional responses to problems. It works that way with me, if I have the presence of mind to use what I know.

Tension flooding appears to be the operative element in psychotherapeutic methods such as systematic desensitization, exposure therapy, aversion therapy, implosion therapy, massed practice, awareness training, and eye movement desensitization and reprocessing (EMDR). None, however, employs the conscious acceptance of muscle tension exclusively, but are occupied instead, diffusely, with the entire range of subjective feelings. Passive tension flooding is closer in concept to a method proposed by British physician Nicholas Malleson, who held that it is necessary to fully experience not only your fears, but also all the bodily sensations that come with them (Malleson 1959, 226).

Psychiatrist Joseph Wolpe defined flooding as the intentional prolonged exposure to relatively strong anxiety. He believed it was similar to *abreaction,* a phenomenon that has a long history in human affairs. In abreaction, you tell about a disturbing memory that is connected to your anxiety or fear. As you describe the event, you experience overpowering emotion and appear to be living through it again. People typically feel great relief after going through an abreaction (Wolpe 1958, 195-198).

Passive tension flooding is similar to abreaction, except that, again, it is concerned exclusively with muscle tension. Because of this mechanical, nonpsychological focus, I believe it can be safely used as a general desensitization procedure to self-treat nervous tension, anxiety, anger, and fear. It's the antithesis of control, and yet it makes the ultimate control of negative emotional states far more certain. It should be used first with fantasized events when you're alone and in a safe, quiet place. In a fantasized event, a kind of daydream, you can safely experience your aversions, fears, phobias, anxieties, resentments, and other things that make you defensive or tense.

Repeated practice of this imaginal experience with passive tension flooding can diminish the intensity of your negative responses and reduce habitual muscle tension. Later, you can gradually introduce passive tension flooding into real situations. I've used this technique for decades and continue to use it, totally without negative consequences.

When using passive tension flooding to temper your tension reaction to a particular problem, divide your attention between the fantasized event and your muscle tension. Work with the least troublesome problem first. If it's a noise, for instance, choose the noise that bothers you the least and progress step-by-step over time to more bothersome noises. You grow stronger by degrees when you choose battles that you can win. If you would like to start the day with good karma, do both passive tension flooding and active tension release first thing in the morning, working with some current problem in an imagined scene. An ability to calmly face the problem in fantasy will improve your response in real situations as you go along through the day.

Expectations

This two-part method of systematic relaxation isn't something that you do a few times and then you're all cured of your nervous tension. Your tension reactions are so much a part of you that it's unreasonable to expect them to ever completely disappear. Stomach tightening in problem situations, for example, can happen so fast that it catches you by surprise, before you even realize what's going on. A lifelong habit of responding to stress with tension in your neck and shoulders can be so insidious that you may be unaware of it most of the time. Sleep is another place where you will inevitably be victimized by old unconscious tension habits.

Even when you're able to make the method work well in a given circumstance, it may take a while to see any overall improvement. If you persist, however, in time you will notice a general decrease in tension and a lowered intensity of reaction to annoyances and perceived threats.

If your motivation is strong enough and if you are capable of applying good information with persistence, I believe systematic relaxation can be learned and implemented without professional help. If your psychological problems are severe, however, or you're leery of the very idea of passive tension flooding, trust your intuition and leave it alone. Or you can find a professional counselor who can help you with it. A professional, in fact, might be very interested in the contents of this chapter. In an exhaustive search of the Internet and the perusal of several dozen books on psychology, I've found no therapy that resembles passive tension flooding in its specific and exclusive focus on muscle tension.

Your success with systematic relaxation will be intimately linked to how much you practice it. It's inevitable that you will fall back into old habitual responses unless you are committed to learning new ones. Systematic relaxation has to become a part of living, something that you do almost without thinking. You will find that, like self-applied trigger point massage, this system is extraordinarily easy once you understand it, develop some skill with it, and integrate it fully into your life.

You shouldn't take any of this to mean that you should aspire to be constantly relaxed. That's not possible and not really desirable either. Tension, even a certain amount of nervous tension in the form of vigorous action, is necessary for a meaningful life. It's only when tension becomes excessive that it makes trouble for you. The main thing here is that if you want to have less physical and emotional pain and fewer and more manageable trigger points, make a commitment to learning to deal with unnecessary habitual muscle tension.

Epilogue

In writing this book, I've put everything I know about trigger points and referred pain into your hands. I trust it will be a constant and reliable resource in your quest to become self-reliant and free of pain. You've seen by now that my methods for combating pain are safe and practical and that the benefits are quick, clear, and undeniable. My goal now—and I hope it will become yours—is to get the word on trigger points to every corner of the earth.

As you continue to gain experience with trigger point therapy, I would encourage you to reach out beyond your own needs and pass on what you learn from this book to other people. Almost everybody hurts, including your friends and neighbors, your parents, your children, the people you see in the grocery store, even your doctor and chiropractor. Most people have some kind of chronic ache or recurrent pain: headaches, low back pain, sore feet—you name it. They all have a need to know what you know about trigger points and referred pain. Seek to share this valuable information.

If someone is headed for surgery because they think they have carpal tunnel syndrome, show them how to search for trigger points in their scalenes and other muscles that may be the source of the pain and numbness in their hands and fingers. If someone complains that the pain in their knees has put an end to their exercising, show them how to find the quadriceps trigger points that may be the cause of the problem. If someone has low back pain and you know how to fix it with trigger point massage to the gluteus medius muscles, don't keep it a secret! What you know about trigger points can save someone not only a lot of misery, but also a lot of money.

Bring up the subject of myofascial pain with your doctor and write letters to your HMO. It's long past time for trigger point therapy to become part of mainstream medical practice, not just another kind of alternative medicine out somewhere on the fringe. When physicians become skilled at diagnosing trigger points and begin prescribing appropriate manual treatment, there will be less need for shotgunlike treatment with pharmaceutical painkillers, with their side effects and exorbitant cost.

Look for opportunities to tell other health care professionals about your success with trigger point therapy. Most chiropractors, osteopaths, physical therapists, and massage therapists know about trigger points and referred pain, but few know how powerful and empowering self-treatment can be as a complement to their own methods.

It's the public that will ultimately bring about the acceptance of trigger point therapy among the healing professions, but it will all depend on individual efforts to get the public informed. Consider writing an article about trigger points and referred pain for your professional association. Give a program about self-treatment of myofascial pain at your club, church, or temple. You'll be surprised at how many silent sufferers there are in every group.

People will be skeptical about trigger points at first, even your best friends and closest relatives. Cure-alls are thrown at us constantly in the media and everyone has grown quite leery of extravagant claims. As a consequence, when good information comes along, the best of us sometimes need to be hit over the head with it sixty or seventy times before it begins to penetrate. Have faith that people will eventually come around and try trigger point therapy if you gently persist. There's a world of pain out there. Join in educating the world about trigger points. You can make a difference.

Resources

Acland, R. 1995. *Video Atlas of Human Anatomy*. Baltimore: Lippincott, Williams and Wilkins.

Netter F. 1989. *Atlas of Human Anatomy*. East Hanover, New Jersey: Novartis.

Backnobber

The Pressure Positive Company
128 Oberholtzer Road
Gilbertsville, PA 19525
800-603-5107
www.backtools.com

Thera Cane

Thera Cane Company
P. O. Box 9220
Denver, CO 80209-0220
www.theracane.com

EDCAT Enterprise
733 North Beach Street
Daytona Beach, FL 32114
800-274-3566

Nedco
7812 N.W. Hampton Road
Kansas City, MO 64152
800-587-1203
www.theracane.net

Knobble

EDCAT Enterprise
733 North Beach Street
Daytona Beach, FL 32114
800-274-3566

Knobble Associates
P. O. Box 450
Occidental, CA 95465
800-959-8342

References

Baker, B. A. 1986. The muscle trigger: Evidence of overload injury. *Journal of Neurol Orthop Med Surg* 7:35–44.

Bates, T., and E. Grunwaldt. 1958. Myofascial pain in childhood. *Journal of Pediatrics* 53:198–209.

Bell, W. E. 1969. Clinical diagnosis of the pain-dysfunction syndrome. *Journal of the American Dental Association* 79:154–160.

Bochetta, A., F. Bernardi, M. Pedditzi, A. Loviselli, F. Velluzzi, E. Martino, and M. Del Zompo. 1991. Thyroid abnormalities during lithium treatment. *Acta Psychiatr Scand* 83:193–198.

Bonica, J. J., and A. E. Sola. 1990. Other painful disorders of the upper limb. Chapter 52 in *The Management of Pain*, 2nd ed, edited by J. J. Bonica, J. D. Loeser, C. R. Chapman, et al. 947–958, 1114–1133. Philadelphia: Lea & Febiger.

Breggin, P., and D. Cohen. 1999. *Your Drug May Be Your Problem: How and Why to Stop Taking Psychiatric Drugs*. Cambridge: Perseus Publishing.

Brody, D. M. 1980. Running injuries. *Clinical Symposia* 32:1–36.

Cailliet, R. 1966. *Shoulder Pain*. Philadelphia: F. A. Davis.

Cantu, R. I., and A. J. Grodin. 1992. *Myofascial Manipulation: Theory and Clinical Application*. Gaithersburg, Maryland: Aspen.

Crow, N. E., and B. G. Brodgon. 1959. The "normal" lumbosac spine. *Radiology* 72:97.

Curl, D. D. 1989. Discovery of a myofascial trigger point in the buccinator muscle: A case report. *Journal of Craniomandibular Practice* 7(4):339–345.

Danneskiold-Samoe, B., E. Christiansen, and R. B. Andersen. 1983. Regional muscle tension and pain ("Fibrositis"). *Scandinavian Journal of Rehabilitation Medicine* 15:17–20.

———. 1986. Myofascial pain and the role of myoglobin. *Scandinavian Journal of Rehabilitation Medicine* 15:174–178.

Dobrik, I. 1989. Disorders of the iliopsoas muscle and its role in gynecological diseases. *Journal of Manual Medicine* 4:130–133.

Epstein, S. E., L. H. Gerber, and J. S. Borer. 1979. Chest wall syndrome, a common cause of unexplained cardiac pain. *Journal of the American Medical Association* 241:2793–2797.

Fassbender, H. G., and K. Wegner. 1973. Morphologie und Pathogenese des Weichteilrheumatismus. *Zeit Rheumaforsch* 33:355–374.

Fishbain, D. S., M. Goldberg, B. R. Meagher, R. Steele, and H. Rosomoff. 1986. Male and female chronic pain patients categorized by DSM-III psychiatric diagnostic criteria. *Pain* 26:181-197.

Foster, D. W., and A. H. Rubenstein. 1980. Hypoglycemia, insulinoma, and other hormone-secreting tumors of the pancreas. Chapter 340 in *Harrison's Principles of Internal Medicine*, 9th ed, edited by K. J. Isselbacher, R. D. Adams, E. Braunwald, et al., 1758–1762. New York: McGraw-Hill.

Frankl, V. E. 1984. *Man's Search for Meaning: An Introduction to Logotherapy.* New York: Simon & Schuster.

———. 1988. *The Will to Meaning: Foundations and Applications of Logotherapy.* New York: Meridian.

Graff-Radford, S., B. Jaeger, and J. L. Reeves. 1986. Myofascial pain may present clinically as occipital neuralgia. *Neurosurgery* 19(4):610–613.

Gerwin, R. D. 1995. A study of 96 subjects examined both for fibromyalgia and myofascial pain (abstract). *Journal of Musculoskeletal Pain* 3(Suppl 1):121.

Good, M. G. 1950. The role of skeletal muscles in the pathogenesis of diseases. *Acta Medica Scandinavea* 138:285–292, 348–353.

Gutstein, R. R. 1944. The role of abdominal fibrositis in functional indigestion. *Mississippi Valley Medical Journal* 66:114–124.

Hackett, R. M. 2000. Personal communication.

Hagberg, M. 1981. Electromyographic signs of shoulder muscular fatigue in two elevated arm positions. *American Journal of Physical Medicine* 60(3):111–121.

Hallin, R. P. 1983. Sciatic pain and the piriformis muscle. *Postgraduate Medicine* 74:69–72.

Hong, C. Z. 1994. Considerations and recommendations regarding myofascial trigger point injection. *Journal of Musculoskeletal Pain* 2(1):29–59.

Jacobson, E. 1938. *Progressive Relaxation.* 2nd ed. Chicago: University of Chicago.

———. 1964. *Anxiety and Tension Control: A Physiological Approach.* Philadelphia: J. B. Lippincott.

———. 1967. *Biology of Emotions.* Springfield, Illinois: Charles C. Thomas.

———. 1970. *You Must Relax.* New York: McGraw-Hill.

Jaeger, B. 1989. Are "cervicogenic" headaches due to myofascial pain and cervical spine dysfunction? *Cephalalgia* 9(3):157–164.

Jeyaseelan, N. 1989. Anatomical basis of compression of common peroneal nerve. *Anat Anz* 169:49–51.

Jonsson, B., and M. Hagberg. 1974. The effect of different working heights on the deltoid muscle: A preliminary methodological study. *Scandinavian Journal of Rehabilitation Medicine*, Suppl. 3:26–32.

Kelley, W. N. 1980. Gout and other disorders of purine metabolism. Chapter 92 in *Harrison's Principles of Internal Medicine*, 9th ed, edited by K. J. Isselbacher, R. D. Adams, E. Braunwald, et al., 479–486. New York: McGraw-Hill

Kendall, F. P., E. K. McCreary, and P. G. Provance. 1993. *Muscles: Testing and Function*. 4th ed. Baltimore: Williams and Wilkins.

Kidd. R. 1988. Pain localization with the innominate upslip dysfunction. *Manual Medicine* 3:103–105.

Kopell, H. P., and W. A. L. Thompson. 1976. *Peripheral Entrapment Neuropathies*. New York: Robert E. Krieger.

Lange, M. 1931. *Die Muskelharten (Myogelosen)*. Munich: J. F. Lehmanns.

Levinson, H. N. 1994. *Smart but Feeling Dumb: The Challenging New Research on Dyslexia—and How It May Help You*. New York: Warner Books.

Lewit, K. 1985. The muscular and articular factor in movement restriction. *Manual Medicine* 1:83–85.

———. 1991. *Manipulative Therapy in Rehabilitation of the Locomotor System*. 2nd ed. Oxford, England: Butterworth Heinemann.

Lilius, H. G., and E. J. Valtonen. 1973. The levator ani spasm syndrome: A clinical analysis of 31 cases. *Ann Chir Gynaecol Fenn* 62:93–97.

Lindgren, K. A., H. Manninen, and H. Rytkonen. 1996. Thoracic outlet syndrome (a reply). *Muscle Nerve* 19:254–256. (Letter.)

Lippitt, S., and F. Matsen. 1993. Mechanisms of glenohumeral joint stability. *Clin Orthop Res* 291:20–28.

Long, C. 1956. Myofascial pain syndromes, part III—some syndromes of the trunk and thigh. *Henry Ford Hospital Medical Bulletin* 4:22–28, 102–106.

Malbohan, I. M., L. Mojisova, and M. Tichy. 1989. The role of coccygeal spasm in low back pain. *Journal of Manual Medicine* 4:140–141.

Malleson, N. 1959. Panic and phobia, a possible method of treatment. *Lancet* 1:225–227.

Marbach, J. J. 1972. Therapy for mandibular dysfunction in adolescents and adults. *American Journal of Orthod* 62:601–605.

Melnick, J. 1954. Treatment of trigger mechanisms in gastrointestinal disease. *New York State Journal of Medicine* 54:1324–1330.

Melzack, R., E. J. Fox, and D. M. Stillwell. 1977. Trigger points and acupuncture points for pain: Correlations and implications. *Pain* 3:3–23.

Mense, S. and D. G. Simons. 2001. *Muscle Pain: Understanding Its Nature, Diagnosis, and Treatment*. Baltimore: Lippincott, Williams, and Wilkins.

Pace, J. B. 1975. Commonly overlooked pain syndromes responsive to simple therapy. *Postgraduate Medicine* 58:107–113.

Pace, J. B., and D. Nagle. 1976. Piriform syndrome. *Western Journal of Medicine* 124:435–439.

Porterfield, J. A. 1985. The sacroiliac joint. Chapter 23 in *Orthopaedic and Sports Physical Therapy*, Vol. 2, edited by J. A. Gould III and G. J. Davies. St. Louis: C. V. Mosby.

Rask, M. R. 1980. Superior gluteal nerve entrapment syndrome. *Muscle Nerve* 3:304–307.

Retzlaff, E. W., A. H. Berry, A. S. Haight, P. A. Parente, H. A. Lichty, D. M. Turner, A. A. Yezbick, J. S. Lapcevic, and D. J. Nowland. 1974. The piriformis muscle sydrome. *Journal of the American Osteopathic Association* 73:799–807.

Reynolds, M. D. 1981. Myofascial trigger point syndromes in the practice of rheumatology. *Archives of Physical Medicine Rehabilitation* 62:111–114.

Rogers, C. 1951. *Client-Centered Therapy: Its Current Practice, Implications and Theory.* Boston: Houghton Mifflin.

———. 1961. *On Becoming a Person: A Therapist's View of Psychotherapy.* Boston: Houghton Mifflin.

Rosomoff, H. L., D. Fishbain, M. Goldberg, and R. S. Rosomoff. 1990. Myofascial findings in patients with "chronic intractable benign pain" of the back and neck. *Pain Management* 3(2):114–118.

Rubin, D. 1981. An approach to the management of myofascial trigger point syndromes. *Archives of Physical Medicine Rehabilitation* 62:107–110.

Sheon, R. P., R. W. Moskowitz, and V. M. Goldberg. 1987. *Soft Tissue Rheumatic Pain.* 2nd ed. Philadelphia: Lea & Febiger.

Sherman, R. A. 1980. Published treatments of phantom limb pain. *American Journal of Physical Medicine Rehabilitation* 59:232–244.

Shordania, J. F. 1936. Die chronischer Entzundung Muysculus piriformis—die piriformitis—eine der Ursachen non Kreuzschmerzen Frauen. *Die Medizinische Welt* 10: 999–1001.

Simons, D. G. 1960. *Man High: A Space Scientist's Account of His Record-Breaking Balloon Flight to 102,000 Feet.* New York: Doubleday & Company.

Simons, D. G., J. G. Travell, and L. S. Simons.* 1999. *Myofascial Pain and Dysfunction: The Trigger Point Manual.* Vol 1, 2nd ed. Baltimore: Lippincott, Williams and Wilkins.

Sola, A. E. 1985. Trigger point therapy. Chapter 47 in *Clinical Procedures in Emergency Medicine,* ed. by J. R. Roberts and J. R. Hedges. Philadelphia: W. B. Saunders.

Sola, A. E., and R. L. Williams. 1956. Myofascial pain syndromes. *Journal of Neurology.* 6:91–95.

Sonkin, L. S. 1994. Myofascial pain due to metabolic disorders: Diagnosis and treatment, Chapter 3 in *Myofascial Pain and Fibromyalgia,* ed. by E. S. Rachlin. St Louis: Mosby-Yearbook, Inc.

---

* Janet Travell was listed first as the senior author in the first edition of *Myofascial Pain and Dysfunction: The Trigger Point Manual* (1983, 1992). Doctor Travell is no longer living, so in accordance with standard practice in publishing she is listed as the second author in the second edition of volume one (1999). Since the authors of the *Trigger Point Manual* are commonly referred to as "Travell and Simons," that is the form of reference used in this book.

Storrow, H. A. 1967. *Introduction to Scientific Psychiatry: A Behavioristic Approach to Diagnosis and Treatment.* New York: Appleton-Century-Crofts.

Thiele, G. H. 1937. Coccygodynia and pain in the superior gluteal region. *Journal of the American Medical Association* 109:1271–1275.

Travell, J. G., and D. G. Simons.** 1992. *Myofascial Pain and Dysfunction: The Trigger Point Manual.* Vol 2, 2nd ed. Baltimore: Lippincott, Williams and Wilkins.

Voss, D. E., M. K. Ionta, and B. J. Myers. 1985. *Proprioceptive Neuromuscular Facilitation.* 3rd ed. Philadelphia: Harper and Row.

Wolfe, S. M., L. D. Sasich, R. E. Hope, and Public Citizen's Health Research Group. 1999. *Worst Pills, Best Pills: A Consumer's Guide to Avoiding Drug-Induced Death or Illness.* New York: Pocket Books.

Wolpe, J. 1958. *Psychotherapy by Reciprocal Inhibition.* Stanford: Stanford University Press.

Yaksh, T. L., and S. E. Abram. 1993. Preemptive analgesia: A popular misnomer, but a clinically relevant truth? *American Pain Society Journal* 2:116–121.

Zohn, D. A. 1988. *Musculoskeletal Pain: Diagnosis and Physical Treatment.* 2nd ed. Boston: Little Brown and Company.

** Janet Travell was listed first as the senior author in the first edition of Myofascial Pain and Dysfunction: The Trigger Point Manual (1983, 1992). Doctor Travell is no longer living, so in accordance with standard practice in publishing she is listed as the second author in the second edition of volume one (1999). Since the authors of the Trigger Point Manual are commonly referred to as "Travell and Simons," that is the form of reference used in this book.

Index

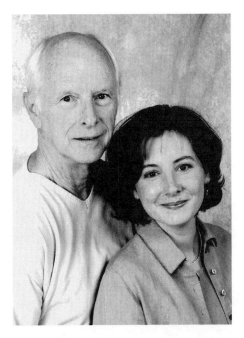

Clair Davies, N.C.T.M.B. (Nationally Certified in Therapeutic Massage and Bodywork), is a member of the American Massage Therapy Association, and a graduate of the Utah College of Massage Therapy. He specializes in trigger point massage for the treatment of pain.

Mr. Davies's interest in massage began when he successfully self-treated a frozen shoulder with trigger point massage. Inspired by the experience, he began an intensive private study of trigger points and referred pain. He subsequently retired from a thriving piano service business to become a professional massage therapist. After tuning pianos for nearly forty years, he now "tunes" people.

From his home base in Lexington, Kentucky, Mr. Davies travels extensively with his daughter Amber, leading workshops and seminars on the self-treatment and clinical treatment of pain using trigger point massage. For information about dates, locations, and workshop format, go to www.TriggerPointBook.com.

Amber Davies, N.C.T.M.B., is a massage therapist specializing in teaching self-treatment to her clients, many of whom travel to her from several surrounding states. She also teaches trigger point massage in massage schools in both Louisville and Lexington. Previously, Amber worked in teen pregnancy prevention, cultural diversity, and violence prevention. She has a degree in Theatre Performance, which has been a benefit in her many roles as a public speaker and as a presenter in the workshops with her father.

Amber suffered a debilitating back injury while doing summer theatre as a teenager. The injury wasn't completely resolved until many years later when her father began treating her as part of the development of his method of trigger point therapy. The success of the treatment inspired her to follow her father into a career as a therapist.

Amber and her husband, James Adler, live in Louisville, Kentucky.

Some Other
New Harbinger Titles

A Cancer Patient's Guide to Overcoming Depression and Anxiety, Item 5044 $19.95

The Diabetes Lifestyle Book, Item 5167 $16.95

Solid to the Core, Item 4305 $14.95

Staying Focused in the Age of Distraction, Item 433X $16.95

Living Beyond Your Pain, Item 4097 $19.95

Fibromyalgia & Chronic Fatigue Syndrome, Item 4593 $14.95

Your Miraculous Back, Item 4526 $18.95

TriEnergetics, Item 4453 $15.95

Emotional Fitness for Couples, Item 4399 $14.95

The MS Workbook, Item 3902 $19.95

Depression & Your Thyroid, Item 4062 $15.95

The Eating Wisely for Hormonal Balance Journal, Item 3945 $15.95

Healing Adult Acne, Item 4151 $15.95

The Memory Doctor, Item 3708 $11.95

The Emotional Wellness Way to Cardiac Health, Item 3740 $16.95

The Cyclothymia Workbook, Item 383X $18.95

The Matrix Repatterning Program for Pain Relief, Item 3910 $18.95

Transforming Stress, Item 397X $10.95

Eating Mindfully, Item 3503 $13.95

Living with RSDS, Item 3554 $16.95

The Ten Hidden Barriers to Weight Loss, Item 3244 $11.95

The Sjogren's Syndrome Survival Guide, Item 3562 $15.95

Stop Feeling Tired, Item 3139 $14.95

Responsible Drinking, Item 2949 $19.95

The Mitral Valve Prolapse/Dysautonomia Survival Guide, Item 3031 $14.95

The Vulvodynia Survival Guide, Item 2914 $16.95

The Multifidus Back Pain Solution, Item 2787 $12.95

Move Your Body, Tone Your Mood, Item 2752 $17.95

The Woman's Book of Sleep, Item 2493 $14.95

The Trigger Point Therapy Workbook, second edition, Item 3759 $19.95

Fibromyalgia and Chronic Myofascial Pain Syndrome, 2nd edition, Item 2388 $19.95

Rosacea, Item 2248 $14.95

Coping with Chronic Fatigue Syndrome, Item 0199 $13.95

Call **toll free, 1-800-748-6273,** or log on to our online bookstore at **www.newharbinger.com** to order. Have your Visa or Mastercard number ready. Or send a check for the titles you want to New Harbinger Publications, Inc., 5674 Shattuck Ave., Oakland, CA 94609. Include $4.50 for the first book and 75¢ for each additional book, to cover shipping and handling. (California residents please include appropriate sales tax.) Allow two to five weeks for delivery.

Prices subject to change without notice.

Quick Muscle Index

These 120 muscles can all be found in the regular index, but this one-page index will help you find them quicker. To make the book even more useful, you may want to have a coil binding put on it at a copy center, which will allow it to open flat to any page, leaving both hands free to do therapy.